A Breath of Cyanide

Factual Account of a Crucial Discovery,
The Heights,
Houston, Texas,
1981-1982,
With Worldwide Significance Today

A Breath of Cyanide

by: Timothy Swiss

*A True and Factual Account
of an Incredible Environmental Discovery*

> *To Kathy D. Smith,
> an Elysian Boss,
> & a Wonderful Woman.
> 7/29/2020*
>
> *Timothy Swiss*

A Breath of Cyanide
Copyright © 2020 by Author. All rights reserved.
Copyright Registration Number TXu 2-185-439
Issued under the seal of the Copyright Office in accordance with title 17, United States Code, and made part of the Copyright Office records.

For nothing is secret, that shall not be made manifest;
neither any thing hid, that shall not be known and come abroad.
Luke 8:17 KJV
Holy Bible

Introduction

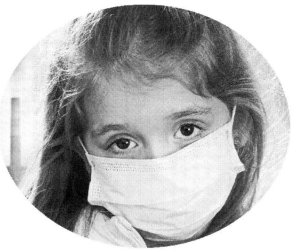

A Matter of Life and Breath

Take a deep breath of air and hold it. The quantity of cyanide that is now inside your lungs depends upon several factors: your location, wind direction, weather inversions, and the time of day. Whether or not you feel any effects from cyanide also depends upon several factors, including your bodily rate of metabolizing cyanide and/or the presence of immunological sensitive to cyanide. The time finally came when airborne lead from using leaded gasoline became recognized as adversely affecting human health; and now the time has come to recognize an airborne poison that plays a preponderant role in human maladies and suffering. Okay then, you may now breathe.

In an article published by the EPA in 1993, namely EPA-454/R-93-041, the emission of cyanide compounds into the air in 1991 in the United States was estimated at 974 tons, or 2,147,299.8 pounds. Production of hydrogen cyanide in the United States in 2003 was 2.019 billion pounds according to TOXICOLOGICAL PROFILE FOR CYANIDE, U.S. Department of Health and Human Services, Agency for Toxic Substance and Disease Registry, July, 2006. This same agency reported the half-life of hydrogen cyanide in the atmosphere as being about 1 to 3 years, and also reported that vehicle exhaust and biomass burning are major sources of cyanide released into the air. At another site in this agency's report, the residence time of hydrogen cyanide in the atmosphere is estimated at about 2.5 years, with a range of 1.3 to 5 years, and it is also reported that only 2% of the tropospheric cyanide is expected to be transported to the stratosphere, meaning that 98% of the cyanide remains in the lowest part of the earth's atmosphere—the air we breathe. And the agency further reports that despite the various ways cyanide is thought to be released into the environment, available monitoring data are limited. It reports that the worldwide emissions of hydrogen cyanide and acetonitrile (most of the cyanide in the atmosphere will be present as hydrogen cyanide) due to biomass burning are based in part on highly uncertain global estimates, but are estimated at about 1.1 to 3.7 billion pounds per year. Notably, polluted air that is generated in China can reach the western coast of the United States within days, and remember that the half-life of airborne cyanide is measured in years.

Over thirty years have passed since composition of the story contained within this book, a story I wrote using an electric typewriter in the early 1980s. Although I am a writer of fiction and fantasy, as found in books such as *Princess Vayle*, this book is strictly factual apart from pseudonyms used for some medical patients who may not want their real names disclosed, or for persons whose real names are not obtainable.

When I first wrote this book, many years ago, quite a number of names and titles were fictionalized due to the fact that a major lawsuit was underway and I did not want to write anything that would be damaging to the suit; but now, I have been able to replace many of those fictional names and titles with the true names and titles. The fact that I typed out this story in the early 1980s, a story that began in 1981, contributes to its authenticity and accuracy. I attempted publishing this book years ago, but to no avail. Thanks to preservation of the typewritten manuscript for over thirty years, this book will now be published.

The contents of this book contain my real name, *Timothy R. Oesch, M.D.*, rather than my pen name, *Timothy Swiss*. Having learned much about airborne cyanide and its effects since first discovering the problem, I will add commentaries from time to time within the main body of the manuscript, but these will always be italicized and contained within brackets [ ] so that readers can differentiate between what was contained within the original text, and what has been added as my commentaries. Note that any comments that are not contained within brackets, or comments contained within parentheses ( ) rather than brackets, are elements of the original manuscript. My prose and grammar were not as polished in the early 1980s as they are now; but for the most part, the text that was typed in the 1980s has been transcribed with little alteration. PS: I have decided, at the end of this book, to disclose the real names of a few notable persons who were given fictitious names within the body of the text, persons who deserve credit and admiration. This, I believe, is something that those individuals would desire and appreciate.

Table of Contents

Prelude to Chapter 1

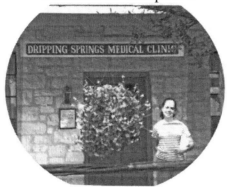

From the Texas Hill Country
17

Chapter 1

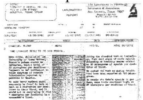

Astounding Discovery
21

Chapter 2

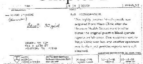

Sewer Vapor
32

Chapter 3

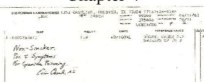

Foul Play
46

Chapter 4

Stalking Death
60

Chapter 5

Note: the above is a copy of cyanide levels reported by Harris County Medical Examiners Toxicology Laboratory from blood drawn 12/2/1981 at Gulf Coast Bible College.

Rottenness Within
80

Chapter 6

Intriguing Information
98

Chapter 7

Clandestine Killer
115

Chapter 8

Underground
136

Chapter 9

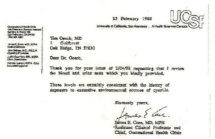

Repressed Disclosure
146

Chapter 10

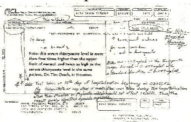

Astounding Rediscovery
172

Chapter 11

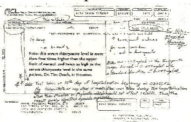

Threat After Threat
185

Chapter 12

Summary and Conclusions:

Dr. Oesch is a bright 28 year old male who demonstrates good creative and intellectual ability, excellent problem-solving and reasoning skills, and exceptional judgement in both social and practical situations. Some denial and/or suppression of negative feelings is evident, but this along with his control of impulses and external expression of affect may be a reflection of the influence of his Christian ethics upon his life. No significant psychopathology is evident, nor any salient personality features which would impede his social, emotional, or intellectual functioning.

Edward G. Daniels
Psychometric Technician

Aaron Bothyl, Ph.D.
Licensed Clinical Psychologist

Frame-Up
199

Chapter 13

Mental Status Examination:

Dr. Oesch was neatly and appropriately dressed in a three piece suit. Initially tense, he relaxed maintaining good eye contact through the interview. He was friendly, warm, and cooperative. Normal in its rate rhythm and tone, his speech was spontaneous, coherent and goal directed. His mood and affect overall was full, expressive and appropriate. There was no evidence of perceptual disturbances, no symptoms of depression, no ideas of reference or influence, no magical thinking or thought incertion or broadcasting. There was no evidence of derealization or depersonalization. He denied suicidal idiation. His sensorium was intact, revealing an above average intelligence and an ability to use abstract thinking and reasoning. There was no impairment in his judgement.

Summary:

Dr. Oesch is a 28 year old white married male. He presents himself in a warm friendly manner. There were no abnormalities in his speech, mood or affect. There was no evidence of a thought disorder nor of an underlying organic process. He manifested above average intelligence and an ability to think and reason abstractly. His judgement ability was intact.

Accessment:

No significant underlying psychopathology detected.

Cheryl L. Sanfacon, M.D.
Psychiatrist

Unnerving Apparition
214

Chapter 14

BILL ARCHER
7th District, Texas

MEMBER:
WAYS AND MEANS
COMMITTEE

Congress of the United States
House of Representatives
Washington, D.C. 20515

July 13, 1983

Dear Mr. Secretary:

I have been contacted by my constituent, Timothy R. Oesch, a former resident of Houston now on active duty with the U.S. Navy as a Lieutenant in the Medical Corps.

Inside Help
237

Chapter 15

Challenge
242

Chapter 16

Accumulated Proof
267

Chapter 17

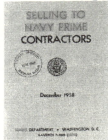

First Hearing
293

Chapter 18

Revelation
329

Chapter 19

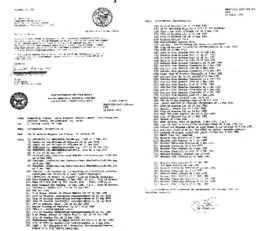

Second Hearing
373

Chapter 20

Present Status
397

Chapter 21

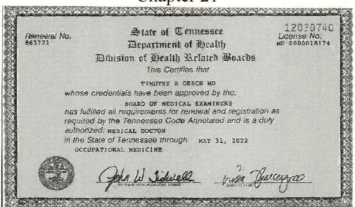

What Happened After That?

Prelude to Chapter 1

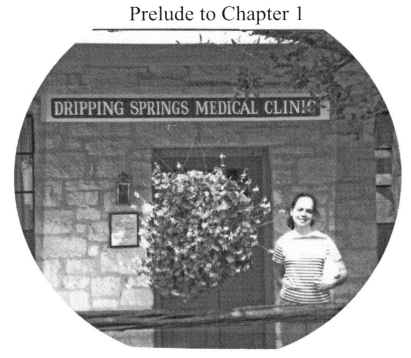

From the Texas Hill Country

To begin with, the following paragraphs are from a submission I made to an editor at *New American Library* in New York, dated January 12, 1986. The editor responded with a kind letter informing me that NAL was no longer considering any unsolicited material for publication, and my manuscript was returned free of charge, even though I had included a check to cover the cost of returning the manuscript:

Dear Michaela Hamilton:
  My name is Timothy Ralph Oesch. About fifteen months ago, I opened a private medical practice in a small town which had been

without a physician for twenty-five years. The practice is doing very well. My wife and I are living normal, happy, healthy lives in the beautiful hills of central Texas. This is very different from the incredible series of discoveries and experiences which dominated our lives from the fall of 1981 to the spring of 1984.

Houston has yet to hear or see the truth, despite heavy news coverage of cyanide pollution first discovered in the fall of 1981. The health department tried to dismiss the issue, and no polluters offered confessions of guilt, but thirty-one lawsuits have now been issued. Since that time, a lawsuit has been filed against a plating plant utilizing cyanide in San Antonio, and I have been requested to furnish information which may help disclose airborne cyanide as the problem for symptoms suffered in a town in California.

In the summer of 1982, after finding at least eighty individuals suffering from cyanide exposure in Houston, the Navy called me to active duty in Philadelphia. I was assigned to work in the industrial shipyard, where again I found the problem of cyanide pollution. An officer in the environmental department threatened my life, but I would not ignore the problem, and I was finally discharged from the Navy with a psychiatric diagnosis—the Navy claiming that there was no cyanide pollution either in Houston or Philadelphia. They claimed this despite objective laboratory tests to the contrary, and despite civilian psychiatric testing which maintained that I was of sound mind.

I have written a book which discloses the shocking truth of the politics surrounding this current environmental issue.

I look forward to hearing from you,
Sincerely,
Timothy R. Oesch, M.D.
Timothy Swiss

Now follows the original introduction to the manuscript that was first entitled *Cyanide City*, penned by Timothy R. Oesch, M.D., in the early 1980s. Following this introduction is the manuscript itself.

At times the truth seems more fantastic than fiction. Most individuals experience episodes during their lives which are incredible and alarming. Now and then such an episode leads to stunning revelations. Unveiled facets of bureaucracy, politics, or social policy may amaze and astound perceiving minds. Furthermore, the unfolded truth of certain matters may initiate solution to baffling problems. Hopefully, though certain proper names of individuals are substituted with fictional titles, the following true story will stimulate alert minds toward redemptive awareness. Details of events and subject matter are accurate to the best of my memory and resources.

A remarkable series of events culminated in my residential habitation of Houston, Texas. After graduating from medical school in May of 1980, I was commissioned to work in a missionary hospital at Nalerigu, Ghana, West Africa. Oddly, after shots, training, and five months of expectant waiting, my visa failed to materialize. Shortly afterwards I returned to school, but for communications training rather than additional medical training. I thought the courses would aid my preaching, which I do from time to time at churches, missions, or wherever I am invited. Little did I suspect the divergent manner in which these courses would soon assist me.

During my additional education I met a lovely young lady at a local church. The following August we married and spent a marvelous honeymoon in the Smoky Mountains. She was young and brilliant, and I strongly desired her opportunity to pursue further education in college. That opportunity presented itself as I was accepted as a staff member at Gulf Coast Bible College. At Gulf Coast Bible College, I would serve as campus physician and study New Testament Greek.

Although our journey to Gulf Coast Bible College moved my wife and me hundreds of miles and several states from both of our families, I knew our destination well. In fact, our future upstairs apartment in Houston, located directly above the medical office, was only about one block from the house where my family resided when I was thirteen. My previous high school was several miles northwest, and my previous college was several miles southwest. Closer by was a swimming pool where I lifeguarded as a city employee for two summers. Later, it would seem quite ironic that the City of Houston had once paid me to guard people's lives.

Chapter 1

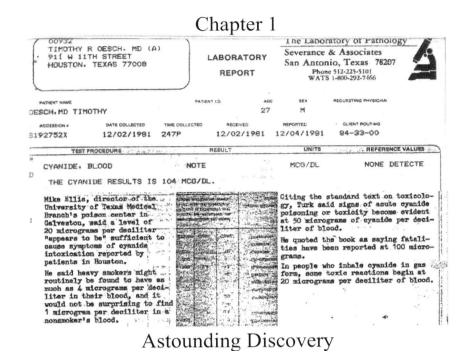

Astounding Discovery

"**O**h! Honey come here, a roach is trying to get me!" a very disconcerted voice erupted from the bathroom. Urgent desperation fairly flung my stomach into my throat. I dashed into the bathroom, and there my wife huddled warily against the rear of a large, old tub. At the opposite end, two long, dark feelers protruded from openings in an overflow drain. I remember contemplating the likelihood that whatever the whisker-like filaments were attached to would surely be too large to squeeze through the drain.

"He won't bother you, just splash a little water and he'll go back in," I explained to my wife. In my mind, however, I formulated an unnerving episode picturing a large roach plummeting into the tub and swimming toward my wife. I even put myself in her position, admitting to myself that an aggressive advancement by the roach would probably compel my evacuation from the tub. The roach retreated quickly when I gave him a few splashes, and I returned to the bedroom.

The bedroom was old with a high ceiling and white walls. Large, twin windows decked adjacent walls on the east and south. The east windows were covered with curtains my mother-in-law mailed to us, and the south windows were draped by a large quilted blanket made by my wife's grandmother. In the middle of the room sat our only piece of new furniture, a queen-sized bed. Several boxes lined the walls and served as drawers, and there was a large end table on my wife's side of the bed which matched another one in the den.

The den was located through a door which was always kept open in the north wall of our bedroom. A huge, old, felt sofa spanned the north wall from its east end to the apartment entrance on the west. An inverted, white box made an attractive stand for my wife's portable television. We carefully positioned wedding gifts and various decorations about the room. Our kitchen adjoined to the west.

The apartment was provided by Gulf Coast Bible College, along with free tuition for my wife and free meals at the school cafeteria. [*Our actual street address was 1119 Lawrence, Houston, Texas, 77008.*] In return, I served as school nurse thirteen hours a week, two and one-half hours Monday, Tuesday, Thursday, Friday, and three hours Saturday. The remainder of the time I was free to see patients in my own practice as a physician. This I did whenever available. I put myself on call twenty-four hours a day as a physician. The arrangement seemed quite satisfactory.

Though our apartment was referred to as a cracker box, my wife and I found it sufficient and developed an enjoyable lifestyle. We ate meals together, studied together, exercised together, and worked together in the office. Our office was about half as large as our small apartment, sharing half the downstairs space with a washateria. Apparently both the washateria and our office had once been a garage. Despite its tiny size, the office was newly refinished and attractive inside. There were two rooms: a front waiting room and a back examining room.

The illness came on us slowly, my wife was affected first. Perhaps the west winds of fall, uncommon in our area, brought heavier doses our way. For weeks I grew to consider the region a mushroom of viruses and bacteria. Frequent illness perplexed me. An astounding percentage of my patients were anemic. I issued thousands of iron tablets to patients who were probably affected by an agent I did not even suspect. Perhaps providence brought John to my office.

"All right, Doc, I want you to find out what's wrong with me," stated John. "I've been to my doctor and he can't figure it out. He gave me some pills to take, but they don't work. It keeps coming back."

"What seems to be bothering you?" I posed.

John was more than glad to describe his ailments to me. He was actually suffering a number of symptoms, but the strangest were painful sensations in his in his hands and fingers. There was no notable joint inflammation, just unexplained pain and tingling. At first I explored conventional etiologies: arthritis, gout, vitamin deficiency, etc. Nothing turned up positive. Finally I decided to stop retracing tests done by prior physicians and move to new ground. I asked John what he was exposed to at work.

"A bunch of things," responded John.

"Like what?"

"I can't remember all of them. I'll have to make you a list at work."

John made his list and brought it back to me. There were various metallic ingredients which caught my eye and drew suspicion, but I decided to investigate each item on the list. As it turned out, only one thing appeared likely to cause John's symptoms in the sparse literature at hand, and that was cyanide. I also screened John for lead and copper, which were within normal limits.

"It's a long shot," I told John, "but I've tried everything else I can think of. I don't know if this will show anything, but nothing else has."

"That's all right," said John, "I've got insurance. Do whatever you think needs to be done. I just want to find out what's wrong."

Blood was drawn and sent to Severance and Associates Laboratory. I felt a little helpless about John's evasive pathogenesis, and was far from certain about the environmental speculation underway. Nonetheless, John's blood cyanide returned at two micrograms per deciliter. This was only a fraction of levels found later, but it was still more than the reference value the laboratory stated, which was *none detected*. I informed John of the result.

By this time my own illness was becoming quite noticeable. I attributed it to recurrent flu and a possible bout of strep throat, and made no connection between my symptoms and John's ailment. Since John worked where cyanide was utilized quite extensively, I surmised that he acquired his cyanide at work. Meanwhile, John's wife was persistently ill, and so were many others in the vicinity. I continued advising dietary iron and gave quite a number of penicillin shots.

From time to time John had his blood retested for cyanide, especially when his illness worsened. Headaches and dizziness began to bother him more than his hands. John decided to do something about the problem, and sought legal advice. Not long afterwards, he approached with a rather interesting request.

"Listen Doc, I've got to get my wife tested for cyanide," said John.
"Your wife? What for?"
"It's to prove I'm getting poisoning at work instead of home, otherwise someone might claim my wife and I were poisoning each other."

This seemed almost amusing. I was not yet aware that a significant percentage of past, reported cyanide poisonings in the United States had domestic origins. Despite the seeming senselessness, I agreed to perform the test.

"All right, have your wife come over and I'll draw her blood."

My brain was jolted. John's wife turned out a positive blood cyanide. [*Her blood cyanide level was 5 mcg/dl on 11/18/81. She later had blood drawn on 12/7/81 that yielded a blood cyanide of 14 mcg/dl, and a serum thiocyanate level of 0.4 mg/dl (thiocyanate is a metabolite of cyanide). Interestingly, her husband (John) also had a blood cyanide level of 14 mcg/dl on 12/7/81, and I think they both came to my office for blood testing at the same time. John's blood was drawn at 10:30 a.m., and there is no time given on his wife's test, which definitely leads me to believe that they were together—I probably put the time on John's test to account for the time of both of their tests. John's serum thiocyanate on 12/7/81 was 0.6 mg/dl, which was 50% higher than that found in his wife. His higher serum thiocyanate indicated more overall exposure to cyanide as compared to his wife, while their exact blood cyanide levels of 14 mcg/dl indicated that they were both breathing the same air and had their blood drawn at the same time. Both John and his wife were nonsmokers.*] Somehow, from that moment on, I knew we were being poisoned. My objective, realistic reasoning did not yet endorse the verdict, but something deeper affirmed it. I contacted John right away.

"Hello, John...listen, we've got a problem."
"A problem? What kind of problem?" John answered on the phone.

"Your wife came back positive."

"Positive! You're kidding!" John exclaimed.

"Does she ever come visit you at work?" I inquired.

"No, she never comes near the place. Could we be getting it in the house?"

"I don't know, but Glenna's been real sick too, for a long time, and I haven't been able to find out what's wrong with her. I think I'll run a test on her."

Glenna was a neighbor who worked for a while in the Gulf Coast Bible College bookstore until her illness grew too burdensome. She was my wife's best friend, and lived in the house in front of our garage apartment. Her husband and children also experienced ill symptoms, but not as severely as Glenna. Other blood tests revealed nothing specifically wrong with Glenna except for mild anemia. This was hardly sufficient to explain the long-term mental depression, headaches, and lack of energy afflicting this previously cheery and exuberant young woman.

"Let me know as soon as you get the results," requested John.

"Okay."

The test for blood cyanide was relatively expensive. I added little to the lab cost, but the figure still approached forty dollars. When I proposed the test to Glenna, however, she welcomed the opportunity. Her illness was trying and frustrating, and an unknown etiology added to her anguish.

By this time, over a month had elapsed since John's first cyanide test. My own health was relentlessly disintegrating. At first, I just seemed to get sick more often than usual; then my athletic ability began dwindling. For many years I ran track, and I competed with collegiate athletes the previous spring. Now I could no longer exercise at all, the exertion was too much, my body too weak, my tolerance too low.

Glenna's test returned positive with a blood cyanide of twenty-three micrograms per deciliter. My stubborn reasoning was satisfied. The cyanide was real. My wife had jokingly suggested that cyanide was making us all sick, but this was no longer a joke. I examined the evidence and the grave effects to my own health, and pondered upon a number of patents with similar and worse symptoms. It was ghastly.

Thanksgiving was approaching. My wife and I were soon leaving for Tulsa to visit my grandmother. Admittedly, I was glad to be leaving, even for three days. There were a few things to do, though, before departing. I contacted a national poison control center and reported the cyanide contamination of persons in Houston. In turn, they contacted a state poison control center in Texas, which in turn contacted a Harris County poison control center, which in turn contacted the health department in Houston.

The health department in Houston elected to handle the problem. This seemed satisfactory, and I expected a quick solution. Besides contacting health authorities before leaving for Tulsa, I informed several of my patients about the cyanide findings. There were many persons whose physical and mental afflictions matched those of the first three persons identified with cyanide intoxication. [*Note:* **cyanide intoxication** *is a two-word phrase that I coined in order to refer to symptoms of cyanide poisoning from doses of cyanide that are very unlikely to be immediately fatal.*] Seven more individuals had their blood drawn for testing.

"What a relief. I can't wait to get out of this city," commented my wife as we departed for Tulsa.

"Maybe it will be gone by the time we get back," I responded, referring to the cyanide. Perhaps my statement was naïve or overly optimistic, but it was still what one might expect.

We stopped to eat at a restaurant several hours after leaving Houston. Severance and Associates Laboratory did not have results for the seven additional blood tests when we departed, but they expected to have them soon. I called from a pay phone while my wife sat awaiting our order. The tests were positive, all seven of them. The levels ranged from sixteen micrograms per deciliter to over twenty micrograms per deciliter.

After calling Houston and relaying the results to John, who was to contact the patients for me, I returned to our table and informed my wife of the results. She is a wonderful, gentle, and lovely creation, but she clearly did not like being poisoned.

[*Melody was among the first to have blood tested for cyanide:*

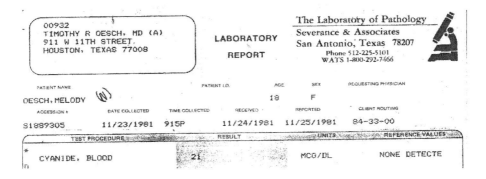

Melody's blood was drawn on 11/23/81 at 9:15 p.m., and the result was highly positive in regard to environmental cyanide exposure with a blood cyanide level of 21 mcg/dl. Melody has never been a smoker.]

There were then ten patients testing positive for cyanide poisoning, and none testing negative. This seemed staunchly significant, but I was not aware that I was stumbling onto a political battlefield.

Some weeks later, I learned that the half-life of cyanide in the blood, after exposure to hydrogen cyanide gas, is about thirty minutes. This means that someone with an exposure to HCN (hydrogen cyanide) which causes a blood cyanide level of three hundred micrograms per deciliter, a level in excess of recorded lethal levels, may yield a blood cyanide level less than five micrograms per deciliter only three hours later. The stark fact that patients were exposed to cyanide shortly before visiting my office, perhaps even in my office, and were exposed constantly and consistently enough to yield positive blood tests morning, noon, and evening of the same day, was still beyond my comprehension. Had my knowledge of cyanide poisoning in November been what it was the following June, things may have progressed differently. What is now history, however, is something bordering a science fiction nightmare.

My grandmother greeted us in Tulsa, and was delighted to meet my new bride for the first time. Our spirits picked up; the depressing effects of cyanide intoxication filtered from our bodies like stagnant filth from a sand-sifted stream. We visited the zoo and played antique, cylindrical records in my grandmother's spare bedroom. By the end of our three-day visit, I felt capable of physical exercise and seemed to possess volition for extracurricular activity. Our temporary rejuvenation, however, was soon spoiled.

Within twenty-four hours of returning to Houston, my wife and I were both miserably ill. Our recent improvement in Tulsa served to contrast how well we could feel against our relentless illness. One thing was certain—the problem still persisted.

"Honey, come here and look at this squirrel!" exclaimed my wife. I was somewhere inside the apartment, and soon joined my wife on the metal porch outside our door. She pointed to a nearby squirrel sitting on a tree limb. "He's really been acting weird," she said, "running back and forth across the tree and standing there shaking."

I observed the squirrel long enough to ascertain that he had a problem. He stood blankly on a limb and intermittently displayed vigorous, convulsive-appearing shivers. Empathetically, I mentally wagered that he and I were both suffering from a common environmental enemy, an enemy that entered our bodies without visual or auditory warning. Some hideous, alien entity seemed suspended in the atmosphere.

After returning to Houston from Tulsa, I was confronted with the question of what to do next. Obviously, something needed done that was not being done. By this time, I had assembled a list of the symptoms that my patients and I experienced. The list included tiredness, depression, headaches, shortness of breath, and forgetfulness. It would be weeks and months before the true extent and severity of cyanide intoxication began perceptively impressing my mind. Until then, I would underestimate and understate the immediate danger to individuals in the community.

At first I envisioned the cyanide as a gradually destructive agent. This was largely due to the effects I personally encountered in myself and my patients. Glenna first became ill nearly two years prior to the cyanide discovery, so the likelihood of her dying within the next few days seemed very remote. This reasoning led me to make a difficult decision in withholding information from the public. I hoped that during a short period of suppressed knowledge, official investigators would gather environmental data identifying the source of poison.

Exactly how long I should withhold information regarding the cyanide discovery was something I never had to decide. Within a couple days, a major newspaper, The Houston Chronicle, revealed the finding to all quadrants of Houston. This triggered a lot of communicative action, but preceding most of the action came a visit from my first, new, outside, cyanide patient.

By outside, cyanide patient, I mean an individual found with cyanide poisoning who did not previously know me, nor my family, and did not attend Gulf Coast Bible College. Such patients were rare initially because my office was very small and off the road, and there was no road sign indicating that an office was even present. I once placed an announcement in a local paper, but I was instructed not to include an address with the announcement. This instruction came from Mr. Saul, an official at Gulf Coast Bible College who had authority over the position I filled as the college nurse. [*Mr. Saul is a fictitious name, and I am not certain of Mr. Saul's title at the college, but I think he was vice president.*]

My first, outside, cyanide patient was Laverne Brown. She was bright, slim, blonde, and looked like a figure from a western soap opera. There were few words wasted in relating the purpose of her visit.

"Are you Doctor Oesch?" posed Laverne, entering the office door. At twenty-seven, I still looked about twenty and was commonly questioned about identification.

"Yes," I acknowledged.

"My name's Laverne, and I've just found out about that cyanide poisoning and I want tested for it."

"All right. This is my wife Melody," I replied, motioning to the young secretary sitting behind the front desk, "and she'll get you a patient information sheet to fill out. You can sit over there."

There were two, black lounge chairs between the front desk and the west wall of the waiting room. The front door to the office opened to the inside from the east, and the examining room was straight through to the west. I often interviewed patients while seated in the black lounge chair beside the desk, with the patient seated in the other lounge chair facing me.

Laverne and I seated ourselves as my wife rose from the desk and handed Laverne a patient information sheet. Melody thoroughly enjoyed working in the office, and took it upon herself to organize medicines and supplies in meticulously neat fashion. There were times when she had classes, and I certainly missed her. Filling roles as receptionist and secretary, as well as physician, gave me an authentic appreciation for office help.

"What kind of symptoms have you been having?" I asked Laverne as she finished writing her name, address, age, and phone number.

"It's been terrible," said Laverne, addressing my wife and me with belabored eyes. "I feel so depressed I just sit down and cry for no reason. The other day I cried for four hours straight and my husband didn't know what to do with me. He kept asking me what was wrong, and I'd say *nothing*, and he finally told me that he was going to call men in white coats to get me if I didn't quit crying."

I knew the feeling, though I never cried for four hours. Cyanide is apparently a direct mental depressant, capable of depressing individuals surrounded by the best of circumstances. Laverne conveyed an aspect of cyanide poisoning that I learned to recognize as a chief demarcation—distraught desperation.

"That's pretty common with the patients I've seen," I explained to Laverne, "the cyanide seems to depress people without any external cause for depression."

Laverne stared at me as though I dropped in from outer space. "That's it. Everyone else thought I was going bananas!"

"What other symptoms have you been having?" I asked.

"I just feel bad all over," resumed Laverne, "and I have these constant headaches."

"How long do they last?"

"Hours, days, lately it's been almost constant."

"Well, you sure have the symptoms. We'll get the blood test, and I may have something to help your headaches."

"I'll try it."

Literature addressing chronic cyanide poisoning is very sparse. I found information regarding acute cyanide poisoning rather easily, and used it to formulate a treatment for chronic cyanide poisoning. For some time the only treatment I offered was sodium thiosulfate, which seems to help the liver metabolize cyanide into thiocyanate. I also had amyl nitrite on hand for inhalation, but this was only for precaution in case of acute cyanide poisoning. Amy nitrite can cause migraine headaches and drop blood pressure drastically, so I decided not to use it except in dire situations.

Acquiring sodium thiosulfate was quite a challenge. In acute, life-threatening cyanide poisoning, emergency rooms use intravenous sodium thiosulfate. I wanted oral sodium thiosulfate which my patients could take at home, and which I could administer in my office without invading a vein. After phoning chemical supply houses, pharmacies, and laboratory suppliers, I finally located a hospital pharmacy in downtown Houston that supplied an oral form of sodium thiosulfate. To date, I know of no one who produces sodium thiosulfate pills, but I was able to obtain sodium thiosulfate crystals.

When Henry Armstrong found out I needed sodium thiosulfate crystals, he soon had them on hand for me. Henry was a local pharmacist who quickly adopted me when I moved into his area. He was very helpful as I initially built my practice. Soon after my request for sodium thiosulfate, Henry had some stocked in his store. This brought Henry into personal contact with many cyanide patients who came to him for medication.

I gave Laverne a sample of sodium thiosulfate and drew some blood in the examination room. Melody watched me perform various medical operations and procedures, and was learning to do some of them herself. She hated to hurt anyone, though, and only drew blood from some of the tougher male volunteers. As I drew Laverne's blood, Melody conversed empathetically. Her own illness, like mine, gave her insight into the suffering that cyanide patients experience.

As Laverne sat writing her check for the office visit and cyanide test, her pen suddenly halted. Sensing her frustration, I instructed Laverne how to finish filling out her check.

"See, I can't remember anything, my mind just goes blank," stated Laverne. "I'm really not normally like this. I'm usually a sane, sensible person."

"I'm like that too," commented Melody, "sometimes I just sit and stare off into space."

"Oh, I'm so glad to hear that. Don't get me wrong," added Laverne, clasping Melody by the arm, "I'm not glad you're sick, I'm just glad to know I'm not going crazy."

"I know what you mean," confirmed Melody. "I was sick a long time before we figured out what was going on."

I informed Laverne that we would contact her when her blood result came back: it was positive. [*Laverne's real name is Linda. Her blood was drawn 11/25/81 and yielded a blood cyanide level of 8 mcg/dl. She was a smoker, but at that time the laboratory simply gave a reference level of "none detected" for blood cyanide levels. I definitely believe that Linda suffered from cyanide intoxication.*]

Chapter 2

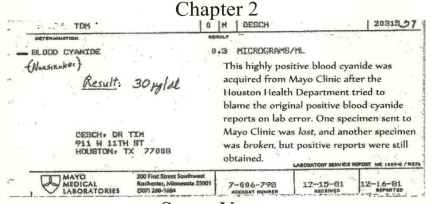

Sewer Vapor

Melody and I were both present when Mr. Blunz came to visit. He represented the Houston Health Department—air division.

"What's your impression of the problem?" inquired Mr. Blunz.

"I think it's in the air," I responded, standing in the concrete driveway before the clinic. "Our symptoms seem much worse when the air comes from the west."

Mr. Blunz seemed somewhat annoyed by my westward indications, but he listened attentively.

"The first patient I found with the problem worked over in that direction, at a plating plant. I tested him several times, and his cyanide levels seemed to go up at work. If you will set up air testers all around the plating plant, I think it will be your best chance of finding the problem."

Mr. Blunz made little comment. He stared toward the west.

"You may be able to test some of the foliage around here too," I added. "If it's in the air, it may settle out of the atmosphere and be absorbed through the roots of trees and grass. We think it may be in the pecans around here."

Mr. Blunz looked interested.

"My wife saw a squirrel acting very strangely." I looked toward Melody, "Tell him about the squirrel."

Melody was engrossed in the entire conversation. Mr. Blunz represented the organizational power we both hoped would soon deliver us from our suffering. "He was right up there on a limb," said Melody, pointing to a lower branch on a huge pecan tree growing north of our apartment. "He just stood there and shook and shook," she explained, holding both arms limply before her and wriggling spasmodically. Having seen the squirrel myself, I noted that her depiction was markedly accurate.

The squirrel pantomime did not seem to impress Mr. Blunz. "Have you noticed any odors?"

"Yes," I replied, and Melody concurred. "It smells rather pungent, and burnt."

I knew that hydrogen cyanide gas is supposed to smell like bitter almonds, to those who are able to smell it, but I did not know what bitter almonds smell like, and I still do not. Therefore, I attempted using language familiar to my mind to describe the odors which drifted in from time to time, most noticeably from the west. To complicate this factor, however, a coffee plant was located to the west. The smell of burnt coffee beans presented difficulty in differentiating whether or not there was also the smell of burnt or bitter almonds.

"All right, if you notice the smell again, give us a call so we can come out and check on it," stated Mr. Blunz.

"Okay."

Mr. Blunz departed. I was not sure what action would be taken, but I expected action soon. The serious nature of the problem demanded a fast and sure solution. It was unthinkable that such a situation would persist, not after being identified. I supposed there were governing forces in society that would quickly deliver ailing citizens from such terrible oppression. I was wrong.

On December 2, 1981, The Houston Chronicle released a front-page article announcing that the Houston Health Department would assign an epidemiologist to investigate cyanide poisoning of several persons in the Heights area of Houston. My name was mentioned as a general practitioner and part-time staff member of Gulf Coast Bible College. The paper stated that tests showed cyanide poisoning in ten patients. Patient symptoms included dizziness, lack of motivation, fatigue, depressions, nausea, and headaches. These facts were quite accurate, but there was additional information that troubled me.

Dr. Herbert McKee, a high-ranking official with the Houston Health Department, said he doubted that the cyanide was airborne because of the limited area affected. This puzzled me: there were no grounds upon which to claim that the area affected by cyanide was limited in the least. Dr. McKee knew of ten persons tested for cyanide, and all ten were positive. I pointed out that patients did better in central air-conditioning than outside air, and that symptoms were worse when winds came from the west, and that a strange odor permeated the atmosphere from time to time; yet an official representative of the Houston Health Department belittled the idea of airborne cyanide. At first, I excused this as a simple lack of knowledge, but later I was forced to think otherwise.

The newspaper article gave several other pieces of information which were probably wrong, but I was not knowledgeable enough to recognize the errors. For example, the paper quoted me affirming that the cyanide poisoning was probably not a life-threatening situation, and I know now that it was. The paper also quoted me agreeing with health officials in stating that once the source of poisoning was located and cut off, there would be no lasting effects from the poisoning. There was no way anyone could be certain of that, and quite to the contrary, most literature dealing with chronic cyanide poisoning concludes that serious, permanent damage may result from repeated exposure to low doses of cyanide. I was not yet familiar with the literature concerning chronic cyanide poisoning, and there were other reasons why I tended to underplay the serious threat of the poisoning.

As alluded to previously, I assumed that the cyanide problem would be corrected rapidly. For this reason, I deemed it unnecessary to arouse the community with details of possible cyanide effects. Imagine how the typical neighborhood would respond to news that an agent in their atmosphere may be capable of inducing blindness, deafness, and sterility. One fact I could not ignore, however, was that hydrogen cyanide may be rapidly fatal. It was my moral obligation to inform citizens in the area about the symptoms of acute cyanide poisoning.

The other primary reason that I tended to understate the cyanide problem was to please the two top officials of Gulf Coast Bible College. Both men seemed vitally concerned about keeping any reports of the problem in check. As a member of the college staff, I certainly wanted to respect their advice as much as possible. Furthermore, I wanted to clarify that the problem was not peculiar to Gulf Coast Bible College, and probably originated a considerable distance away from Gulf Coast Bible College. This proved very difficult to do.

Before the December second news release, a news conference was held at Gulf Coast Bible College. Quite a number of news reporters contacted college officials to inquire about the poisoning, and the college administrators decided to host an organized news conference. The Gulf Coast Bible College Chancellor contacted me [*this was the President of Gulf Coast Bible College—I used the term chancellor, when writing this manuscript, to disguise his identity*] and requested that I prepare a report to present to the student body of Gulf Coast Bible College. The student body was to meet in a chapel service the following day, so I worked into the early morning hours to prepare a report that was educational, morally acceptable, and as unalarming as my conscience would allow. I was to meet with the college chancellor early the next morning so that he could look over my report.

At about 2 am on December 2, 1981, my paper was completed as follows:

There is understandably a great deal of concern over the recent discovery of cyanide in this community. Although this discovery is a recent one, the accumulated evidence indicates the cyanide pollutant has been present for at least eight to nine months, and perhaps as long as two years. Therefore, we have not so much experienced a recent poisoning, as we have the recent discovery of a chronic, persisting problem. It is now inevitable that the source of the contamination be sought out and corrected, hopefully very soon.

A major symptom among those with positive blood tests has been tiredness, with depression and lack of motivation. Nauseous headaches with dizziness have also been prominent. Children in these families tend to sleep excessively and complain of headaches and stomach aches. Research and resources indicate that the effects of cyanide disappear once exposure to cyanide is halted. My personal experience, and data obtained from affected patients, supports this information. Individuals vacationing away from the contaminated area as long as two days have generally reported complete recovery from the bothersome symptoms the cyanide imposes.

A Breath of Cyanide

When my suspicions concerning cyanide were confirmed a week ago with a third positive blood level, I dialed the National Poison Control Center and also contacted local health officials. Subsequently, state and county health personnel were notified. Soon afterwards, seven additional blood levels proved positive, and thus far no negative report has been obtained from an individual known to live in the Heights area.

The poison control center was very helpful in supplying reference values for cyanide blood levels. In instances of chronic cyanide poisoning, which is what we are now dealing with, toxic levels were reported from 2 to 36 micrograms per deciliter, with an average of 18 micrograms per deciliter. The average blood level among those tested thus far is about 17 micrograms per deciliter, varying from 2 to 28 micrograms per deciliter. One patient, who has completed six blood tests, yielded levels of 2, 10, 28, 5, 20, and 24 micrograms per deciliter in that sequence, the last two levels being drawn only three and one-half hours apart. This demonstrates that cyanide blood levels may rise and fall over short periods of time, and it is important to note that hydrogen cyanide gas can enter the bloodstream very rapidly. There were no deaths reported, by my resource, from cases of chronic cyanide poisoning. In events of death from acute cyanide poisoning, blood levels range from 100 to 1500 micrograms per deciliter, which is approximately four to sixty times greater than the upper levels discovered so far. Acute poisoning by lethal doses of cyanide may be specifically treated in an emergency room, but time is an important factor. I suggest that anyone developing the following symptoms be transported to an emergency room immediately. The symptoms are as follows: a nauseous headache with rapid breathing, dizziness, and semiconsciousness. Anyone with a history of these symptoms who is found unconscious should be rushed to an emergency room, informing the emergency room personnel of likely cyanide poisoning. Bear in mind that I give these precautions as a safety measure, and that no such incidents have occurred in this area to my knowledge.

As I mentioned previously, this is evidently an old problem just surfacing. The general health and emotional status among members of this community should significantly improve in the near future, as the source of the problem is discovered and altered. I encourage each of you to cooperate with city and government officials in tracking down the origin of this contaminant. I will be available for questioning in the foyer at the conclusion of this service.

At about 7:00 am that same morning, I sat in conference with the Chancellor of Gulf Coast Bible College as he reviewed my paper. He seemed to think the paper exaggerated the problem too much, but I assured him that I played the problem down as much as I could. He finally conceded, and I looked forward to sharing the report with the students.

Shortly before chapel service, I was informed of a change in plans. Several press agents were planning to attend the service in order to hear my report, but the chapel report was cancelled. Instead, a news conference was held in an upstairs foyer inside the administrative building of Gulf Coast Bible College. As I reflect back, I realize that this was only one of many actions that disallowed firsthand confrontation between the community and the facts. Dr. McKee was positioned directly after me in speaking order, and he very authoritatively stated that no evidence of cyanide poisoning had been found by Houston health officials and that the problem was confined to a very small area.

Soon after the report, I confronted the Chancellor of Gulf Coast Bible College, Dr. Fields [*the name Dr. Fields is fictionalized*], personally: "Could I speak with you a minute?" I asked.

"Sure Tim, come on in. Well, I thought the conference went rather well. What about you?"

A lump grew at the base of my throat. Having been raised to respect authority, I possessed a subconscious aversion to disagreeing with someone in a position of authority over me.

"I think we should get someone else to investigate this problem, I don't really trust Dr. McKee. He seemed set on dismissing the whole matter, and he said something that he had no way of knowing."

Dr. Fields responded with a look of inquisition. "What was that?"

"He claimed that his health department found absolutely nothing, and yet he was able to use that information to specify the confines of the contamination. Now how can you specify something by using nothing?"

Dr. Fields looked away. "Yes, we'll have to take that into consideration."

About that time someone barged into the office with us. I soon departed.

Later that afternoon, The Houston Chronicle publicized information from the news conference. They also mentioned that the first patient diagnosed with cyanide poisoning worked at an electroplating plant in the area. Mr. Blunz was quoted defending the electroplating plant, stating that the plant was too far away from the neighborhood where the first patient and the others lived. Indeed, the plant was about two miles west of the college. Later on, however, patients would be diagnosed with cyanide poisoning several miles west of the electroplating plant, as well as east. [*In fairness to this electroplating plant, it is now my understanding that they were using a state-of-the-art system to destroy cyanide in their industrial effluent through superchlorination, and readers may want to google a publication from January of 2019 entitled:* **Cyanide Destruction, A New Look at an Age-Old Problem**. *In addition, there is little doubt that there were other sources of airborne cyanide contributing to the poisoned atmosphere in the Heights. And furthermore, it may be that cyanogen chloride, a toxic war gas, could be found in the effluent of any plating facility that utilizes cyanide compounds for plating purposes and then incorporates a treating system featuring superchlorination to accomplish, or attempt to accomplish, destruction of cyanide. Also, I would not consider it the fault of this electroplating plant that the sanitary sewer system was apparently old and leaked into the storm sewer system, something that may have contributed to the local release of cyanogen chloride into the air. Having said that, however, I definitely believe that cyanogen chloride was released into the atmosphere through the operating system of this electroplating facility, and that this cyanogen chloride greatly contributed to "above average" levels of airborne cyanide in the vicinity of the plating plant, and that this cyanogen chloride also contributed to significant illness, probably even deaths, in persons who worked or resided in the vicinity of the plating plant. Note that cyanogen chloride, when inhaled, causes cyanide poisoning and contributes to positive findings for blood cyanide, serum thiocyanate, and urine thiocyanate. One finds a description of chronic poisoning from cyanogen chloride in* **handbook of POISONING: Diagnosis & Treatment, EIGHTH EDITION, by ROBERT H. DREISBACH, MD, PhD, Clinical Professor of Environmental Health, School of Public Health and Community Medicine, University of Washington, Seattle, and Professor (Emeritus) of Pharmacology, Stanford University School of Medicine, Stanford, California, Lange Medical**

Publications, Los Altos, California, 1974; *and the description is as follows:* **inhaling small amounts of cyanogen chloride repeatedly causes dizziness, weakness, congestion of lungs, hoarseness, conjunctivitis, loss of appetite, weight loss, and mental deterioration. Similar symptoms have also been reported from inhaling cyanide in low concentrations for one year or more.** *Years would pass before I would find out that cyanogen chloride was being discharged into the sanitary sewer system from whence it escaped into the atmosphere; so then, back to the story written in the 1980s.]*

Many things were happening, things I would not comprehend until later. My wife and I went to sleep in our queen-sized bed with uneasy misgivings about the events that transpired on December 2, 1981. Perhaps the next day would be better: perhaps someone from the Houston Health Department would recognize the problem that wracked people's health and mentality. If nothing else, we could hope and pray.

The next day, seven more patients visited my office for cyanide testing. Linda Blausen was the first. [*Linda's real is Shirley. She was actually the second patient tested for blood cyanide on 12/3/81, since a man named Larrie had blood drawn at 2:17 a.m., and Shirley had her blood drawn at 8:55 a.m. And I also need to make another correction— there were actually ten persons who had blood drawn for cyanide testing in my office on 12/3/81. This testing of 12/3/81 is covered in much more detail later in this book, in chapter 9.*] She had a long history of illness, and was dying. Her weight had gradually decreased to where she was almost unrecognizable from what she had been a year before. Her son, who lived with her in the same house, experienced terrible headaches. Upon questioning, I discovered that her son slept with his bedroom window open at night.

"I've been to doctors, in the hospital, everything!" exclaimed Linda. "And they couldn't find anything wrong with me, but I'm dying!"

"Has your appetite been decreased?" I asked.

"Yes! I can hardly eat at all."

"Do you feel like eating, but after a couple of bites, suddenly you're full and can't take another bite?" I further questioned. This was a symptom that I experienced myself that was notably distinct from symptoms I had previously experienced with stomach viruses.

"Yes, exactly."

"Well, with your headaches, depression, difficulty remembering things, decreased appetite, and weight loss, you definitely seem to fit in with the other patients that report the same symptoms. All of them tested so far have had positive blood cyanide tests." [*I want to mention, at this point, that persons with milder symptoms of cyanide intoxication may gain weight, rather than lose weight.*]

"Then let's get one."

Linda was not to be denied a blood test; that was for certain. Her interest in the situation, though, extended far beyond a blood test.

"Do you know where this stuff is coming from?" she inquired.

"Not for sure, but my wife and I are sicker when the wind comes from the west. I think it may be coming from a couple miles west of here."

Linda looked at me intensely. "Just what I thought. I live just north of that area, and when the wind blows out of the south, am I ever sick!"

A long pause followed.

"Is anyone doing anything about it?" asked Linda.

That was a good question. As I look back, I realize there was quite a bit being done about it, but not what an honest person would expect. As of December 3, 1981, I still had hopes that the Houston Health Department would solve the problem. I assumed, perhaps, that they were groping in ignorance, and that additional information would cause them to realize and alleviate the pollution. That is why I responded to Linda's question as follows:

"The next time you get ill, just call Mr. Blunz. He works with the Houston Health Department. He said he will send someone out to test the air if someone will just notify him when they get ill."

Two days later, Linda was brought to my office by her daughter, Ann. Ann was married and lived in a different part of town. Both women were obviously ill when they arrived at my office. They were breathing rapidly and their eyes were tearing.

"Hello, come on in," I said, gesturing for them to enter my office. "What brings you back to see me?"

Linda did most of the talking. "We found it. There was this white steam coming out of the ground at the corner of Greengrass and Overmyer." [*The intersection of Greengrass and Overmyer is located about 1,200 feet northwest of Jaycee Park in Houston.*]

"The ground?"

"Some sewer or drain opening."

I was amazed by the women's initiative. "Did you call the Houston Health Department?"

"Yes, but they would not come out. They told me they had already checked in that area and that there were no elevated cyanide levels there."

I was stunned. It seemed like the Houston Health Department was a malicious, uncaring monster. Only days before, Dr. McKee had stated that the poison could be dumped sporadically and may not always be present. This directly disputed the denial to investigate Linda's complaint on grounds that a prior test had been run. I shook my head in regretful disgust.

Linda assumed speaking, "Since they wouldn't come and test the air, we decided to test it ourselves."

"Really," I returned, quite convinced that there was more to this woman than met the eye.

"Yes. My son works with some folks that might be able to test the air. We went out and got some in a plastic bag."

"Where's the bag now?"

"I've got it in my garage."

Noting that both women were quite miserable with acute symptoms of cyanide intoxication, I offered them the usual treatment with sodium thiosulfate crystals. I had been using the treatment for some time with John and other patients, and it seemed to greatly relieve the headaches and depression accompanying chronic cyanide poisoning. Both women seemed to do all right at the time, but Linda, possibly with additional exposure to hydrogen cyanide gas [*or cyanogen chloride gas*], was in the hospital soon afterwards. She was admitted with severe disorientation, a symptom noted in acute cyanide poisoning.

Back in my office the two women seemed fairly stable.

"I really got sick when we reached the corner with steam coming up," explained Linda.

"So did I," added Ann. "My eyes started burning and watering, and I could hardly breathe. It was like I was suffocating."

"Maybe we should get another cyanide test," stated Linda.

Here I made a regretful mistake. My knowledge of chronic cyanide poisoning was still very limited, and due to the first ten blood cyanide tests being positive, I mistakably assumed that patients with symptoms of chronic cyanide poisoning would always yield positive blood cyanide tests. This was far from correct. Cyanide is attracted to body tissues, rather than blood, and may remain in the blood for only a short time with each exposure to hydrogen cyanide gas. Furthermore, cyanide that does remain in the blood is quite rapidly converted to thiocyanate or otherwise metabolized so that it would not show up on a blood cyanide test. An individual who is ill with chronic cyanide intoxication may yield a completely negative blood cyanide test more often than not, and still be desperately ill from cyanide intoxication. Not knowing this, I advised Linda and Ann against an additional cyanide test:

"Listen Linda, we already have plenty of positive blood cyanide tests on other patients, and even though yours is not back yet, I'm sure it will probably be positive. I don't want to waste your money."

"Well, they are rather expensive," she conferred, "maybe we should just check Ann." [*The blood cyanide tests, back then, cost me $35.00, and I charged the patients $38.00.*]

"I agree with that. She has been healthy up until now, and a positive test should reveal a recent exposure. But I don't want to test her for cyanide, I want to check her for copper."

"Copper!" returned Linda. "Why?"

"We have plenty of proof that people are getting exposed to cyanide, and your symptoms are obviously from cyanide exposure, so I think we should test for something that may narrow down the source. The electroplating plant uses copper cyanide, and they are bound to be dumping copper as well as cyanide."

Linda was obviously interested. "But would copper be in the air?"

"If the steam was coming out as thick as you say, then I imagine it could have carried some copper ions with it," I surmised. "How about it?"

Linda and Ann both agreed to the test and Ann was tested for blood copper. Her blood level came back high at 220 mcg/dl, normal being from 87 to 153 mcg/dl. This helped confirm my suspicions, at least in my own mind, but I was certainly consternated when Linda's previous blood cyanide test came back negative. [*Of note, Linda, whose real name is Shirley, was a smoker. I definitely believe that she suffered from environmental cyanide intoxication.*] In fact, four out of seven patients tested for blood cyanide on December 3, 1981, yielded blood cyanide levels of zero. [*Make that 7 out of 10 patients tested for blood cyanide on December 3, 1981, yielded blood cyanide levels of zero; and an eighth patient, who had a level reported as "less than 10 mcg/dl", probably also had a blood cyanide level of zero.*] The wife of one of these patients was later positive for cyanide poisoning by testing for thiocyanate, a metabolite of cyanide that is not as short-lived. Probably all four of those missed cases were victims of chronic cyanide poisoning. I had a lot to learn.

Of several patients tested on December third, only two had blood cyanide levels above 4 mcg/dl. One was a young man whose mental depression had been so severe that at one point he had actually placed a gun barrel in his mouth. [*One of my maternal uncles, who served in the United States Coast Guard, told me that suicides among* **stack inspectors** *were attributed to their exposures to cyanide.*] Like many of the patients, he expressed how unlike him it was to be depressed, much less to have thoughts of suicide. [*This young man, a nonsmoker, had a blood cyanide level of 8 mcg/dl.*]

The other patient with a blood cyanide above 4 mcg/dl on December third was a young lady accompanied by her mother. She complained of worrisome shortness of breath, and of burdensome depression. She became quite short of breath in my office just from speaking. One may not usually notice it, but one does not breathe regularly while speaking.

The young lady accepted a dose of sodium thiosulfate and was able to breathe much better in a few minutes. When able to speak, she definitely carried her share of the conversation. Her name was Jennifer.

"Oh, I can breathe!" exclaimed Jennifer. "This is unbelievable. I walked in here just a few minutes ago about to die of suffocation, and then you give me some little salt crystals to drink, and now I can breathe! [*I dissolved the sodium thiosulfate crystals in water, and then patients drank the solution.*] And my head—I can think! I feel like a different person."

"I'm glad I could help."

Jennifer eyed me with a look of excited discovery. "Help! Do you realize what I've been through? First I went to doctors, and they couldn't find anything wrong, and now I've been seeing a psychiatrist. I keep telling everybody I'm not crazy, but until now no one could tell me what was making me sick."

Jennifer was only one of several patients suffering from chronic cyanide poisoning who had been directed to a psychologist or psychiatrist. I decided to see if she shared another common characteristic.

"Do you notice any difference in your symptoms when you leave the area?" I posed.

"Yes, I've been telling my mother that whenever I go down to Galveston for the weekend, I feel fine."

This pretty much sealed Jennifer's diagnosis. She had extensive symptoms of chronic cyanide poisoning that were dramatically alleviated by a specific antidote for cyanide, and she also experienced marked improvement within a day or so of leaving the area of cyanide contamination. Her blood cyanide test would only be topping on the pudding, as far as I was concerned, but then I realized that without positive laboratory data the problem might escape public recognition. In fact, at least to that point in time, the problem was persisting quite menacingly despite positive laboratory data. [*Jennifer's real name is Robin, and she had a blood cyanide level of 5 mcg/dl. Robin was a nonsmoker.*]

The Houston Chronicle carried front page articles about the cyanide problem in both their morning and evening editions on December 3, 1981. The other major newspaper, The Houston Post, also got into the act with a front page story in their evening edition. Radio and television coverage was also blooming, and my phone was ringing nearly every time I put down the receiver. As news reports flowed forth, I began to realize that the news media held public opinion in the palm of their hand to a large degree. The facts that reached the public could be screened or preened at the media's option.

I was fairly displeased when I read the first article in The Houston Post. After the effort I had expended to downplay the seriousness of the cyanide contamination, mainly to protect the interests of my friends at Gulf Coast Bible College, the newspaper actually depicted a map which supposedly outlined the area of cyanide contamination, featuring Gulf Coast Bible College right in the middle of the map. I realized that Gulf Coast Bible College was probably being used as a scapegoat, for whatever reason, by the Houston Health Department. What made it worse, I knew that the two top Gulf Coast Bible College officials were bending over backwards to cooperate with the Houston Health Department.

I examined the map on the front page of The Houston Post and noted that an area six blocks from north to south, and five blocks from east to west, was circumscribed. Considering my persisting belief that the source of the poisoning was about two miles away, I found the little map quite incredible. A few other statements in the article also drew my interest. Dr. McKee was quoted saying that the problem was extremely localized, that a community problem from cyanide has been rather unlikely historically, and that cyanide that is used by industry does not generally escape into the atmosphere. It was obvious to me that all of these statements, along with the distinctly circumscribed map, served to place the origin I most suspected safely out of the picture.

The Houston Chronicle did not provoke me quite as much as The Houston Post. They included many of the same statements by the Houston Health Department, but they also mentioned that people living outside the neighborhood were also complaining of symptoms which could be caused by cyanide poisoning. The fact is, the sickest cyanide victims I would ever find during my work in Houston would be patients who lived outside the boundaries depicted in The Houston Post. There would even be tangible evidence that individuals as far as fifteen miles west of Gulf Coast Bible College suffered from chronic cyanide poisoning. This information, though, would be tiresomely long in coming.

Linda Blausen moved to a different part of town and her health improved tremendously.

Chapter 3

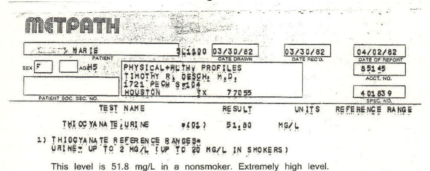

Foul Play

Before moving on to December 4, 1981, allow me to backtrack to December second. Besides being the morning of my first news conference, it was the afternoon when the Houston Health Department rechecked my cyanide patients for cyanide. At that time, I did not realize how ridiculous it was to look for cyanide in the blood of patients who were positive for blood cyanide several days earlier. Cyanide disappears from blood in minutes or hours, much less days. Besides the time element, the Houston Health Department elected to draw the blood samples in the upstairs room of a centrally air-conditioned building.

There were several other individuals, besides my previously diagnosed patients, who wished to have their blood tested by the Houston Health Department. The upstairs room was fairly populated.

"We would be glad to test the other individuals," remarked Dr. Noble, a representative of the Houston Health Department, "but I'm afraid we did not bring enough blood specimen tubes."

"I've got some in my office," I returned.

"All right," consented Dr. Noble, "if you can get us more tubes, then we will test as many of the others as we can."

What bothered me the most was testing the patients inside a centrally air-conditioned building. [*My medical office was small and had no central air conditioning.*] To make matters worse, the patients had to wait quite a long time and have an interview before their blood was drawn for testing. As I look back on the situation, I do not know whether the Houston Health Department was ignorant or criminal in its strategy. It would have been much better to test patients over an extended period of time, and to draw their blood right in their homes or at their jobs where they experienced the worst symptoms of cyanide poisoning. One factor gave me a glint of hope; the wind was blowing from the west.

    I walked briskly to my office and picked up several specimen tubes. My office was only a short distance from the building where the tests were taken. No sooner had I returned to the building than it became evident that still more tubes were needed. Exactly how many trips I made between my office and the neighboring building I cannot remember, but I managed to inhale a sizeable quantity of outside air.

    What I have not yet mentioned, up to this point, is that on Wednesday, December 2, 1981, many people who lived in my neighborhood were ill. Low doses of cyanide tend to sicken some people and symptomatically spare others, but this particular Wednesday was seemingly cyanide plagued. I fully expected some of the tests taken by the Houston Health Department to be positive despite the central air conditioning. Still, I had a wary mistrust of the health department, and decided to have an additional blood test performed on myself to double-check them.

    I was one of the first volunteers to have blood drawn in the centrally air-conditioned building. My waiting period was shorter than for those who followed me: only fifteen to twenty minutes. I worked with the Houston Health Department officials, encouraging my ailing patients to go through with the needle jab that preceded extracting three tubes of blood. It was only about thirty minutes after my blood was drawn when I summoned a college professor named Mrs. Bland to redraw my blood in my medical clinic. This followed several trips back and forth between my office and the college administration building to deliver blood specimen tubes. It would be long afterward before I gained sufficient knowledge to realize the unperceived wisdom in this action.

    In the back room of my medical clinic, Mrs. Bland adeptly pierced my vein with a 21 gauge needle. Then, to my surprise, we both observed bright red blood spurt into the vacuum tube. Earlier, when my blood was drawn in the air-conditioned building, it was purplish-blue, a normal color for venous blood. Now the blood appeared like arterial blood. I decided to show the blood to Dr. Noble.

As the bright red blood spouted into the collection tube, my mind flashed back to another occasion when I saw blood of that color. It occurred nine days earlier, shortly before my wife and I left on our trip to Tulsa. Peter Minowsky [*fictitious name*] came to my apartment; something was obviously wrong.

"I hate to bother you, doc," Peter spoke rapidly, standing outside my door, "but my wife is so sick she can't stand up. She nearly passed out onto the floor. I think she's got that cyanide stuff like Glenna."

Glenna and Jan, Peter's wife, were close acquaintances. Jan was probably aware of the cyanide problem from conversing with Glenna. I dashed down to my office, grabbed some supplies, and quickly accompanied Peter to his tiny, upstairs apartment a little over a block away. When we entered the door, Janet was collapsed in a large, old lounge chair. She was in obvious distress; she appeared feverish, breathed rapidly, and conveyed significant pain without speaking a word.

Jan responded satisfactorily to antidote therapy with sodium thiosulfate. What caught my eye, though, was the color of her venous blood; it was bright red. When her lab results returned with a blood cyanide of 27 mcg/dl, I recollected that John [*the first patient found to have blood cyanide, who worked at the electroplating plant*] previously had a higher blood cyanide without having bright red venous blood. Sometime later, I learned that the bright red color is not caused by cyanide in the blood, but rather by cyanide in the body tissues. When enough cyanide binds to the body tissues, then oxygen is not used from the blood as it flows through capillaries, and the venous blood remains bright red due to a high oxygen content.

I left my office with the blood Mrs. Bland had drawn and walked directly to the administration building where Dr. Noble was still supervising blood-collecting for the Houston Health Department.

"Look at the color of this blood. It was just drawn in my office," I said, holding the blood up for Dr. Noble's inspection.

Dr. Noble examined the blood with interest. "Yes," he remarked, "the bright red color is caused by cyanide blocking oxygen uptake in the tissues."

I was surprised, not by the scientific data, but by Doctor Noble's openness and honesty. He did not seem like the other officials I had met from the Houston Health Department, there was something genuine and trustworthy about him. Even with his notably foreign accent and Asian look, I felt much more confidence in this man than his fellow employees.

In retrospect, I realize that circumstances were almost ideal for finding a positive level of blood cyanide when Mrs. Bland drew my blood. The wind was from the west, I had been walking vigorously out-of-doors, and my blood was drawn almost immediately after entering an office without central air-conditioning. The level of cyanide in my blood was 104 mcg/dl. The average lethal level is notably higher, but the minimal lethal level is generally stated at 100 mcg/dl. It is rather sobering to discover that one's blood had more than a minimal lethal level of poison in it. The same laboratory found only a blood cyanide of 21 mcg/dl from my blood that was drawn earlier that day after spending fifteen to twenty minutes in the centrally air-conditioned building.

One may wonder how I felt with a blood cyanide of 104 mcg/dl. That is a reasonable question. I had a dizzy headache, was a little short of breath, and felt achy all over. Sounds a lot like the flu, doesn't it? It is not unlikely that many doctors in Houston were treating patients for the flu when they actually had cyanide poisoning.

The fact is, I was much sicker at other times than on the afternoon of December second. It is not the amount of cyanide in the blood that causes illness, but rather, the amount of cyanide in muscle, heart, brain, and other body tissues. Some of the patients who sat for hours in the centrally air-conditioned building did not have positive cyanide blood levels at all, even though they were pitifully ill with chronic cyanide poisoning. One should realize, though, that chronic cyanide poisoning must indeed be very elusive, very insidious, and very vague diagnostically, or else someone would have discovered and defined the problem long ago. The fact that it causes symptoms in some people while sparing others, flees the blood quickly invading body tissues, and causes illnesses which mimic viral diseases, heart diseases, and psychiatric problems, has enabled chronic cyanide poisoning to plague myriads of human beings for years, without recognition.

It was some time before any results were released by the Houston Health Department. Personally, I don't think they liked what was discovered. Each patient had three blood samples taken, and one of the samples was sent to each of three different laboratories: the City of Houston Health Department Laboratory, Harris County Medical Examiners Toxicology Laboratory, and Severance and Associates Laboratory in San Antonio. I did not receive blood levels on all of the patients, but I did receive reports on those individuals who were assumed to be my patients. There were twenty-two such individuals.

Of the twenty-two individuals I received reports on who were tested through the Houston Health Department, sixteen of them had positive blood cyanide levels greater than 10 mcg/dl found by at least one of the three laboratories. Interestingly, I was able to get an estimate from eighteen of the twenty-two individuals as to how long they had to wait in the central air conditioning before having their blood drawn. Four of them waited less than 30 minutes, eight of them waited 30 minutes to an hour, and six of them waited over an hour. All four of those who waited less than 30 minutes had positive blood cyanide levels, seven out of the eight who waited 30 minutes to an hour had positive cyanide levels, and only three out of the six who waited over an hour had positive blood cyanide levels. Notably, the Houston Health Department did not find a single positive cyanide level in any of these patients. Was it any wonder that they also failed to find cyanide in the air or water?

The most notable correlation between time spent waiting in the central air conditioning and blood cyanide levels was demonstrated by Severance and Associates Laboratory. They found 75% of those who waited less than 30 minutes positive for cyanide, 37.5% of those who waited from 30 minutes to an hour positive for cyanide, and none of those who waited over an hour positive for cyanide. The Harris County Medical Examiners Toxicology Laboratory found a larger number of patients with positive blood cyanide levels than Severance and Associates Laboratory, but they found as large a percentage of positive results in those who waited over an hour as in those who waited less than 30 minutes. From all indications, Severance and Associates Laboratory did the most accurate testing.

One may assume that the Houston Health Department would have to admit the reality of cyanide contamination after collecting so much positive evidence. This would be a reasonable assumption, but there are forces at work in our society other than the power of reason. During my stay in Houston, I received quite an education about some of the more nefarious forces in modern civilization and how they operate. Sometime after the blood tests were taken by the Houston Health Department, each patient received a copy of their results along with some carefully constructed propaganda.

The report that the Houston Health Department sent to the previously-tested individuals was absurdly misleading. They referred to reference values given by a committee of experts from the school of the health department. [*I do not remember the exact name of the school.*] Using this committee as grounds of authority, they conveyed that normal healthy people could have blood cyanide levels ranging from 0-31 mcg/dl, and that smokers could have levels from 1-52 mcg/dl. Not only were these levels far above any reference values I had obtained from several different sources, they were blatantly inconsistent with the blood cyanide levels found by the Houston Health Department. Of the twenty-two patients tested by the Houston Health Department whose results I received, the Houston Health Department did not find a single positive blood cyanide in any one of them, including at least one smoker.

As I looked back over the report issued by the Houston Health Department, I noticed an intriguing play on words. They did not state that the reference values presented were normal values; but rather, that they could be found in normal, healthy people. The same levels could also be found in people sick with cyanide poisoning! In other words, the report did not give normal values at all, it gave an observation that there are individuals in this world who can have elevated blood cyanide levels without demonstrating illness. Big deal—there may also be individuals who can hold their breath for three minutes or drink a pint of gasoline without demonstrating illness. The report was signed by a high-ranking official of the Houston Health Department.

With environmental conditions lending extensive potential for positive cyanide testing, I regret that only one patient besides me was tested in my office on December second. Mrs. Patterson was a vivid example of the crushing personality changes assaulting many individuals suffering from the poison, and her particular case yielded a great deal of ecological information. One of my wife's favorite teachers at Gulf Coast Bible College, Mrs. Patterson was well known for her uplifting enthusiasm and energetic lectures. As the poison began affecting her, however, the students noticed a change in their teacher. Her face grew haggard, her usually sparkling eyes looked dull, and her bubbly energy changed to dragging fatigue.

Unlike most of my cyanide patients up to that time, Mrs. Patterson did not actually live in Houston, she lived about eighteen miles northwest of the Heights area. By the time she learned about the cyanide contamination, her illness had progressed to the point where she was missing quite a bit of school. It was evident to her that her symptoms were better at home and grew worse whenever she came to work at school, but she did not know why. It was during a sick leave from school that she learned about the cyanide problem and made a special trip to my office for evaluation. She waited in my office for nearly an hour before I saw her, and was not feeling well when I arrived.

"Hello, I'm sorry you had to wait, someone just now told me you were here," I apologized as I entered the office.

"Don't worry about that, I'm glad someone may have finally figured out what's wrong with me. I've only been in town about an hour, and I'm already having a terrible headache. Oh, I haven't even introduced myself, I'm Mrs. Patterson."

"Mrs. Patterson!" I returned. "My wife's teacher?"

"Yes, Melody is a lovely student."

"Melody talks about you all the time. She really likes you."

Mrs. Patterson flashed a thankful smile. "I like teaching too, but lately I haven't felt much like it."

"What's been the matter?" I inquired, seating myself leisurely in a swivel chair.

"For some time now I've noticed myself growing weaker and less motivated. Lately it's become so bad that I can hardly lift my head, and I have to force myself to do anything. When I'm here at work I get headaches so bad it feels like the top of my head is going to pop off."

I listened to the symptoms with interest. They were very much like those of other patients, but Mrs. Patterson just came from eighteen miles away. She was having a headache after only one hour in the affected area.

"You say you're having one of those headaches right how?" I questioned.

"I sure am."

"Have you had anything to eat since coming into town?"

"No."

"Where do you get your groceries?"

"Out at a grocery store near my home."

This was exactly what I hoped to hear. It seemed apparent to me that the poison was airborne, but after reading the newspaper, I knew the proof would probably be dependent on private investigation. There remained one further question:

"Have you had anything to drink since coming to town?"

"Nothing."

"All right, I'd like to get a blood cyanide on you."

Mrs. Patterson looked pleased, if not relieved. "Please do, that's what I'm here for."

After being home several days, and returning to Houston for only about one hour, Mrs. Patterson yielded a blood cyanide of 55 mcg/dl. This solidified an already certain point in my mind: the cyanide was airborne. There were still some major questions to answer, like how cyanide at such levels could come from a source miles away without killing several people in between. Eventually the answers would come. Meanwhile, I had to stick to evidence in the face of coolly desperate denial from the Houston Health Department.

One other incident took place December second that looms significantly among the events which followed the early publication of cyanide contamination in Houston. It was a phone call. Initially, the call seemed insignificant. It was a strange call, once I began thinking about it, but it came at a busy time. I was probably hoodwinked. In my mind, I can still hear the warmly confidential voice that sounded from a distant origin:

"Hello, this is Dick Parker. I'm calling from Connecticut."

"Connecticut!" I responded. I did not know anyone named Dick Parker, and although calls were streaming through my telephone, none had come from outside my own state.

"That's right. I keep up with the news quite a bit, and just happened to read about the cyanide poisoning down there. I understand you're the doctor that first discovered it."

"Yea, it was sort of providential luck, I guess you could say," I returned. Considering the events which fit together in disclosing the cyanide poisoning, I thought taking too much credit would be a mistake. I know God is still in business, and I believe he must have had more to do with the disclosure than I did.

"Well, congratulations, you've made quite a name for yourself. I work around a little cyanide myself, working with precious metals, and when I came across the article about your discovery, I was intrigued. That's just the way I am. From time to time I see something that interests me and I like to find out all about it. Tell me, where do you think this cyanide stuff is coming from?"

As I look back, I realize I should have been suspicious. How many times do people call over a thousand miles away to talk with someone they do not even know about something they read in the newspaper? Perhaps I can partly blame the cyanide for depressing my brain cells, but I still confess that I was probably badly suckered.

"I'm pretty sure it's coming through the air," I commented. "There don't seem to be any foods all of my patients share in common, and some of them don't drink hardly any water at all, they drink mostly pop, or tea, or coffee, but not water."

"Well they have to put water in their tea or coffee, don't they?"

"I suppose so," I concurred, though I knew that a couple of my patients with cyanide intoxication drank very little besides diet soda, despite my disapproval.

"You still haven't satisfied my curiosity," Mr. Parker persisted. "What do you think is the origin of the cyanide poisoning?"

"Well, I…"

Mr. Parker had called at a busy time in my office, and regardless of my excessive willingness to answer questions, circumstances beyond my control again proved educational.

"I'm sorry, I have to take care of a patient. Thank you for calling, it's really something to talk with someone who takes such an interest in things as you do," I said to Mr. Parker. We had conversed for quite some time.

"Wait, I'm not through yet," interjected Mr. Parker. "I'd still like to talk with you more about this. Can I call later?"

"Sure, I'm not certain when I'll be here. My office hours have been pretty irregular lately."

"Well, why don't you call me when you get a chance? I can leave my number."

"Well…um…can I call collect?"

I still remained unsuspecting. Realizing my financial situation, though, I was not anxious to call long distance, especially to someone so long-winded as this man. My gross, monetary income for 1981 was less than seven thousand dollars, and at that rate a little money can make a big difference.

"Oh, sure," responded Mr. Parker, though he sounded surprised by my question.

"All right then, what's your number?"

Mr. Parker gave me his number, and after taking care of the business at hand I called him right back. The second round of conversation almost succeeded in drawing an inkling of wariness from my mind. Mr. Parker got right back to the subject:

"Okay, now where were we," directed Mr. Parker. "I think you were about to tell me where you thought the cyanide was coming from."

"It's kind of a touchy issue down here," I said, somewhat hesitant to comment. Talking to someone who seemed truly interested and willing to listen, though, was a refreshing change from dealing with the Houston Health Department. "The place I think it's coming from is the same place I suspected from the very start."

"What's that?" coaxed Mr. Parker.

"An electroplating plant about two miles west of here. They use cyanide bound to metals, like copper cyanide or silver cyanide, and after the electroplating takes place, the cyanide is a by-product."

"Two miles away! Don't you think it's more likely something local. It seems like lots of people would be dead if the source was two miles away, especially employees at the plant."

The similarity of Mr. Parker's arguments to those of the Houston Health Department was probably more than coincidence. Still, considering that the call was from Connecticut, I did not make any connection between the two at the time.

"What you're saying might be true if the cyanide went directly into the air," I conceded, "but I don't believe that is what's happening."

"Oh really, what do you mean?"

"Well, in the first place, there may be some people between here and the plant who have died from cyanide poisoning. Death from cyanide poisoning could easily pass for a heart attack or a stroke."

"Do you think there have been any deaths?

"Well, I imagine there probably have been, especially with older people or people who are already ill. Someone with heart disease may get pushed on over the edge with a dose of cyanide that would only make a normal person feel a little sick."

"But there haven't been any proven deaths from the poisoning," Mr. Parker posed.

"No, but then they haven't been checking people who died in this area for cyanide. It's not the kind of thing that anyone would find without looking directly for it."

"Getting back to the plant you mentioned," redirected Mr. Parker, "you said the cyanide is not going into the air. Do you think it's in the drinking water?"

"No, I think the cyanide is in the air, but I think it's in water first. The plant dumps their discharge into the sewer or drainage ditches, and from there it flows along in the public sewers or storm sewers. The cyanide is not stable in the water, though, and comes back out as hydrogen cyanide gas. [*It was several years before I was informed about the cyanogen chloride in the discharge water from the electroplating plant.*]

"I see," said Mr. Parker. It seemed as though a notable change of tone colored his voice. "That still doesn't sound very likely to me. You know where I would check if I were you?"

"Where?" I responded. By this time I had a strange feeling about Mr. Parker. He expended too much energy trying to reshape my thinking.

"They make a lot of cheap jewelry in Mexico using cyanide solutions. I bet someone has dumped some of that jewelry into your drinking water. I would check there if I were you."

For a man with such a professional, sensible-sounding voice, Mr. Parker's suggestion sure was far-fetched. For a second I was speechless, not wanting to be rude or belittle the man's suggestion.

"Well," I finally conjured, "I'll keep that in mind."

"You do that, that's probably your culprit."

"Thanks for calling."

"It was a pleasure. Keep up the good work."

"Okay."

"Bye now."

"Goodbye."

The conversation was not alarming to me. There were quite a number of people giving their opinions about the source of the contamination. It was awesome to receive a call from more than a thousand miles away, but I thought little of it. Little, that is, until a few days later.

There were a couple of employees from the electroplating plant who delivered some interesting information from time to time. One of them, who I'll refer to as Mr. Z, relayed a message that jostled my memory and aroused my mind. He approached me with obvious concern:

"Say, doctor, can I talk with you a minute?"
"Sure, what is it?"
"How about in your office?"
"Fine."

My apartment and office were in such close proximity, with my office below my apartment, that patients often found me in transit between the two. Mr. Z apparently wanted to talk in private. Once confident of privacy, he quickly addressed the matter concerning him:

"I think there's something fishy going on over at the plant. Some big shots showed up at the beginning of the week from Connecticut, and they've been meeting together with officials from the Houston Health Department."

Something in my mind starting clicking. "Did you say Connecticut?"

"Right. That's where the national headquarters of General Electric is located." [*General Electric happened to own the electroplating plant; and at that time, a national headquarters for General Electric was in Plainville, Connecticut.*]

"That's interesting."

Mr. Z looked at me inquisitively. There were probably messages written all over my face.

"Why's that?" asked Mr. Z.

"I got a phone call during the middle of the week from Connecticut. Whoever it was said that the only reason he called was because he read about the cyanide poisoning and was interested in finding out about it."

"Likely story," Mr. Z replied. "They're up to something, and it's probably no good. The big shots met with officials of the Houston Health Department today, then left. They've gone back to Connecticut now. I wouldn't be surprised if there were a few bucks passed back and forth."

Suddenly I felt rather sickened about all the information I passed over the telephone. "Thanks, if you hear anything else, let me know."

Mr. Z left my office with the same conviction as me: it would be a royal battle to get anything done about the poison that was plaguing our neighborhood.

Sometime later an idea crossed my mind. I found out from Mr. Z the name of the town where the headquarters for General Electric was located, namely Plainville. Next, I asked a favor of one of my patients,

James Marshal. In short, I asked James to dial the phone number Dick Parker had given me and to find out where Mr. Parker had called from.

James Marshal was a gracious patient. Between diagnosing a small parasite in his skin, and finding that he also suffered from chronic cyanide poisoning, I was privileged to help explain and alleviate some very annoying symptoms. Besides this, James was a helpful, cooperative person, and he definitely wanted to see the end of the cyanide poisoning. When I confronted him with my request, he was more than willing to comply.

Not long afterward, James informed me of a successful mission. As I remember it, he first called me on the phone:

"Hello, Doctor Oesch?"

"Yes."

"This is James."

"Oh, hi James." I was anxious to hear whether or not James had called Connecticut, but I refrained from asking for fear of intimidating or pressuring him. After all, he may have called for an entirely different purpose.

"I called the number you wanted me to."

"And?"

"The call came from Avon, Connecticut."

"Good work," I commended, but I was curious to find out more details. "What happened when you called?"

"A lady answered the phone, and I asked her if Ginger Parker was there. She told me it was the Parker residence, but that she did not know any Ginger Parker. Then I asked her if she knew of any Ginger Parker in her town, and she told me that there were several other Parkers in Avon, but she did not know of any named Ginger. So then, I thanked her and hung up. I called from a pay phone."

"Fantastic!" I further lauded. Playing detective can be fairly tricky, and I certainly appreciated James's smooth work. "Thanks a lot for your help."

"If you need me for anything else, just let me know."

"All right."

"Bye."

"Goodbye."

After the call, I headed straight for a map. Avon was easy to locate. It was situated about ten miles north of Plainville. The circumstantial evidence was plain. Besides calls within my own state, the only call I received as of December 3, 1981, regarding the cyanide poisoning, came from a town over a thousand miles away which sat about ten miles north of Plainville, headquarters of General Electric.

Assimilating the information gained through James Marshall and Mr. Z, along with the phone call I received from Dick Parker, it was easy to deduce that foul play was likely underway. A more difficult question was what to do about it. Surely there were at least a few decent, honest individuals working within the Houston Health Department. Considering the size of the organization, it was unthinkable that they could all be crooked. Even so, it was only a small minority who ruled the organization, and I had reason enough to believe they were a threat to the citizens who paid their salaries.

Actually, the last hope I held for some measure of integrity in the Houston Health Department was crushed a day or so before the visit from Mr. Z, on the evening of December fourth. After what happened on that day and that evening, my eyes were opened to an evil deeper than ignorance. It may be folly for a foolish man to instruct others, but for a knowledgeable man to direct amiss is criminal.

Chapter 4

```
BIO-SCIENCE LABORATORIES 5303 CAROLINE, HOUSTON, TX 77004 (713)528-6346
,JOE                        OESCH        ACCOUNT #   99998    DATE RECEIVED  05/11/82
                                         BIL SPEC. # D75686   DATE COLLECTED 05/11
                                         VOL/24 HR  UNSTATED  PAGE    1

     TEST              RESULT          UNITS           REFERENCE RANGE
U THIOCYANATE           1.8            MG/100ML       NORMAL UNDER 0.2            A
                                                      SMOKERS UP TO 3
```

Non-Smoker.
Pos. c̄ Symptoms
For Cyanide Poisoning.

Stalking Death

December fourth was another busy day. Eleven additional patients were tested for blood cyanide in my office. Six of them yielded levels of zero, but positive blood cyanide levels stretched as high as 18 mcg/dl. Again, most or all of the eleven patients probably suffered from chronic cyanide poisoning, but blood levels of cyanide are short-lived. I was in the process of obtaining any information on chronic cyanide poisoning I could acquire, but the information was sparse and came from widely diverse origins.

It was around noontime that I received a request to meet with a group of officials from the Houston Health Department. Among them would be Dr. Judith Craven, Director of the Houston Health Department. Bear in mind that at this point in time I was not aware of the information Mr. Z would shortly make known to me. I had hopes for a productive and informative meeting. [*For persons who would like to see the newspaper articles regarding the cyanide reports in the Heights, the Houston Public Library has the Houston Post on microfilm from 1880 to 1995, as does the M.D. Anderson Library at the University of Houston. I would assume that The Houston Chronicle could also be found on microfilm at the Houston Public Library, and it is also available on microfilm, 1969-1984, at the Texas State Library and Archives, 1201 Brazos St., Austin, TX.*]

The gathering in my office filled the front room to capacity. [*I likely borrowed some folding chairs to accommodate my visitors.*] There were about five distinguishably dressed persons occupying the room with me. Three of them have escaped my memory, but the other two are still memorably distinct. I think the two I remember did most of the talking. Dr. Craven was one of them, and the other was an older, middle-aged man with gray streaks running through carefully groomed hair.

Dr. Craven initiated conversation. "As you know, Doctor Oesch, we're meeting together today to discuss the recent reports of cyanide poisoning in this area. I'm Doctor Craven, and with me are several of my associates."

"Welcome to my office."

Dr. Craven maintained a stern and professional countenance. "To be frank, Doctor Oesch, we are a little concerned about the way this problem has been published. Don't you think the Houston Health Department should have been notified before the news media?"

The question rather startled me. It was far from a constructive discussion of the cyanide problem.

"Well, actually, I was not the one who contacted the news media," I replied.

"You are not the one who contacted the news media?" spoke up the gray-haired gentleman.

"No. Apparently one of my patients lives down the street from a newspaper reporter…"

"So that person told the reporter and the reporter took it from there," interjected the same gentleman.

"Right."

The gentleman settled back in his chair and faced the other members of the group. "Yes, that's the way it usually happens."

"Besides the news media," resumed Doctor Craven, "we don't feel you have been handling this investigation properly. I understand you have been having your tests run at Severance and Associates Laboratory."

"That's right."

"Is that the only laboratory you have been using?"

Severance and Associates Laboratory was a large, established, and well-respected laboratory. Up to the time of that meeting on December fourth, it was indeed the only laboratory I had used. It is not customary for physicians to use more than one laboratory for doing blood tests, taking X-rays, or diagnosing patients prior to surgery. Generally a physician uses a lab and depends on that lab for accurate results. Each lab has the responsibility of checking their own procedures and guaranteeing dependable testing.

"Yes," I replied, with the distinct feeling I was being backed into a corner.

"Testing individuals for a problem of this nature should be conducted in an organized, scientific manner. Several different laboratories should be used so that results can be double-checked between the different laboratories."

"I have no objection to using different laboratories," I responded. "In fact, I think that's a real good idea. What I think would be a good idea would be for the Houston Health Department to test people at various points farther and farther away in all directions from this area. That way you could find out how far the problem extends. So far, no one has done that."

An uneasy silence lingered for several awkward seconds. Before anyone replied, I resumed speaking. "I would be glad to run the tests myself, if the Houston Health Department could supply funds. I just don't have enough money to run tests like that myself."

By the end of my resumed discourse, there was detectably regained composure among my listeners.

"We will certainly take your suggestions into consideration," offered Dr. Craven. "Of course, we have already collected quite a number of tests from your patients, plus a number of other people in this area."

"You mean the tests you took last Wednesday?" I inquired. [*By* **last Wednesday**, *I was referring to two days before, on 12/2/81.*]

"Yes, the tests were taken in full cooperation with the college administrators here."

"That's good," I conceded, "but that still doesn't show the boundaries of the contamination. Besides that, the levels of contamination seem higher on some days and lower on others. They also seem worse in instances where people do not have central air conditioning. I think the best way to test people for blood cyanide would be right in their homes. By keeping track of the locations and wind direction, you may be able to get a good idea of where the poison is coming from."

The data and suggestions I shared with the officials in my office were drawn from toilsome experience in dealing with my own illness and that of my patients. It was almost disconcerting when my sincere suggestions were all but ignored, seemingly given audience only to pacify my desire to share them.

"Is that your diploma?" questioned the gray-haired gentleman. The change of subject was avidly supported by the eyes and body language of his comrades. He glanced toward the large certificate that hung on the south wall of the office.

"Yes, it is."

"Looks like you graduated from…where?"

The diploma was huge, definitely Texas-sized, but the gentleman was sitting some distance away, against the west wall of the office.

"From the University of Texas Medical Branch in Galveston," I conferred.

"That's supposed to be a pretty good school, from what I hear," proceeded the gentleman. "When did you graduate?"

"I graduated in nineteen eighty."

"Nineteen eighty, and this is only eight-one. Sounds like you are a pretty young doctor."

"Yes. I'm twenty-seven, and people tell me I look younger than that."

The gentleman stared at my diploma, but his mind seemed otherwise occupied. It was a number of seconds before he posed his next question. "Do you feel comfortable working in your own practice like this, especially being such a young doctor?"

By this time I began surmising that the central topic of discussion was not the cyanide problem, it was me. An unmistakable impression that the veracity and reality of the cyanide contamination was more dependent on my personal qualifications and personality than on objective laboratory testing was definitely cast by the interrogative group gathered about me.

"I've been working with people in different jobs and programs for years," I replied. "I don't have any problem relating to people at all."

"I see, but what about the medical side of your practice? Do you feel you have enough knowledge to carry on your own practice?"

Obviously I was being sized up, but I did not know why. "I do a lot of reading. If a patient comes in with a problem I find puzzling, then I do some research on it. Of course I refer patients when necessary, but it's rarely necessary."

"Did you do an internship after you graduated?"

"Well, I finished the basic requirements for graduation during the first three years of medical school, then I did a year of externships: emergency room, family practice clinic, dermatology, labor and delivery, various studies I thought would be handy for practicing where no other doctors were available. I thought I might practice in a small town or overseas as a missionary. In fact, I was commissioned as a missionary, but my visa never came through."

The gray-haired gentleman looked intently about the office, at me, and at the diploma hanging above our heads.

"What do your associates say about the cyanide problem?" he posed.

Having just started my practice about three months before, operating out of a small, secluded office some distance off the road, I really did not have any medical associates. "Well, as far as I know, I'm the only one who has been testing anyone for cyanide poisoning. I haven't met any of the other doctors in this area yet."

"So you are the only doctor who has been testing for cyanide?" the gentleman reiterated inquiringly.

"As far as I know."

Placing both hands on his knees, the gentleman straightened and looked about at the other individuals in the group, especially at Dr. Craven. He seemed ready to leave. Doctor Craven took the gentleman's cue and tersely summarized the meeting:

"Basically, Doctor Oesch, we feel that this type of problem is rather complicated and ought to be handled by the proper authorities, which in this case is the Houston Health Department. To this point, we don't feel that any conclusive studies have been performed, and we are worried about the community becoming overly alarmed."

Listening to Dr. Craven speak, I remember being impressed by her seeming ignorance: a profound community problem devastated many people's lives. I imagined that, with time, if I were patient with them, the Houston Health Department would probably deduce the presence of such a plainly evident plight. I was not yet positive that they were part of the problem.

"I'll be glad to have all the help I can get," I responded. "I don't mind your handling the problem at all. In fact, I've been trying to get some help for some time now."

"It sounds like you intend to keep testing patients on your own then," stated Dr. Craven.

"If a patient comes to my office sick, and wants tested for cyanide, I probably won't refuse to test him."

Dr. Craven turned her head, facing the others in the group. "I guess that's about all we had to say. Does anyone else have something to add?"

There were no additions, and the meeting was ended. It was not the scientific discourse I had expected. I walked up the steps to my apartment feeling that little, if anything, had been accomplished. My wife liked to keep tab on events; she was especially curious concerning how long the poisoning would continue.

"Hi honey, how did the meeting go?" inquired Melody. "Are they going to do anything?"

Melody often sat at a small, wooden table in the kitchen to study. Small stacks of books, poster board, and numerous colored markers bedecked the tabletop. These were cleared to one side from time to time for meals. My seat of study was nearby, on the large sofa in the den. I plopped there and kept my books handy upon or below the coffee table before the sofa. We often communicated with one another between these two points of academic ardor.

"I'm not sure. They said they would take the matter into consideration," I replied.

Sometimes when I am communicating with my wife, I can almost see her face without looking at it. On this occasion, there was a pause before she responded to my statement, and I still can visualize her probable facial characteristics. Glittering and sparkling erupt within her eyes like live wires touched together before a Fourth of July sparkler. Her lips close firmly together above a tightened jaw, and her dimples engrave her prominent cheeks deeply. Here is what she said:

"Take it into consideration! People are being poisoned in their own homes and they're going to take it into consideration! Why don't you tell them they can come and live here for a while, then we'll see if they want to take it into consideration!"

What could I say? She said what I dared not, because if I did, I might lose my relations with the press, with the Houston Health Department, and with officials at Gulf Coast Bible College. I knew that the wrong public image on my part might endanger the lives and health of thousands of others. It was a constantly present challenge to relate a horrifying truth, and yet to remain calm, assuring, and unemotional. I admired Melody's simple, straightforward frankness.

"You have a point, dear," I concurred.

As the day wore on, the time soon approached for the six o'clock news. From December second to December fourth, my wife and I found ourselves the focal object of quite a few camera lenses. All the major television stations were making a production of the cyanide discovery. Also interviewed were patients, college students, and various officials. It caused quite a bit of excitement among the more camera-loving individuals in the neighborhood.

Ultimately, the news coverage may have helped bring aid to the community. On the other hand, there were ways the media was used to thwart the facts and hinder expeditious solution of the cyanide pollution. At first my wife and I attempted to follow the news fairly closely, but after a while we decided to work with known information and let the news go as it may. So, when the six o'clock news came around on December fourth, we both found other things to do besides watch television. When the ten o'clock news followed later, however, we were both before a television set. The reason was a message we received from our closest neighbors, Fred [*fictitious name*] and Glenna.

We were invited by Fred and Glenna to watch the late edition of the news in their home. Perhaps they wanted to see what our reaction would be when we saw and heard what they did at six. There were quite a number of people telling me that the Houston Health Department was crooked, and that they were out to disprove the existence of cyanide poisoning regardless of the facts, but I like to give people the benefit of a doubt. So, until I saw the news report for myself, I still hoped for respectable action from the Houston Health Department. Following the report, however, I realized that the Houston Health Department was capable both of mispresenting facts and of blatant prevarication. A little ignorance I could accept, but not purposeful dishonesty.

We were gathered in Fred and Glenna's living room. They had several children, so there was quite a crowd. That is where I received a shock I could hardly believe.

"Here it comes," announced Glenna, "they're going to show it."

Chatter ceased and all ears perked toward the set. A newsman interviewed Dr. Craven, and soon I perceived why Fred and Glenna were so upset. Dr. Craven's basic approach was to apologize for the alarm the public was experiencing due to the reported cyanide poisoning. In other words, she insinuated that no reason for alarm existed, and that an injustice against the community had been imposed by the young doctor who reported the poisoning, namely me. She even stated that I had acted prematurely in contacting the news media.

I could conceivably attribute much of Dr. Craven's discourse to lack of information. But one thing was plain, and that was Dr. Craven's accusation that I contacted the news media before I should have. Only a short time before delivering her news report, Dr. Craven sat in my office where I was questioned about that very matter. There, I clearly explained that it was someone else who contacted the news media. This added up to a single conclusion, Dr. Craven presented data to the public that she must have known was untrue. Therefore, I could not trust any information given out by the Houston Health Department. Furthermore, since the Houston Health Department was the agency responsible for investigating the cyanide pollution, the chances of solving the problem seemed threatened.

Night after night my wife and I suffered ills that constantly reminded us of the poison's reality. Meanwhile, I received literature which convinced me that prolongation of the cyanide contamination could cost lives as well as cause illness. I realized the neighborhood I lived in was quite a distance from the probable source of contamination, and that there could be other individuals far sicker than most of my patients. On the night of December 4, 1981, I conceded to myself that the Houston Health Department was a dangerous threat to my patients and the community. Their major concern was obviously politics, not humanity.

It would take time for me to apprehend the far-reaching effects of the Houston Health Department's propaganda. A sudden decline in patients requesting cyanide testing occurred, dropping from eleven on December fourth to none on December fifth. [*Note: this is not quite correct—although no one was tested for cyanide on December 5th, it is the day that Linda Blausen returned to my office and a blood test for copper was performed.*] Fortunately, though I did not know it, there were other private physicians courageous enough to submit tests for cyanide poisoning. Later on, a couple patients who were found positive for the poisoning by other doctors using laboratories other than Severance and Associates would seek me out. Until then, I would have to hold fast to my findings in the face of practically debilitating illness and increasing public denouncement.

Nonetheless, truth is truth. The following morning, December fifth, I posted a news release on the front door to my office. It was a slow morning all around; the news personnel, like the patients, had practically vanished. Matt Star, a writer for The Houston Chronicle, was the only one I remember coming by. When he came, he discovered the following message on my door:

News Release:

Due to the manner of investigation and attitude of concern being demonstrated by the Houston Health Department, I can only conclude that the welfare of the people in this community does not have proper priority in the Houston Health Department's investigation, as compared to other factors that I elect not to mention. Furthermore, in light of the urgency of this grave situation, indicated to be even more serious than I previously suspected through information I received from the Poison Control Center, I request on behalf of this community that an experienced government agency, without ties to the Houston Health Department, be immediately called upon to search for the source of the poison in our neighborhoods.

Sincerely,
Tim Oesch, M.D.

P.S.
I expect to announce
results of further blood
testing by Monday afternoon.

P.S.S.
I plan to be in my office
off & on tomorrow.

Despite the media, the Houston Health Department, and social ridicule, most of my patients remained faithful and supportive. Those who endured the pains of cyanide poisoning were not always easily persuaded to deny the poison's existence. It was December fifth that Linda Blausen came to my office after attempting to capture cyanide from a sewer or drainage outlet, as conveyed in chapter two. It was also around this time, as I remember, that a college official paid a visit to my office. I was alone, sitting at my desk.

"Hello Doctor Oesch, do you have a minute?" inquired Mr. Saul, poking his head through my door.

"Sure, come on in. Would you like to sit down?"

"No, I'll just stand," replied Mr. Saul as he closed the door and stood before my desk. "I don't want you talking to any more news reporters. If any reporters show up, don't answer any questions, and notify my office."

Previously, I had agreed not to make any statement on behalf of Gulf Coast Bible College. I had retained, however, the right to make statements as an individual physician.

"I haven't made any statements for the college," I responded. "In fact, I've been trying to take the focus of the problem off the college. It's the Houston Health Department that has made the college look like the center of the problem."

"Well, I just want you so stop all communication with the news media, all right?"

"I won't say anything on behalf of the college. When it comes to my private practice, though, I have a responsibility to my patients and this community. It's not just the college involved."

Once Mr. Saul ascertained that I was not going to comply with his request, his disposition changed quickly for the worse:

"Look, I don't know whether you are purposely trying to destroy this college, or if you are just ignorant. Just what are you trying to do?"

I was having definite misgivings about Mr. Saul. He may have done more to associate Gulf Coast Bible College with the cyanide problem than anyone else on earth. Besides closely associating himself with the Houston Health Department, he practically invited newsmen covering the cyanide investigation to inhabit Gulf Coast Bible College as a home base. In my efforts to divert pubic focus away from Gulf Coast Bible College as the center of the problem, Mr. Saul was a major obstacle.

"I'm not trying to hurt the college," I replied. "In fact, I played the whole problem down as much as I could for the sake of the college. Unless this problem is solved, though, no one will be safe here. The best thing that could happen for the college is for the source of the cyanide to be found and the contamination stopped. This area should be safe within a few days, once the output of cyanide is stopped."

My exhortation did not seem to pacify Mr. Saul in the slightest. "Why is it that you're working so hard on this? Night and day you never seem to stop and rest. You're just like your dad, you're trying to be some kind of knight in shining armor, a savior of the people."

My dad is a preacher, so he does work to direct people toward salvation—spiritual salvation. My dad is a man I trust and respect. From the tone of Mr. Saul's voice, however, I detected that he was not purposefully paying me a compliment.

"Right now I'm not so sure how popular I am," I returned, "but I intend to do what is right, regardless of whether it makes me a knight in shining armor or a social outcast."

Seeing that I held my ground, Mr. Saul grew visibly angry. "I know some things about you and your dad that I could make public, if you don't decide to cooperate."

I had no idea what Mr. Saul was talking about, though later I realized that he was threatening me with blackmail.

"You can make anything about me or my dad public that you want to," I replied. "But I still need to do what's right."

Mr. Saul grew so furious that his face flushed red with rage. He turned, pulled open the door, and then faced me tersely. "We won't let you do this!" he declared.

I wondered who Mr. Saul meant by *we*, and I also wondered what it was that he did not intend to let me do. At that particular time, however, I was growing bleakly ill from chronic cyanide poisoning. I decided just to forget about Mr. Saul's visit, figuring that I had more important things to worry about. Time would allow me to reflect upon my decision, and I experienced a change of mind.

Also somewhere along this period of time, I received a phone call from Henry Armstrong, my pharmacist:

"Hello Doctor Oesch, how are things going?"

"Well, I'm pretty sick today."

"I've been listening to the news. It sounds like the Houston Health Department isn't going to be any help."

I appreciated Henry's perception. "I think you're right. I think they're trying to sweep the whole thing under the carpet."

"That's pretty obvious," returned Henry. "If we're going to get anything accomplished, we may need some help."

"Some help?"

"Some political help. It's obvious these people are sick, but we need more than medical proof, we need some political push. I have a friend who may be able to help us. Would you be willing to meet with him?"

Considering all the opposition stacking up, I was in no position to discourage help.

"Sure. When would he like me to meet him?"

"How about three o'clock, here at my store?"

"Okay, see you then."

I drove to the store where Henry introduced me to Buddy Adams. Buddy instructed me to call him by his first name. He was neatly dressed, with a strong western flavor to his attire. Sometime during our conversation, I learned that he was an attorney. We met in a small side room within the pharmacy.

"Pull up a chair, Doctor Oesch. Would you like a soda?"

"I'll take a little," I accepted.

Buddy poured some coke and set it before me, then sat down with Henry and me at the table. Buddy was quite talkative and commented on a variety of topics. I'll attempt to reconstruct come of the more pertinent segments of our conversation.

"Henry has filled me in on most of the details regarding this cyanide contamination," commented Buddy, "and it sounds to me like someone is trying to pull a snow job."

"It's beginning to look that way," I affirmed. The simple manner of Buddy's speech seemed like revelation. After all the double-talk, deception, and silver-tongued propaganda displayed by the Houston Health Department, Buddy's words were almost therapeutic.

"I knew something fishy was going on before Henry even contacted me. It was obvious that the Health Department was trying to hide something, just listening to their reports tipped me off to that. What they said didn't make any sense. They had no grounds to make the claims they did, and they certainly did drag you through the mud. That's something they wouldn't do unless they were desperate," stated Buddy.

"Well, I was trying to cooperate with them," I explained, "but in their last news report they said something that wasn't true. I mean, they said several things that weren't true, but they said one thing that they knew was not true."

"That's not too surprising," returned Buddy. "Now, let's get down to the real point of this meeting. I grew up in the Heights, Doctor Oesch, and I have a personal interest in the people of this community. Henry is a good friend of mine, and he is convinced that there is a real problem with this poisoning. He tells me you have been doing a lot of research about cyanide, and that you have some ideas about approaching this problem. Is that right?"

"Yes," I responded, "but unfortunately I'm not in much of a financial position to carry out many ideas."

"Well, Doctor Oesch, that's where we might be able to help you. I'm going to talk with my partner, Phil Stevens, and see what we might be able to agree on."

"I'm willing to put up some money too," interjected Henry. "You can count me in on this thing."

My mind was racing. Most of my patients, like me, did not have much money. It was rare for an individual to request more than one laboratory test, and sometimes a cyanide test would return negative when I was sure the patient suffered from chronic cyanide poisoning. Asking patients to put up more money for a retest was difficult for me to do.

"That sounds great," I said, and soon one thousand dollars were allotted solely for the purpose of paying laboratory costs.

After returning to my office with the knowledge that funds were available, I began considering the use of additional laboratories. It would still be weeks before I switched to the preferable test, thiocyanate, but I decided that multiple laboratory testing would aid in the political battle with the Houston Health Department. Newspaper coverage on December sixth denoted Severance and Associates Laboratory standing firmly behind their findings, but I sensed that someone was putting quite a bit of pressure on them. The laboratory even changed their reference value for blood cyanide from *none detected* to *up to 20 mcg/dl*. Considering the number of zero levels the laboratory turned out, I was inclined to believe that their first reference value was the more accurate. [*This reference level for blood cyanide of* **up to 20 mcg/dl** *included smokers as well as nonsmokers, though the printed laboratory reports failed to mention this fact. On one such printed report, I wrote that the reference level for blood cyanide in a nonsmoker was less than 5 mcg/dl, and I assume that I acquired this reference level by calling the laboratory. I think it would be unlikely to test a smoker and find a blood cyanide level as high as 20 mcg/dl that resulted from simply smoking, unless blood was drawn during or immediately after smoking. Furthermore, I think any positive test for blood cyanide, even as low as 1 mcg/dl, should be considered significant when investigating the possibility of airborne cyanide* *intoxication; and furthermore, a negative test for blood cyanide certainly does not rule out the possibility of serious environmental intoxication from airborne cyanide.]*

December sixth was a Sunday, and both major newspapers made an issue of my dissatisfaction with the Houston Health Department. One caption indicated that I wanted a federal agency to help check out the illness. Being federal does not necessarily make someone honest, but I was beginning to suspect that the Houston Health Department somehow shared responsibility for the cyanide contamination, so they were hardly fit to be investigating the problem. A public city agency indicated that a company west of the Heights was licensed to dump discharge water into the public sewer system. That permit was probably condoned by the Houston Health Department. [*A report on pages 1 and 16 of The Houston Chronicle on December sixth, 1981, quoted the director of the University of Texas Medical Branch poison center, namely Mike Ellis, as saying that it is not uncommon to find one microgram per deciliter of cyanide in healthy people and as much as four micrograms per deciliter in heavy smokers. He also said that—**it appears the levels found in Oesch's patients are sufficient to cause problems for the patients**. Of note, and probably due to some sort of political pressure, Severance and Associates Laboratories, after reporting several positive blood cyanide levels including one as low as 2 mcg/dl, starting reporting any levels less than 10 mcg/dl as simply **less than 10 mcg/dl**. I was still able to call the laboratory and find out if blood cyanide levels from 1 to 9 mcg/dl were found, but such levels did not appear on the initial, printed reports. I am not certain on what date Severance and Associates Laboratories stopped reporting blood cyanide levels less than 10 mcg/dl, but I know for certain that in the testing for blood cyanide done in the Gulf Coast Bible College administration building on December 2, 1981, Severance and Associates did not report any blood cyanide levels that were less than 10 mcg/dl as being anything other than **less than 10 mcg/dl**. In contrast, I received a report for a blood cyanide level from Metpath Laboratories for blood collected from a **smoker** on May 14, 1982, with the level reported being only **1.4 mcg/dl**. The very first positive blood cyanide reported by Severance and Associates Laboratories, which was from blood collected in September of 1981, was only **2 mcg/dl**. Thank goodness the laboratory was not reporting levels less than 10 mcg/dl as simply **less than 10 mcg/dl** at* that time, or I may have concluded that John's blood test for cyanide was negative. And one more note before continuing—the same newspaper article published on December sixth, 1981, also stated that the only company in north Houston licensed to dump cyanide compounds was a General Electric distribution assembly plant at 3530 W 12th Street; and the article went on to say that the manager of employee relations at the plant stated that the city had given the plant's waste treatment facility a **clean bill of health**. The article further stated that GE discharged into a city sanitary sewer system.

Reportedly, the GE plant at 3530 W 12th Street was licensed, by the City of Houston, to discharge up to 38,000 gallons of wastewater into the public sewer system per day, at up to 2 ppm cyanide. This, then, could legally release enough cyanide, on a daily basis, to produce about forty million cubic feet of air with 0.2 ppm cyanide—enough air to fill the entire inner volume of the Houston Jones Hall for the Performing Arts about forty times. At forty hours of exposure per week, industrial workers have been found to develop symptoms of cyanide intoxication at air levels from 0.2 to 0.8 ppm (**see Chandra et al. {1980} studied the effects of HCN exposure on 23 male workers**); and in the case of individuals living in polluted cities, exposure to airborne cyanide may be twenty-four hours per day, and I certainly believe that there are individuals with greater sensitivity to cyanide than the industrial workers who were tested.

An INTER OFFICE CORRESPONDENCE of the CITY OF HOUSTON corroborates that General Electric was permitted to discharge up to 2 ppm cyanide in the sewer water insofar as an engineer employed by GE claimed that the treatment system would reduce a reported cyanide spill to about 2 mg/L (milligrams per liter), and 2 mg/L is equal to 2 ppm (parts per million). The report, dated January 7, 1982, follows:

CITY OF HOUSTON
INTER OFFICE CORRESPONDENCE

To: File

From: William R. Osborne

Date: January 7, 1982

Subject: Cyanide upset at
General Electric
3530 West 12th
77008

Roger Grebing, facilities and process engineer with G. E., called today to report that a metal rack that is used to dip parts into their plating bath fell into and punctured the cyanide tank, resulting in a spill of about forty (40) gallons of cyanide into their waste treatment system. Grebing said that the concentration of CN going into the system was about 550 mg/l and that their cyanide destruction system should have reduced the concentration to about 2 mg/l. I recommended to Grebing that he contact P. W. to report the incident.

William R. Osborne
William R. Osborne
Northwest District Supervisor

Before moving on with the manuscript, and in light of the fact that it was publicized that the City of Houston gave GE a clean bill of health, I am going to insert an affidavit taken in 1988:

AFFIDAVIT
THE STATE OF ARKANSAS $
COUNTY OF **CLARK** $

My name is JOHN MICHAEL SHEARIN, SR., and I am over twenty-one (21) years of age. I have personal knowledge of everything stated herein. Everything stated is true and correct.

I worked for the General Electric Company on West 12th Street in Houston, Texas from September, 1978 until February, 1982. I worked in the Box Department under Mr. Taylor. On occasions, I assisted in the Plating Department when they were short of personnel or needed someone to work overtime. I worked in the Copper Department operating drill presses, punches, lay-out and metal cutting machines.

I worked on both the old and new plating system. The old system had very poor ventilation and did not work properly most of the time. This system was outdated and hazardous. The overflow from the various tanks (vats) went onto a concrete slab, into the company pipes and then into the Houston sewer lines. On several occasions, we had acid leaks that were not properly monitored or adequately repaired. Periodically, all the vats were drained, cleaned, and re-serviced with new liquids. All the contents from the vats, including acids and other chemicals, were drained down the sewer system without any filtering during that process.

I heard from several other plating department personnel that the City of Houston had complained and even fined the General Electric Company for the discharge tests being above the allowable limits to the permit. It was standard practice to drain, rinse, and clean the copper plating system tanks on certain days when the city's sewer inspectors were not checking the discharge readings.

My understanding was that General Electric was forced to build a new plating system with its own wastewater treatment system. Work began in approximately November, 1980 and continued through January, 1981. From the beginning the new system had a lot of problems. Several of the (vats) tanks developed cracks and leaks. It seemed like it took forever to get the leaks repaired. The waste treatment portion of the plating system was a bigger headache. It was always malfunctioning or being shut down to have work done on it. The system was often run without the treatment system operating.

Correct procedures for testing the water discharged into the city sewer system was neither taught nor followed. Required readings and logging were not monitored by supervisors.

Chemicals were added too, periodically without adequate training or supervision and often without proper equipment (safety devices) readily available.

On several occasions as I came to work, alarms on the monitoring control panels were buzzing with no one paying any attention. Sometimes, the alarms would be stopped by placing a rubber stopper in the alarm button to keep the alarm system off.

On at least two occasions, the waste treatment storage basement became flooded. It was pumped out with a submission pump directly outside and onto the parking lot and into the ditch in front of the plant on W. 12 Street.

John Michael Shearin, Sr.
MICHAEL SHEARIN, SR.

Mr. Shearin verified the above affidavit, and it was signed by a Notary Public in and for the State of Arkansas on the 28th day of March,

1988. The notary public's signature appears to be either Enga Gail Neagle or Enga Gail Reagle, and her notary expiration date was given as 7-21-90.]

It was not long after the cyanide discovery reached the press before General Electric Company was given a clean bill of health by the Houston Health Department. The company even sent me three of their employees to be tested for blood cyanide. One employee had been home on a long weekend and came to my office before going to work. The other two, at my request, went to work before coming to my office, but they were only at work for thirty to forty-five minutes before leaving and coming to my office. With a half-life for cyanide of about thirty minutes in the bloodstream, these were not very meaningful tests. I mentioned to the company nurse that the best time to test an employee would be after the employee spent the whole day at work, but for some reason the company did not choose to follow that procedure. All three tests were negative, and all three employees lived a considerable distance from their job.

The church I attended was several miles northwest of the Heights. I generally made both services on Sunday, and went early for choir practice on Sunday evenings. Singing was quite enjoyable; I stood between the bases and tenors where I could reach some of the notes in both parts. On this particular evening, December sixth, I was having an embarrassing problem. Whenever I tried to sustain a note, I nearly passed out. I had to stop singing and breathe while everyone else was singing.

I decided to drive home while I was still capable. Having been a quarter-mile sprinter in college, I was not used to shortness of breath from singing. My wife was ill at home, and I joined her earlier than she expected.

"Is church over already?" posed my wife as I entered the apartment.

"No, I got sick in choir and decided to come home. I was afraid that if I waited much longer I wouldn't be able to drive. How are you doing?"

"Not so good. My head hurts so bad it feels like it's about to burst open. I think I could use a Percogesic."

Doctors have access to quite a myriad of medications. Personally, I don't like to take medicine unless there's a pressing reason for it, and it is very rare that I even take an aspirin. With the cyanide intoxication, however, I thankfully took frequent doses of thiosulfate, and on a couple of occasions took two Percogesic tablets. Percogesic is a little stronger than plain Tylenol, and is supposed to be especially helpful when sore or achy muscles accompany a headache. My wife and I both qualified for the treatment.

"All right, honey, I'll go down and see if I can find some."

I stepped down to the dispensary and walked to a closet in the far wall of the examining room. The medications were neatly arranged and labeled, thanks to my wife, so it took little time to locate the Percogesic tablets. Soon I was upstairs with four tablets.

The night that followed was one that lingers frightfully in my memory. My wife and I lay awake in bed with pain in almost every part of our bodies. Foggy-mindedness deadened my senses, taking the edge off a shattering headache and lessening my awareness of lower back and neck pain. One of my muscles twitched involuntarily, keeping me awake even after my pain yielded somewhat to treatment with Percogesic. Unlike any other night of my life up to that point, I truly wondered whether or not I would awaken on earth the next morning.

My breathing was desperate. Though air passed in and out of my lungs, I felt as though I never got quite enough oxygen. For a short while as I lay gazing at the ceiling, it seemed as though I began floating upward out of my body. Somehow, I finally drifted into a restless sleep.

At three o'clock in the morning I awoke, gasping for air. Rising dizzily from the bed, I stumbled into the kitchen and leaned heavily on the sink. By placing both hands solidly against the front edge of the sink, I was able to engage my thoracic musculature to aid in respiration. Time after time my mouth filled rapidly with saliva. I spat and spat into the sink until the volume of saliva expectorated impressed even my stunned cerebrum.

"Are you all right, dear?" my wife's voice sounded from the bedroom. I had not bothered with waking her.

"I had to spit," I responded. I had never gotten out of bed to spit during our entire marriage.

"Are you okay? Are you coming back to bed?"

"I'll be there in a little while, I need to finish spitting."

A nearby container served to collect a sizeable sample of saliva. The sample was turned over to a seemingly concerned television reporter, but I never heard what became of it. The reporter, though, seemed genuinely interested in helping, and I suspect the saliva was tested somewhere. Perhaps someday I will find out.

When I returned to bed, my wife's eyes related her apprehension through the dim darkness of a fearful night. I lay beside her and realized I was probably nearer death than with any illness I had ever experienced. It seemed sinisterly ironic that my life was endangered by an agent that public authorities denied altogether. I figured that if I died, they would probably claim I had been poisoned by some prankster, or else that I poisoned myself.

Other thoughts passed through my mind too. Thoughts like: how many other people are suffering symptoms similar to mine, and are being told they have heart trouble, migraine headaches, a virus, or a mental disorder? What will happen to the investigation if I am no longer around? Will someone else step in to take my place? Then finally, an inescapably profound question dawned in my thinking: what on earth was I doing lying around breathing cyanide until it almost killed me?

Without turning my head, I made a simple, but firm announcement to my wife. One that proved true from that time forward: "This is the last night we're spending in this apartment."

Chapter 5

**HARRIS COUNTY MEDICAL EXAMINERS
TOXICOLOGY LABORATORY**

SAMPLE #	CN(mcg/dl)
10001	25
10004	15
10007	Less than 10
10010	Less than 10
10013	15
10016	15
10019	15
10022	Less than 10
10025	15
10028	Less than 10
10031	15
10034	Less than 10
10037	Less than 10
10040	Less than 10
10043	Less than 10
10046	15
10049	15
10052	36
10055	15
10058	23
10061	15

Note: the above is a copy of cyanide levels reported by Harris County Medical Examiners Toxicology Laboratory from blood drawn 12/2/1981 at Gulf Coast Bible College.

Rottenness Within

With additional test results returning from the laboratory, patients again began frequenting my office for cyanide evaluation and treatment. A couple of the blood cyanide levels were too high for any manner of dispute or denial, except to blame the results on lab error. The Houston Health Department did just that, as was recorded in The Houston Chronicle. It looked as though facts were stacking up favorably, and they were, but a major battle was only beginning.

The Director of Health Services for the Houston Health Department publicized that an ad hoc committee was being assigned to determine whether or not there was any cyanide problem. The committee consisted of several doctors from the University of Texas School of Public Health—all faculty members. Since this was a state university, it represented a step upward from mere city-sanctioned inquiry. However, I was wary of any group or organization solicited or condoned by the Houston Health Department, and the ad hoc committee seemed too closely associated. Nonetheless, considering that the committee had to work with information given to them by the Houston Health Department, some of the comments they issued were interesting and helpful.

The Houston Chronicle recorded several suggestions and statements by members of the ad hoc committee. For one thing, the committee strongly suggested testing future patients for thiocyanate, which eventually helped acquire a much higher percentage of positive tests. Furthermore, one of the committee members pointed out that the higher levels of blood cyanide were unexplained. He said that sampling of the environment should continue with the help of state and federal agencies, and he also ruled out the possibility that a disease was causing the symptoms being credited to cyanide poisoning.

On the other hand, the committee certainly had its drawbacks. The head of the committee, Doctor Marcus Key, produced a written statement claiming that blood cyanide levels ranging from 0 to 31 mcg/dl in nonsmokers, and 1 to 52 mcg/dl in smokers, are found in normal, healthy people. This statement, absurdly misleading as explained in chapter three, was printed in propaganda sent by the Houston Health Department to patients they tested for blood cyanide on December second. Doctor Key also claimed that cyanide was found in people who ate certain foods or smoked. His arguments sounded suspiciously in keeping with those of the Houston Health Department.

Another interesting fact about the ad hoc committee was the time when they were selected. Dissatisfied with the sole handling of the investigation by the Houston Health Department, I contacted state authorities to see if state intervention was possible. The response I received was promising; it sounded as though state health personnel would look into the matter. The very next day, Doctor Craven announced that she asked for state aid and the ad hoc committee was commissioned. Perhaps this timing was coincidence, and perhaps it was not. A state employee confided with me later, saying that the state basically only did environmental testing when and where the Houston Health Department dictated. It definitely did not sound like the type of intervention I wanted.

News coverage, around the time that the ad hoc committee was forming, featured a provocative sideline. A family in the Heights, afflicted by the cyanide poisoning, received word from out of state that one of their relatives became ill after consuming a large number pecans they had mailed as a gift. The pecans came from a tree in their yard. The sick relative was taken to an emergency room. The cause of the illness was unknown, though it resembled an acute, severe bout of flu. The Heights family directed their relative to be tested for blood cyanide, but unfortunately the test was done about a week after her illness. The blood level at that time was less than one microgram per deciliter.

The story was definitely interesting. Hydrogen cyanide in the air could theoretically settle in rain, and roots from trees might venture down to sewer lines. One industrious newsman retrieved a bag of pecans allegedly grown from the same tree as those mailed out of state. He had them tested at a laboratory, but they contained only 900 parts per billion cyanide, hardly enough to cause acute poisoning. [*To my knowledge, pecans should not contain any cyanide at all.*]

The idea of cyanide collecting in plants or fruit prompted further investigation. A patient ill with chronic cyanide poisoning had tomato leaves tested from his garden. This time the result was significant, the leaves contained approximately 4.8 parts per million. There are some plants known to produce cyanide naturally, but in speaking to a specialist on the subject, I learned that tomato plants are not among that group. The tomato plants must have absorbed the cyanide from the environment.

Airborne cyanide was still the apparent mode of poisoning, even after plant testing began. Another thing I learned from the plant specialist [*to the best of my memory, I contacted someone at Texas A&M University*] was that cyanide is not stable in plants. It reportedly does not persist in grass or tomato leaves more than several hours. The tomato leaves tested for cyanide probably absorbed the cyanide only a short time before they were collected. Chances are that whoever harvested the tomato leaves inhaled a little cyanide himself.

While on the subject of reports from out of state, another patient, Mary Gibbs, brought some intriguing news to my office. She suffered typical cyanide symptoms of tiredness, headaches, decreased appetite, and she had a notable case of anemia. She developed a case of pneumonia shortly before traveling to Arizona on vacation. After returning from Arizona, she paid me a visit:

"Come in," I said, after light knocking sounded from my office door.

Mary entered the office stealthily, closing the door quietly behind her. She obviously wished to say something discreetly.

"I've got some news I thought you might want to know," conversed Mary, leaning slightly forward over the desk in my office.

I deduced from Mary's carriage that she had information regarding cyanide.

"What's that?"

"Before I left on vacation I got sick, and when I got to Arizona I felt so bad I went to a doctor. I told the doctor about the cyanide problem here."

"What did the doctor say?" I questioned. Chronic cyanide poisoning is a newly recognized entity, and I am always inquisitive to hear how individual doctors respond when they first hear of it. In this case, I was in for a surprise.

"The doctor said I had fluid on my lungs from pneumonia, and that he wanted to draw some of the fluid out and test it. Well, when he tested the fluid for cyanide, it came out positive."

"He tested fluid from your lungs?"

"Right. It was called pleural effusion."

This was a new slant. I knew that pneumonia was a fairly common complication among my patients with cyanide intoxication, but I had never heard of testing pleural fluid for cyanide.

"That's pretty impressive, Mary. Do you think you could have the doctor send me a copy of the report?"

"I'll see," she obliged.

"Thanks. I'd sure like to see it."

Mary contacted the doctor who agreed to send the report, but I never received it. Verification was made that the report was mailed, so something must have happened in transit, most likely near my end of the line. There was enough happening, though, to keep my mind occupied with matters other than lost mail from Arizona. [*Considering what I've learned since that time, I have to wonder if Mary was exposed to additional cyanide in Arizona that accounted for the cyanide found in her pleural fluid. Nonetheless, she likely contracted pneumonia after exposure to cyanogen chloride in Houston.*] I received a phone call from Mr. Saul, who stated that he wished to speak with me again. This I would do so long as Mr. Chandler, another college official, was present with us. Soon a meeting time was arranged.

We met in an office at the same building where the Houston Health Department collected blood samples. There were four of us: me, Mr. Chandler, Mr. Saul, and an additional college official named Mr. Roberts. Mr. Roberts greeted me when I first arrived, and escorted me to the office where Mr. Saul wished to meet. We engaged in informal conversation while waiting for everyone to assemble, but after Mr. Saul arrived we quickly settled into serious discussion. Mr. Saul was last to arrive.

"Let's get to the point of this meeting," directed Mr. Saul, bringing a halt to less tedious dialogue. "As you know, we had a meeting some time back with Chancellor Fields, and we agreed not to release any report to the news media without the assigned committee agreeing on it, namely Mister Roberts, Doctor Oesch, and myself."

"That's right," I agreed, "pertaining to information released on behalf of the college. The Chancellor said, however, that I was free to release information in regard to my private practice without consulting the committee."

Mr. Chandler, sensing a confrontation between Mr. Saul and me, interrupted the dialogue and addressed Mr. Roberts. "You were in the meeting, Mr. Roberts, what was your understanding of this matter?"

Mr. Roberts was considerably younger than the other two men, and I sensed that the nature of the meeting made him a little nervous. He seemed to have a resolute courage, however, that would not yield to any measure of anxiety.

"I understood Chancellor Fields to say basically what Doctor Oesch has conveyed, that any announcement on behalf of the college must be approved by the committee, and that Doctor Oesch was free to make comments regarding his private practice," Mr. Roberts replied smoothly.

"Well, I don't think that's such a good idea," remarked Mr. Saul. "This entire situation has gotten entirely out of hand. Here Doctor Oesch is, trying to take on the Houston Health Department single-handed, when they're trying as hard as they can to help us."

"They've made public announcements that were not true. They've made the college look like the center of the problem, when there is no reason for it, and now they're accusing the laboratory of giving falsely positive readings," I refuted.

"How do you know the laboratory didn't make a mistake," posed Mr. Saul.

"Because I've been sick, and so have a lot of other people."

Mr. Saul did not demonstrate much sympathy. "You're fighting a losing battle, there's no way you can win. By the time the big shots with the city get through with you, you'll be wallowing around in the gutter."

I found Mr. Saul's statement rather curious. How did he know what the big shots with the city would do to me? Furthermore, why should it matter to an official of a Christian institution? Are not Christians to do what is right regardless of threats or persecution?

"That may be true," I replied. "I don't know what may happen to me. The decisions I make are not based on whether or not I end up in the gutter, they are based on what I believe is right, on what I believe God would have me do."

"It takes money to carry on an investigation," commenced Mr. Saul.

"Well, I've got a lawyer helping me…"

"A lawyer! Don't tell me some lawyer has you eating out of his hand now. You don't have a lawyer, he has you. You're just a puppet around his little finger. How much is he getting you to pay him?"

Mr. Saul's speech was becoming quite heated. Mr. Chandler maintained a composed face, but I think he was slightly angry about the verbal lashing Mr. Saul dished out. Mr. Roberts displayed a slightly befuddled expression.

"I'm not having to pay him anything. In fact, he is giving me some money to pay for blood tests."

"He's paying you money! Ah, ha, ha….that's a laugh."

A Breath of Cyanide

Mr. Saul seemed almost beside himself. He was definitely the only one laughing. At that particular time, Chancellor Fields was away on a speaking engagement. That left Mr. Saul in charge of the college.

"The fact is, Doctor Oesch, that until Chancellor Fields returns, I'm the one in charge here. I'm in a position of authority, and the Bible says to subject yourself to those who are in authority over you."

I wondered whether or not Mr. Saul would behave in the presence of Mr. Chandler as he did when we were alone. Obviously, he did not find the added company very hindering. Once he started quoting Scripture, I had heard enough.

"The Bible says there is no authority except from God," I replied. "Some men try to use the Scripture you mentioned to condone rule over others, regardless of how wicked that rule is, but I don't believe there is any authority with those who are out of line with God and what is right. Let me ask you a question, are you a Christian?"

Considering the content of our discussion, with Mr. Saul's emphasis for decision-making placed on money and politics, I was all but daring him to call himself a Christian.

"I claim Christianity, just like most other people around here," responded Mr. Saul.

This was not satisfactory. Claiming Christianity is something the worst of villains might find beneficial. Furthermore, there were quite a number of contributors to Gulf Coast Bible College who would not like the idea of the Chancellor's Aid not affirming Christianity. After all, it was a Christian institution with a primary goal of educating preachers.

"But are you a Christian?" I reiterated. "Is Jesus Christ your lord?"

Mr. Saul looked taken back considerably. It seemed as though he jostled his mind a bit before delivering a reply. "I would rather not comment on that at this time."

Silence exploded and flooded the room. None of the threats or belittling by Mr. Saul seemed to dumfound Mr. Chandler and Mr. Roberts like this evasion. It was simply unthinkable that a man should achieve the position of Chancellor's Aid at Gulf Coast Bible College who would not unashamedly attest the lordship of Jesus Christ.

Mr. Saul himself broke the silence, which in actuality was brief. "Besides, that's not the issue here. The issue's your unwillingness to cooperate with Chancellor Fields' request. You're trying to be a one man show and get all the attention and limelight you can, regardless of what effect you're having on everyone else, and you're going to end up destroying yourself too."

At this point I realized that Mr. Saul's argument presented a double standard. I had not done anything Chancellor Fields had forbidden, but Mr. Saul certainly had.

"Now that you mention it," I inserted, "nothing was supposed to be said publicly on behalf of the college by any of us unless the committee met first and agreed on what should be said. You've been saying all kinds of things as if you were the official college spokesman, and we haven't met together once to okay what you had to say. You are the one who has not done as Chancellor Fields instructed."

"I don't need you to okay what I have to say," blustered Mr. Saul. "I think it's rather obvious that you're not going to listen to anyone's advice. I see no point in carrying this meeting on any further."

My memory seems almost blank as to what happened next. I think Mr. Chandler closed the meeting with prayer. Whatever the case, we soon departed company. I walked from the office building and back to my apartment. As usual, my wife wanted to know everything that happened.

Not long thereafter, Mr. Saul appeared on public television again. As always, he did so without consulting the committee that Chancellor Fields appointed. Though I did not see his interview myself, some friends related his remarks to me. In brief, Mr. Saul pointed out my financial inadequacies and lowly estate, claiming that I would be unable to carry out any further investigation. He also lauded the Houston Health Department for their concern and admirable work in dealing with the cyanide *scare*. The Houston Health Department and Mr. Saul seemed closely knitted: Gulf Coast Bible College received a superb rating from the Houston Health Department for freedom from occupational or environmental hazards.

As the mudslinging increased, Ruth SoRelle decided to pull me from beneath mounting debris. She was a sharp reporter who wrote medical articles for The Houston Chronicle. Initially, she called me by phone:

"Hello, Doctor Oesch," I answered after picking up the receiver.

"Hello Doctor Oesch, this is Ruth SoRelle, reporter for The Houston Chronicle. I've been covering your problem with cyanide poisoning," she spoke crisply. Her diction clarified every word she pronounced.

"Oh yes, I've read some of your articles. They seem a lot closer to the truth than articles in the other newspaper," I replied. Both papers carried a lot of misleading information issued by the Houston Health Department, but The Houston Chronicle tended to include both sides of the story more accurately than the Houston Post.

"Listen Doctor Oesch, I think it's about time to get a personal profile on you. I would like to interview you and write an article about you as a person—your background, training, hobbies, and beliefs."

Ruth's suggestion sounded flatteringly attractive, but I feared having an article written about me. There were a number of people accusing me of monetary pursuit, or pursuit of fame, and they were claiming that the cyanide problem was artificially fabricated. I knew some of the individuals who were probably fostering the gossip, and I did not want to add fuel to their flame.

"Thanks for the offer, maybe after this problem with cyanide is solved and taken care of we can get together on that. For right now, though, I think I'd better hold off. I don't want to do anything that might hinder things."

When Ruth replied, her voice contained evident determination. "Do you think a story about you will hinder things Doctor Oesch?"

"Well, I'd rather just stick with the problem until it's solved," I answered, hesitant to reveal the real fears that detained me.

"Are you aware of all the things the Houston Health Department is saying about you? We can't just sit back and let them undermine your reputation or no one will listen to you. What good would that accomplish? It's only fair to all the patients depending on you that you allow me to write the truth about you."

Despite my fears, Ruth's reasoning seemed sound. I agreed to meet with her, and we held an interesting conversation in company with a tape recorder. She wrote a very nice article that appeared in the Sunday newspaper on December thirteenth. [*The front-page article was entitled,* **Doctor at odds with city…Heights physician has faith in cyanide diagnosis, God**.]

Going back a little, the preceding Monday afternoon I drove my wife eighteen miles to Mr. and Mrs. Pattersons' residence. We stayed there a night or two before I made arrangements to move in with some old friends I knew from high school days. [*I attended Cypress Fairbanks High School, and these were old friends I knew from church.*] As we stepped from the apartment in the Heights carrying suitcases, a news camera filmed our descent and pictorially recorded our departure. It was depicted as if we were making some sort of getaway, though in actuality I returned to my office that same day and worked until about 11:00 p.m. At 10:40 p.m. I drew my own blood so it could be tested for serum thiocyanate.

Drawing my own blood was quite an experience in itself. There was little choice as to whether I would watch or not, and manipulating the vacutube with one hand proved interesting. My serum thiocyanate level returned at 0.9 mg/dl. This was considerably higher than the average for adult males, namely 0.244 mg/dl, and represented an intake of roughly forty milligrams of cyanide. Forty milligrams is a respectable quantity of cyanide.

My wife and I spent a very pleasant night at the Pattersons' home, and I think that I stayed there the entire next day without returning to work. The phone rang much less often than at my office, and my wife and I both quickly ascertained that the air quality was superior to that at our prior abode. Among other things, cyanide intoxication has a direct effect on both emotional state and libido. Both entities are improved when cyanide is absent from the environment. December ninth I returned to my office.

Two new cyanide patients came to my office on the ninth. The first reported diarrhea, nausea, headache, stomach cramps, dizziness, burning eyes, flushed feelings, dimmed vision, and muscle aches. She yielded a blood cyanide of 18 mcg/dl. The second patient complained of similar symptoms, which her husband experienced also, and yielded a borderline positive test for serum thiocyanate, later followed by a definitely positive test for urine thiocyanate. Meantime, public reports from the Houston Health Department continued to disparage the reality of the cyanide poisoning, and many uninformed or uncaring physicians belittled the idea of cyanide exposure when their own patients inquired about it. I was informed that most physicians would not take the necessary political risks entailed in getting involved with the issue, and unfortunately that seemed to be true. There were, however, some thankworthy exceptions.

Mr. Shawsten was an aquatic expert specializing in cyanide effects upon fish. He sent me several articles dealing with cyanide poisoning in fish, and these coincided surprisingly well with symptoms occurring in human beings. Behavioral change was noted as the *number one* effect of cyanide on fish, and I remember wondering how Mr. Shawsten knew when a fish was behaving wrongly. As time passed, Mr. Shawsten grew quite interested in the work I was doing, and he agreed to meet me at a nearby bayou. I hoped to net some small fish and have Mr. Shawsten check them for cyanide contamination.

My wife accompanied me to the bayou where we met Mr. Shawsten. I purchased a seine for the occasion. We met at the bank of a large, church parking lot that backed up to the bayou. Mr. Shawsten arrived soon after my wife and me. He was a tall, friendly-appearing man with silver hair.

"Hello, you must be Doctor Oesch," spoke Mr. Shawsten as we met on the parking lot.

"Yes, and this is my wife Melody. She decided to come watch."

Mr. Shawsten smiled and nodded. Melody wore her white tennis shoes, but later declined when it came to descending the steep bank of the bayou. I retrieved the seine from my car as Mr. Shawsten looked on with an experienced eye.

"Do you have any poles?"

"Poles?" I returned.

"Yes, you have to tie the seine to poles which you use to push the seine beneath the water," explained Mr. Shawsten. "Otherwise the net will just float in a fast moving stream like this."

I examined the seine; it had two loose ropes at each end, one at the top and one at the bottom. Obviously Mr. Shawsten was right. Looking quickly about, I noted some wild cane growing in some nearby brush.

"Look, there's some bamboo stalks over there," I said, pointing toward the cane.

"That might work, if it's strong enough."

I strode to the bamboo grove and selected two sturdier-appearing stalks. They looked like something Huckleberry Finn would hoist above the Mississippi. We attached these to the seine, and then I walked to a nearby bridge and crossed to the opposite side of the bayou. When I reached the bank opposite Mr. Shawsten, he handed me one of the bamboo poles with the seine attached.

The sweeping water was almost torrential. Mr. Shawsten and I jousted the bamboo poles into the water on each side of the bayou. The bayou was walled with concrete and the sides steeped vertically downward.

"Look out! Here comes a log!" I exclaimed, and we lifted the seine just in time to avoid destruction. There was nothing in the net but oily grime and debris.

Hoping to work the seine nearer the bottom of the bayou, I lay on my stomach and pressed the pole downward. Years before, when I had previously lived in Houston, there were quite a variety of fish to be netted from the bayou, including beautiful green mollies and what my friends called sheepsheads. The net bulged outward and the pole bent farther and farther as I pushed downward.

"Snap!"

Startled by the sound, I hung to both broken ends of the pole, one end in each hand. With my hands thus engaged, there was no way to stop myself as the tug on the net drug my body to the edge of the bayou. My body stopped sliding with only inches to spare.

Mr. Shawsten said nothing, he just looked at me with seemingly amused interest. I think he appreciated my determination. We lifted the seine from the bayou: still nothing.

"These poles just aren't strong enough," remarked Mr. Shawsten.

I offered no argument. "You're right. I've got a friend who lives up the bank. His yard backs down to the bayou. He probably has some shovel handles or something we can use. I'll be right back."

Not far behind and to my right sat the residence of Dr. David Prince. Dr. Prince was one of the first patients found positive for blood cyanide. On two occasions I evaluated Dr. Prince before the cyanide poisoning was discovered. Both times I was puzzled, but settled upon the diagnoses that I considered most likely.

The first time I evaluated Dr. Prince was during a customary office visit on October 16, 1981. He complained of tiredness, sore muscles, sore throat, and mild chest pain. On examination, he had slight injection of his pharynx and some crackling in his right lung. His temperature was normal, as was his blood pressure and pulse. I thought he might have walking pneumonia, and I treated him with an antibiotic called erythromycin.

Ten days later, Dr. Prince still felt fluish symptoms, and also complained of some back pain. On examination, his lungs were clear, but he seemed to have slight liver tenderness as well as generalized muscle tenderness. Suspecting hepatitis, I did blood and urine studies. His urine was okay, but his blood studies revealed that he was borderline anemic and showed a slightly elevated blood potassium. This probably resulted from mild lactic acidosis caused by cyanide in his body tissues. The liver enzyme tests were normal, ruling against hepatitis.

Puzzled by Dr. Prince's symptoms and laboratory studies, I diagnosed him with possible Coxsackie virus. To be honest, there were several people diagnosed with possible Coxsackie virus along that time; I even diagnosed myself with possible Coxsackie virus. There were no laboratory tests to confirm such a diagnosis, but it was about the only thing I could think of to try and explain all of the strange symptoms my patients were experiencing. Finally, on November 24, 1981, Dr. Prince submitted blood for a cyanide test that revealed that he suffered from cyanide intoxication. As with many other patients, a myriad of persisting symptoms were finally explained.

Dr. Prince allowed me to use whatever I could find in his garage to reinforce the seine. Two sturdy wooden handles about one inch in diameter proved sufficient; soon Mr. Shawsten and I were again busily sifting oily slime from the badly polluted bayou. My wife watched for some time from the brink of the bank, her long, dark hair dancing on the wind like a pony's tail. After a while, though, the chilly wind compelled her to seek refuge in our car. Efforts to capture fish were futile; I did not see a hint of aquatic life beyond mossy vegetation.

"Looks like there's nothing in here alive," I finally remarked. "The only thing we'll catch here is driftwood and slime."

"I think you're right," returned Mr. Shawsten. "This bayou is apparently too contaminated to support aquatic life."

"Well, thanks for coming out," I commented, a little embarrassed for putting Mr. Shawsten to such efforts without catching a single fish. "I guess I'll just have to keep testing people, and maybe plants."

"I enjoyed it," Mr. Shawsten asserted encouragingly, "and I wish you all the luck in the world."

"Thanks."

"You may notice fewer people sick when the weather really turns cold, and then more people sick when things thaw out and warmer weather returns," Mr. Shawsten pointed out.

"Why is that?" I inquired, having already noted some decline in new patients following the onset of midwinter coldness.

"Cyanide has less tendency to escape into the atmosphere in freezing weather, but next spring it will be back again."

Mr. Shawsten's statement seemed to prove somewhat true as time passed on, though there were patients whose symptoms continued straight through the winter, and a few cases of outstanding, acute cyanide intoxication despite cold weather. After bidding farewell to Mr. Shawsten, I carried the seine to Dr. Prince's house and hung it on a clothesline in his back yard. Dr. Prince did not seem surprised by the absence of aquatic life in the bayou. He mentioned seeing small fish in the bayou years before, but none recently. To my knowledge, Dr. Prince still has an oil-stained seine somewhere about his house.

The front page article that appeared in the December thirteenth edition of The Houston Chronicle was naturally my favorite. It was nice to hear that old college and medical school friends were pulling for me, and as Chancellor Fields expressed, the article presented me as *a white knight in shining armor*. It was definitely a contrast to many other reports issued by the media, and I certainly did not regret permitting Ruth to interview me. She did a lot of homework besides our interview, as was obvious in the report, and she was courageous enough to mention God and the primary role he plays in my life. As with anyone who is willing to stand for truth and right, God meets a great deal of opposition on this earth. Nonetheless, his name is nothing to be ashamed of, and I was honored by Ruth's commendable report.

As time passed, I learned more and more about chronic cyanide poisoning. One woman complained of a metallic taste in her mouth associated with headaches and depression that had occurred repeatedly during the last two years. Since she said the metallic taste was like having a penny in her mouth, I tested her for blood copper which turned out at 144 mcg/dl, a level in the upper normal range, normal being 87 to 153 mcg/dl. Later, however, I learned that chronic cyanide intoxication can cause changes in taste including the presence of a metallic taste. The taste of cigarettes can also be altered by chronic cyanide poisoning. [*Cigarette smoke, itself, contains a significant amount of cyanide.*]

Facts began collecting that explained many of the symptoms my patients experienced. Cyanide prevents cells from using oxygen, actually asphyxiating them on the cellular level, which reveals why cyanide is such a potent mental depressant. [*Also, cyanide decreases levels of serotonin in the brain, something associated with depression.*] It also explains why chronic cyanide victims fatigue easily, feel exhausted, get sore muscles, have chest palpitations, and are sometimes short of breath. Destruction of intestinal mucous cells may also occur, resulting in gastroenteritis which gives a patient stomach cramps and decreased appetite. Nausea and vomiting may also result.

Other symptoms such as itchy skin rashes and burning eyes occur from direct contact with hydrogen cyanide gas in humid atmospheres. [*The skin rashes and burning eyes may be expected to be notably worse when airborne cyanide is in the form of cyanogen chloride.*] Blood clotting can be affected, so patients may bruise easily and bleed more profusely than normal. Forgetfulness and incoordination are secondary to neurological depression from cyanide in the brain and nerve tissues. Hair loss likely occurs from asphyxiation of the hair roots, and temporarily blurred vision may result from cyanide affecting either the eyes or brain. Increased salivation occurs, but would probably go unnoticed unless poisoning was severe.

Additional information about chronic cyanide poisoning is very sobering. Miscarriages and birth defects may occur. After prolonged illness, patients may suffer permanent neurological damage such as decreased vision and hearing, incoordination, and weakness of arms and legs. Sterility in females may occur, and cyanide may affect the heart, giving patients chest pain and symptoms of a heart attack. Death may occur following these symptoms, or occur suddenly from an acutely increased exposure to cyanide.

As the data regarding chronic cyanide poisoning was assembled, the grave importance of somehow solving the problem grew apparent. December fourteenth brought yet another cyanide patient to my attention, a patient I had previously treated for six weeks while suspecting a chronic kidney infection. About nineteen years of age, intelligent, and a very neat dresser, Kevin Bradley was studying for the ministry at Gulf Coast Bible College.

"Are you busy?" posed Kevin as he edged open the office door after first knocking.

"No, come on in. How's your back doing?"

"It's better, I think those pills are helping."

Later evidence suggested that cyanide may destroy cells in the kidney and urinary tract, increasing the likelihood of urinary tract infections. This may have occurred in Kevin's case, but he had many symptoms besides back pain.

"Listen Doctor Oesch, or Tim, what do you prefer to be called?"

"Tim is fine," I responded.

"Well Tim," resumed Kevin, "I guess you know a lot of people are talking about this cyanide poisoning. Some say they believe it, and some just make a joke out of it."

"Yes, I know."

Kevin seemed to know what he wanted to say, but he wanted to say it carefully. "Well, I was talking to one of your patients who has the poisoning, and I think I may have it. What does it cost to be tested?"

"The blood cyanide test is thirty-eight dollars, but there's another test that may be better, and it's only twenty-seven dollars."

"Another test?" posed Kevin, walking to one of the chairs beside my desk. "Do you mind if I sit down?"

"No, make yourself comfortable. There's another test called a serum thiocyanate test. Thiocyanate is a metabolite of cyanide, and it stays in your bloodstream much longer than cyanide does. It ought to be a better test for finding whether or not you've been exposed to cyanide."

"I see. Well, if you're sure it's a good test, I'm a little short on money right now, and I wouldn't mind saving a few bucks if the cheaper test is as good as the other one. What was the other one?"

"Blood cyanide. It costs thirty-eight dollars."

"And this other test is better because it stays in the blood longer?"

"Right. Cyanide itself is only in the blood a very short time. About the only way you can find it in chronic cyanide poisoning is if someone is being poisoned at the time you test the blood, or shortly before you test them."

"Okay," Kevin pronounced decisively, "I'll get the twenty-seven dollar test then, but there's a few more things I wanted to talk to you about." [*Kevin's serum thiocyanate level was the same as mine, namely 0.9 mg/dl.*]

It was evident that Kevin was deeply concerned. "Sure, go ahead," I responded.

"I've been sick for several months now, and whenever I go back home up north I feel fine, but when I get back down here I feel sick again," stated Kevin, watching attentively for my reactions.

"That's the same way I am. When my wife and I went to Tulsa we felt a lot better, but we got sick within twenty-four hours of returning to Houston."

"Really?" queried Kevin, as if I were taking a burden off his mind.

"Yes, my wife and I both."

"So your wife gets this too?"

"Yes."

Kevin looked relieved, yet puzzled. His forehead wrinkled slightly as he delivered his next question. "My roommate, Bob...you know Bob Hastings don't you?"

"Yes, I've known him for years," I replied. Bob Hastings and I attended the same church, and had also attended the same church during previous years when I lived in Houston.

"Well, Bob and I both live in the same house, and I'm sick nearly all the time, but Bob almost never gets sick. Now, how could I be getting this stuff and Bob not get it?"

"It's not that you're getting it and he's not," I explained. "It's just that different people have different tolerances for cyanide exposure. It may be that his body metabolizes cyanide faster than yours, so at a given air level of hydrogen cyanide gas, your body actually has a higher level of cyanide in it than his. The cyanide builds up faster than your body can handle it, but his body changes it into something else before it gets to a high enough level to make him sick."

Kevin was bright, but he liked to make sure he understood things. "So what you're saying is that two people can be exposed to the same amount of cyanide, and one person will get sick while the other person doesn't."

"Right."

The pieces were fitting together in Kevin's mind, which was obvious from his facial expressions. "All right then, can this stuff affect animals as well as people?"

"Sure. My wife and I saw a squirrel that may have had cyanide poisoning. He sure was acting weird."

"The reason I ask is because Bob's dog, Caleb, a Labrador retriever that Bob raised from a puppy..."

"Right, I've seen Bob taking Caleb for walks," I adjoined. Sometimes Bob walked Caleb down to the college.

"So you've seen how frisky Caleb is?"

"Yes."

Kevin expostulated further. "When Bob comes home from work, Caleb usually almost tears the fence down trying to get Bob to take him for a walk. He runs back and forth along the fence and jumps up and down and barks, he nearly goes crazy!"

"He sounds pretty vivacious," I conferred.

"But here's the thing, other days when Bob comes home Caleb just lies there like he doesn't' have enough energy to get up. If dogs could only talk, I bet Caleb feels just like I do when I have this stuff."

There was no problem believing Kevin's story. Caleb spent very little time in centrally air-conditioned air, if any at all. Dogs depend on respiration to cool their blood, since they lack sweat glands, and rapid respiration would increase cyanide intake. As I contemplated the situation, an idea popped into my mind.

"Have you ever drawn blood?" I asked Kevin.

"Yes, some. Why?"

I think Kevin knew what I was going to ask before I asked it. "If I give you a needle and syringe, do you think you could draw some of Caleb's blood the next time he acts sluggish?"

"Well, if Bob helps me I might. I don't know if Bob will let me stick Caleb, though. He's pretty particular about Caleb."

"He may want to find out if Caleb has cyanide poisoning, and Caleb would be pretty good evidence if he has the poisoning."

Kevin was interested. He obviously wanted Caleb tested for his own curiosity's sake as well as for the investigation. "All right, I'll see what I can do."

Chapter 6

CITY OF HOUSTON
INTER OFFICE CORRESPONDENCE

To E.M. Quevedo   From William R. Osborne

                        Date 2/22/82

                        Subject Cyanogen chloride literature search

I am requesting permission and support for a literature search of references on cyanogen chloride. The service is provided by Toxline, sponsored by the National Library of Medicine and available from the Jesse H. Jones Library in the Medical Center (797-1230, ext. 61). The fee is 90c/minute for the computer time and 30c per printout page. A typical job is about $20; we expect this to be less because the number of references is likely to be small.

William R. Osborne
William R. Osborne
Northwest District Supervisor

cc: W.M. Lee
M.W. Aspan
H.H. Branham

Intriguing Information

December fifteenth and sixteenth marked the last two days that either of the two major newspapers reported anything about the cyanide problem until months later. These last reports basically recapped prior information and stated the Houston Health Department's denial of any significant problem. There was also some objective data and comments by a member of the special ad hoc panel that indicated that the Houston Health Department was not adequately explaining patient symptoms and laboratory findings. This encouraging factor, however, was overshadowed by intimidating propaganda supplied by the Houston Health Department.

Christmas crept closer. Using money from lab fees, I flew my wife to her parents' home for the holidays. I felt compelled to remain in Houston due to the urgency of the cyanide problem, and also due to my ingrained belief in paying rightful bills. The cyanide struggle in the

Heights left me about two thousand dollars in debt, most to Severance and Associates Laboratory. Nearly four months later, I would finally manage to emerge from debt.

It was harsh spending our first Christmas apart, but I feared for my wife's health. It was comforting just to know she was far away from the dreadful pollution. Meanwhile, I migrated to my adopted parents' home where I spent Christmas. Bob and Verdi Daniels were close friends. They had been like family to me for many years. I remember many Sunday evenings spent in a cozy apartment where they lived during my college years. Not only did they provide company and transportation to church—I consumed quite a number of steaks and tacos prepared with Verdi's delectable cooking. Due to the Daniels' graciousness in helping others, part of my stay was shared with Ted and Nancy Buchani, returning missionaries from Guam. Even their son, Scott, joined us for a while from the Air Force.

It was a little over one week past Christmas, January 3, 1982, when I received a call from Barbara Preskin. Between December sixteenth and January third, I visited the office only occasionally. I spent more time recuperating some health and strength at the Daniels'. When Verdi handed me the phone, I heard a voice completely unfamiliar to me. That same voice would become ingrained within my mind; Barbara was a determined woman.

"Hello," said Barbara.

"Hello, Doctor Oesch."

"Doctor Oesch, thank goodness I've finally gotten ahold of you. You're about the toughest person to track down that I've ever come across," Barbara expressed fervently.

"Yes, I'm sort of hiding out for a while, trying to regain a little health. I really got sick there in the Heights, so I figured I'd better recover a little or I wouldn't be much help to anyone."

"Doctor Oesch, you don't know me, my name is Barbara Preskin, but the reason I've called is because I need your help, not for myself, but for a friend, and we don't know anybody else we can turn to," Barbara stated pleadingly.

"My help?"

"My friend's name is Marsha Cheshire, we've known each other for years, and right now she's so sick I'm afraid she might die if someone doesn't do something. I'd take her to the emergency room, but the doctors there don't know anything about this cyanide poisoning, and they wouldn't believe me if I told them that's what she has. I've read all your reports in the newspaper about the symptoms of the poisoning, and I'm sure that's what Marsha has. I even stuck her finger with a needle, and the blood looks brighter than it should. I've stuck plenty of fingers, too, I used to be a lab technician"

Barbara's discourse more than won my cooperation. There was sparse traffic on this early Sunday afternoon, and I arrived at my quaint office about half an hour after hanging up the phone. Already parked on the bank of the gravelly, blacktop road sat an attractive, roomy van. Three people began moving inside the van as I stepped from my car. The side door was already open on the van.

"Doctor Oesch?" posed an aggressive yet polite voice. It was unmistakably the same woman I spoke to on the phone.

"Yes," I replied as I came closer.

"I thought it was you," Barbara announced. "This is my good friend Marsha Cheshire, and a friend of hers named Ron Volker."

I nodded to Marsha and Ron as Barbara spoke. She was lean and active, a certain social catalyst. As she spoke, Barbara helped Ron escort Marsha from the van. Marsha hung like a ragdoll as Ron and Barbara propped her up beneath her armpits.

"Come on to my office," I directed, stepping across the driveway to the office door. Marsha's legs moved like dampened straw, obviously failing to support her weight. I opened the door and the patient was deposited in one of the black swivel chairs beside my desk. She sank in the chair as if merely holding her head up would exert her beyond her resources.

"How are you feeling?" I asked. Sometimes it seems proper to ask questions even when the answers are evident.

"I feel like I'd have to get better to die," Marsha answered laboriously. It was not a very long nor detailed reply, but she communicated convincingly. Small beads of sweat broke out about her neck and above her collar as she grasped her chest.

"She got sick last Thursday, and she's been sick ever since, but she got a lot worse yesterday," Barbara commenced. As she continued speaking, I began checking Marsha's pulse, blood pressure, and temperature. "Her brother got sick too, especially after he came over to visit her last Friday evening. Yesterday they took him to the hospital and he's been on 100% oxygen ever since. I wouldn't trust them with

Marsha, though, because they don't know anything about this. They don't even believe the cyanide exists."

Marsha's pulse was rapid, 100 beats per minute. Her blood pressure was 130/88 mm/Hg.

"What was it?" questioned Barbara, who happened to be an ex-paramedic.

"Her pulse is one hundred. She looks like she could have it," I responded.

"I'm sure she does," affirmed Barbara.

Marsha still had a thermometer in her mouth, and Ron stood by silently.

Barbara spoke again, "An ambulance came after a man that lives across the street from her yesterday, Doctor Oesch. They diagnosed him as having a stroke. Do you think this stuff could cause a stroke? Her bird died yesterday too. Its cage was right beside an open window, and her brother had a bird that died yesterday. He lives several blocks from Marsha."

Barbara's story was definitely arousing my interest. Marsha and her brother both ill on the same weekend, and both with birds that died, plus a man across the street taken to the hospital with the diagnosis of a stroke. I knew that cyanide could affect the heart or brain and could probably cause illness or death that would appear as a heart attack or stroke. The dying birds made me consider psittacosis, but the series of events seemed more compatible with a large discharge of environmental cyanide.

Looking at Marsha, I could not help but notice the similarity to previous patients who tested positive for blood cyanide.

"What's her temperature?" asked Barbara as I retrieved the thermometer.

"Ninety-nine point eight," I stated. Then I addressed Marsha directly. "Can you tell me what kind of symptoms you have been having?"

Marsha did not appear to feel like talking, but she managed to converse quite plainly. "Ever since last Thursday, I couldn't eat, couldn't breathe, and I just feel awful."

"Any change in your memory?" I posed.

"Yes! I can't remember anything. I'm lucky I don't forget my own name."

"Any change in your vision or hearing?"

Marsha looked at Barbara as if I were some sort of mind-reader or magician. "Yes, I've been complaining about my eyes for several months now. My vision seems to be blurring."

"Any itching?"

"Yes! My shins have been itching on both legs. They get these red bumps on them. My eyes have been burning too."

I could hardly have imagined a patient that fit the description for exposure to hydrogen cyanide gas in a humid atmosphere more precisely. [*Or, of course, exposure to cyanogen chloride gas.*] I definitely wanted to acquire a blood test. Considering all the events that surrounded Marsha's illness, I thought a positive blood test would provide the strongest evidence for cyanide contamination that any one individual had yet contributed.

"I'd like to get a blood test," I stated.

Barbara was visibly consoled. "Whatever you say, Doctor Oesch. Is there anything we can do for her? I've never seen her like this in her whole life. She's usually a healthy, vibrant woman. You usually can't even slow her down long enough to say hello. She's got to be dying to carry on this way, Doctor Oesch."

"Sure, I'll give her one cc of sodium thiosulfate, but I want to draw her blood first."

"Fine."

Marsha's venous blood was bright red, much the same as mine had been with a cyanide content of 104 mcg/dl. By this time, early January, I had started testing for thiocyanate rather than cyanide, but I had never missed finding a positive blood cyanide when the venous blood was bright red.

"I was going to test her blood for thiocyanate, a metabolite of cyanide," I commented, "but look at the color of this blood."

"That's just like arterial blood, like when you do an arterial stick on somebody," commented Barbara. "That doesn't look like venous blood at all."

"Right, I think I'll check for blood cyanide rather than thiocyanate," I decided aloud.

"Why not get both?" inquired Barbara.

"Well, they're rather expensive," I explained. It was not common for patients to request additional lab tests from me; in fact, I often had to persuade individuals to acquire a minimal quantity of laboratory testing. Low cost was definitely associated with my practice.

"We don't care about the money," returned Barbara. "Marsha is one of our very best friends, and we want to make sure she is taken care of. Are there any other tests that may be helpful?"

Barbara's discourse was definitely encouraging, it was like arming a soldier with a bazooka when he was used to fighting with a stone-tipped spear.

"Well, it would be nice to have a CBC [*complete blood count*], and it's not very expensive," I coaxed.

"Fine, anything else?"

"I have gotten an elevated blood copper on a couple of patients. The plant that's probably contaminating the area with cyanide uses copper also."

"All right, let's get a blood copper test too."

After months of research, I would learn that cyanide may increase blood copper levels by ionically extracting copper from the liver and other storage sites in the body. Thus, the elevated blood copper levels in the patients tested in Houston may have been due to cyanide exposure alone, rather than to inhalation of mist-borne, ionic copper. Interestingly, my hair was analyzed and found to contain an extremely elevated quantity of copper.

Marsha was forlornly cooperative as she stretched out an arm and permitted three additional tubes of blood to pass through a needle from her vein. Then after fetching a large, plastic tumbler from the upstairs apartment, I instructed Marsha to swallow about one gram of sodium thiosulfate crystals with water. This she accomplished willingly, and probably would have succumbed to more drastic treatment had I advised it. The simple treatment, however, was satisfactory.

"I feel like a human being again," remarked Marsha, about half an hour after receiving the sodium thiosulfate.

Barbara was ecstatic. "You're a miracle worker Doctor Oesch. I don't know how we can ever thank you."

I was flattered. The complimentary words were a welcome contrast to those the health department allotted me. Marsha's recovery was quite dramatic, even more so than I expected. Her pulse slowed, her fever dropped, her symptoms cleared, and yet another blood sample drawn from her arm revealed that her venous blood returned to a more natural, bluish color. A thankful, relieved expression erased Marsha's former look of anguish. It was one of the most satisfying treatments I ever administered.

"Believe me, the pleasure is mine," I replied to Barbara.

"What do we owe you? I know you've gone to a lot of trouble coming out here, so don't be bashful," said Barbara.

I considered the trip so productive toward investigating the cyanide poisoning that I would have paid for the opportunity. "I usually charge ten dollars," I responded.

"Ten dollars! You're about fifty years behind times!" exclaimed Barbara. "We can talk about charges later, I'd like you to come see my laboratory. I'm going to run a test on Marsha's buccal cells and see if anything unusual shows up."

Ron did the driving; I think it was his van. Since Marsha lived just a few blocks from my office, we decided to leave my car and that I would ride back with Ron and Marsha. Barbara lived on the south side of town. It was about a twenty minute drive with light traffic, though during rush hours it would take much longer.

Barbara's house was interestingly decked [*the word should be bedecked*] with artwork and unusual artifacts. She brought Marsha and me into her medical laboratory, a converted bathroom, and scraped some cells from the inside of Marsha's cheek. There she examined the scraping under a microscope, and found something unusual relating to certain types of blood cells. This notably excited her, and soon she invited several of my patients to her home, free of charge, to examine effects of cyanide on cheek cells. After finishing in the laboratory, we sat down for a while in Barbara's living room.

Ron wasted little time finding the kitchen. Barbara treated us all to herb tea. I rarely drink tea at all, but the brew she served was quite tasty. We discussed my impressions of the cyanide problem at some length, and Marsha wrote me out a check for the laboratory tests plus one hundred dollars. They told me it was the going rate for a two hour house call, if not less, and insisted I accept it. It was the only time in my life that a patient paid me ten times more than I requested.

When the day was over, I felt certain that substantial laboratory evidence would be forthcoming with the return of Marsha's blood tests. Her tests returned conclusively positive, but I was surprised that her blood cyanide level was only 14 mcg/dl. The lowest level on any other patient having bright red venous blood was 27 mcg/dl. This impressed my mind with the realization that patients could be seriously ill with cyanide poisoning, and yet have relatively low levels of blood cyanide. It is the intracellular quantity of cyanide that causes illness, not the blood quantity.

Marsha's serum thiocyanate was definitely elevated for a nonsmoker [*she was a nonsmoker, and her real first name is Norma*] at 0.7 mg/dl. Her blood copper was high at 200 mcg/dl, and she was anemic with hyperchromic, normocytic red blood cells. Her red blood cells were decreased in number, too dark in color, but of normal size. Other patients with cyanide intoxication had anemia with small, dark red blood cells. This is different from anemia caused by iron deficiency, because in iron deficiency the red blood cells are too light in color rather than too dark. Marsha continued using sodium thiosulfate at her home, and managed satisfactorily. She eventually moved.

Meanwhile, Marsha's brother remained in the hospital in critical condition for weeks. He suffered from pneumonia which may have developed after damage to lung cells by cyanide [*likely cyanogen chloride*]. Another problem associated with chronic cyanide poisoning, namely urinary tract and kidney infections, may also result from damage to cells by cyanide. Attempts were made to have Marsha's brother evaluated for cyanide poisoning, but I do not know what action was taken. The political furor associated with the cyanide contamination made dealings with other physicians difficult.

During the first few weeks after the initial, publicized cyanide reports, I received a number of phone calls and letters with tips or suggestions. One attorney in Houston, who I never met or spoke to, mailed me a copied page from *Science News, Vol. 120*. The letter he mailed with the article was very brief, simply stating the enclosed article might be of some help in regard to my problem with cyanide poisoning. The article mentioned several potential modern hazards lending to the possibility of widespread contamination. Industries mentioned in the article included electroplating, iron and steel, tanning and coal industries. Pollutant substances mentioned included arsenic, lead, mercury, and cyanide. Of particular interest, of course, was the mentioning of electroplating and cyanide.

Another tip I received was from a woman who definitely wished to keep her name confidential. I was not in my office when she called, but a professor at the Bible college took her call for me. The professor delivered me a note with the following message written down: *General Electric Plating Plant, Sewer eye completely corroded, some chemical corroded it, General Electric only installed was 11/2-2yr, city too liberal in its permits, General Electric dumps cyanide into sewage, waste disposal in sewer cyanide—city works documentation, sewer system, city replaced it, file on General Electric.* Although no name or phone number appeared on the note, there was a date preceding the message: July 20, '81. I think the professor was ill at the time she received the message; both she and her husband evidently suffered from cyanide intoxication. Nonetheless, the message was sufficient when combined with the professor's verbal translation to inform me that some sort of city record on General Electric, filed on July 20, 1981, might give helpful information. I passed this information to my attorney.

Still another note I received came by way of a college student serving as switchboard operator for Gulf Coast Bible College. Melody Brown was an old friend; she was one of my youngest brother's first girlfriends. Miss Brown recorded a message [*in writing*] she received from Walter Davis, one of several calls that came to the college from individuals attempting to contact me. The message read as follows: *He is backing you 100%. He has a confirmed case (18.7) from an independent doctor. He had been sick for two months. He has 21 rent units throughout the Heights area (70% within the area of the cyanide) & he had been working in his rent units. However, he went to work in the Richfield area & he now feels fine.* [Richfield is a fictitious name: I cannot remember the real name of the area where Walter felt better.]

Miss Brown also recorded a phone number for Walter Davis. When I contacted him, Walter had more to say than was written on his note.

"Hello," Walter answered his phone.

"Hello, this is Doctor Oesch."

"Doctor Oesch, you must have received my message."

"Yes, I did. You had a positive test for cyanide…"

"Right, Doctor Yalten tested me over at the Heights Medical Center. He didn't know what to make of it, though. He doesn't know much about cyanide poisoning."

"Neither did I when all this started," I returned. "They didn't teach us about this in medical school. It's a recently discovered problem."

"Well, I'm glad someone knows about it. Let me explain something, Doctor Oesch, I had a real hard time deciding whether to even call you or not. You see, I own a lot of rent houses in the Heights, and if everyone finds out about this poison, my business could really be damaged."

I listened to Walter with interest. On the one hand, he was telling me how damaging verification of the poisoning could be to his business. On the other hand, he had already disclosed a positive blood test from another physician, which was substantial support to the reality of the pollution. Perhaps I was speaking to someone with some genuine moral conscience.

"I decided to go ahead and call you, though," resumed Walter, "because that stuff is terrible. I never felt so awful in my whole life. I must have been in the clinic a dozen times, but no one knew why I was sick."

Walter's language in describing his illness was actually coarser than I wish to transcribe, but I admired the way he esteemed human suffering as a graver problem than financial insecurity. There were some silver-tongued health officials who might learn something from Walter, something about human life taking precedence over dollar bills. I decided to further inquire about Walter's illness.

"Did you get headaches?" I asked.

"Yea I had headaches, but that was only part of it. I was tired, achy, totally exhausted, sometimes I had a sore throat, and my stomach acted up too. I think the exhaustion was the worst part. I just didn't feel like lifting a finger, it was awful."

"How long did your headaches last? Were they thirty minutes, an hour, several hours, or what?"

"More like four and five days a stretch," conveyed Walter. "I was working on my rent houses in the Heights during this time. I've got some other houses in Richfield, and when I left the Heights and started working in Richfield, I was okay. It's just when I work in the Heights that this stuff bothers me."

Walter's illness and laboratory test sounded like significant evidence, especially since another physician besides me ordered the test. I appreciated his phone call, and hoped he would consider allowing others to know about his case. Another factor that added importance to his laboratory result was that SmithKline Laboratory made the finding, rather than Severance and Associates Laboratory.

"Listen, Walter, I think you have some information and evidence that could be very helpful. I won't use it, of course, without your permission, but it might be very helpful to a lot of people who are sick."

I think Walter made up his mind about getting involved before he ever contacted me, but his voice still wavered slightly as he consented to my request. "All right Doctor Oesch, you can use my report, but keep me informed about what happens. I'd sure like to catch whoever is doing this."

"So would I," I concurred. "Feel free to call me anytime if you have any questions."

"All right. I might even stop by sometime."

"Fine."

Sometime later Walter did stop by. His appearance matched his voice perfectly; his clothes and hair demarked a staunch young man who earned his own living by the labor of his own hands. His visit, which was very brief, left me with the impression that he wanted to see me face to face, as if to size up who he was working with.

When I first opened the door after hearing Walter's knocking, I had no idea who was standing there:

"Hello Doctor Oesch, I'm Walter Davis."

"Walter Davis," I returned with recognition, "come on in."

"No, I'm too dirty to come in," replied Walter, gesturing toward his soiled attire. "I just stopped by while I was in the neighborhood. I've found out a couple of things you might want to know."

Like Barbara Preskin, Walter proved to be a catalyst toward investigating the cyanide pollution. He had some ideas of his own:

"Down at one of the houses I work on, I noticed some white steam coming out of a storm sewer drain. It was really gushing out of there, and those drains are just supposed to be for rainwater."

I nodded. "I've had some other people tell me about steam coming out of sewer or drainage openings. The thing is, though, the bayou runs between the General Electric plating plant and the Heights. Sewer lines run from west to east, but if cyanide is getting dumped into storm sewers, someone must be dumping it on the east side of the bayou."

"They could be dumping it anywhere," conferred Walter, "but there's another way it could be getting into the storm sewers too."

"What's that?"

"I've talked to some friends of mine who have access to inside information [*I think Walter may have mentioned the EPA*]. Some of the sewer lines in the Heights are old, real old, and from time to time a line will collapse. If it happens to collapse beneath a road, or a house, it can be expensive and difficult to repair. In some areas these sewer lines fill with rain water and actually back up into houses. When that happens, rather than repair the line, they often just make a bypass into the storm sewer. The only ones who know about this are the people who do it."

For some time I had tried to figure out whether the regular sewer or the storm sewer was the source of hydrogen cyanide gas [*cyanogen chloride gas was likely causing more cyanide poisoning in the Heights than hydrogen cyanide gas, although hydrogen cyanide gas is very probably the greater offender in regard to worldwide cyanide pollution and the worldwide illnesses that airborne cyanide causes*]. Evidence led me to suspect both, but I had decided the regular sewer was the most logical suspect. Walter's additional information finally revealed how both sewers could be involved, even without actual dumping east of the bayou.

Well, that explains a lot," I responded. "That way cyanide dumped into the regular sewer could end up in the storm sewer."

"Right, or they could just dump it in the storm sewer to begin with. What I really want to talk to you about, though, is this—we're not going to be able to stop anybody from dumping cyanide unless we have proof that they're doing it."

"Well, I think a lot of the problem might be the actual process at the plant itself," I explained to Walter. "The discharge water from the electroplating process goes right into the sewer there at the plant. I think the cyanide in that water floats along until it's generated into the atmosphere as hydrogen cyanide gas."

"That may be the case," returned Walter, "but your attorney seems to think there's some illegal dumping going on, and I tend to agree."

"Oh, you could be right," I assured Walter. "In fact, dumping might explain the bad spells of cyanide intoxication that patients experience from time to time."

"Then it would probably be worth checking out."

At this point, I deduced that Walter had something in mind. "Sure," I replied.

"I know these three ladies who will stake out the plating plant for hire. They're professionals—they get pictures and everything. I can assure you they're good at their work."

By this time I had arranged contact between Walter and one of the attorneys involved with the problem. I thought Walter's testimony might be helpful.

"Do you think your attorney might be interested in this?" questioned Walter.

"Well, possibly. It certainly sounds reasonable to me."

"Then I can say I discussed it with you and you were for the idea?"

"Sure."

"All right," said Walter, stepping forward and shaking my hand. "I certainly appreciate all you're doing, Doctor Oesch. I know you're catching a lot of trouble over this, but I'm behind you one hundred percent."

"Thanks."

As Walter departed, just one man who earned his living repairing homes, I could not help but feel encouraged. Somehow, I felt certain that this one man's involvement would make a difference.

It did not take long to spend the thousand dollars Buddy Adams and Phil Stevens gave me for additional patient testing. I sent the specimens to Mayo Clinic, hundreds of miles and several states away. The specimens were sent by certified mail, yet one was reportedly lost and another broken. I soon learned that a representative from the Houston Health Department arrived at Mayo Clinic about the same time as my blood specimens. That did nothing to better my opinion of the Houston Health Department.

Seven persons tested by Mayo Clinic received results. Two were positive, one with a blood cyanide of 30 mcg/dl, and the other with a serum thiocyanate of 0.48 mg/dl. Both were nonsmokers. Regarding the lost and broken specimens, one can only wonder what results they may have afforded. [*Note: the patient with a positive blood cyanide of 30 mcg/dl per Mayo Clinic, also had a second positive blood cyanide of 20 mcg/dl per Mayo Clinic. This patient's first positive blood cyanide was received by Mayo Clinic on 12/15/81, and his second positive blood cyanide was received by Mayo Clinic on 12/21/81. Also note that Mayo Clinic did not report any blood cyanide levels less than 10 mcg/dl; but rather, simply reported such blood cyanide levels as <0.1 MICROGRAMS/ML, which is equal to **less than 10 mcg/dl**. Whether this failure to report levels less than 10 mcg/dl was due to a lack of ability on the part of Mayo Clinic, or due to input from the Houston Health Department, I do not know. But also note, as previously stated* *in this book, that I later received a report for a blood cyanide level in a **smoker** from Metpath Laboratories, with the level reported as only **1.4 mcg/dl**. Since Severance and Associates Laboratory was originally able to report a blood cyanide level of **2 mcg/dl**, and since Metpath Laboratories was able to report a level of **1.4 mcg/dl**, then it would seem likely that an organization as prestigious as Mayo Clinic should have been able to report levels of blood cyanide that were less than **10 mcg/dl**.]*

Not long after sending the additional blood tests to Mayo Clinic, I approached Buddy and Phil with another idea. Perhaps foliage in the Heights area, as well as in the vicinity of the plating plant, could be tested for cyanide content. Buddy and Phil were both quite open-minded. They agreed to finance the operation, and Southwestern Laboratories was commissioned to perform the testing. I accompanied two representatives from Southwestern Laboratories and directed them to testing areas.

Leaves, grass, and moss were collected from several different sites and evaluated for cyanide content. Some types of grass, such as arrowgrass and Johnson grass, may normally generate quantities of cyanide. Other types of vegetation, such as crabgrass and tomato leaves, are better for investigating environmental cyanide contamination. All of the specimens yielded positive findings, with cyanide levels up to 5.60 parts per million. A specialist at Texas A&M University, who I contacted by phone, told me that the detected levels of cyanide sounded unusually high for the types of vegetation evaluated.

Grass in the ditch that ran in front of the plating plant was tested at three different points; the west end of the ditch, the east end of the ditch, and the center of the ditch in front of the plating plant. Water flowing into the ditch drained from west to east, so any discharge reaching the ditch from the plating plant was more likely to accumulate in the east end of the ditch than the west end of the ditch. Interestingly, the cyanide content of grass at the east end of the ditch was more than twice that at the west end, with approximate levels of 2.81 parts per million and 1.33 parts per million respectively. The grass in the center of the ditch was about 1.52 parts per million. Notably, levels of cyanide were even higher in plants as far as two miles from the plating plant. This seemed to indicate that larger quantities of cyanide were dumped into sewers or elsewhere than were discharged into the ditch before the plating plant.

A Breath of Cyanide

The agricultural specialist told me that cyanide that is absorbed into plants from the atmosphere may only remain in the plants around twelve hours. Thus, the environmental testing on plants that Southwestern Laboratories performed likely indicated recent contamination rather than long-term trends. In other words, testing foliage for cyanide may have served to reveal the most recently polluted areas without necessarily showing where most polluting had occurred in the past. I searched my mind for some means of acquiring more specific and permanent evidence of polluting from an industry such as the plating plant. Then a new idea came to me—the plating plant electroplated with copper cyanide and silver cyanide. Copper and silver are more permanent contaminants.

With success testing foliage for cyanide, Buddy and Phil were amiable to my new idea. Soil was collected from several sites where foliage containing cyanide was acquired previously. By contacting a soil specialist, namely Dr. Lloyd Hossner of Texas A&M University, I obtained normal levels for copper and silver in soil: 5 to 40 parts per million and 0.05 to 1.5 parts per million respectively. The soil was collected by a laboratory employee so that any resultant evidence would be legally permissible. The results were impressively positive, with copper levels ranging from 25 to 130 parts per million, and silver levels ranging from 6.9 to 20 parts per million.

Soil from the east end of the ditch before the plating plant yielded by far the highest levels of copper and silver, about twice as high as any soil tested elsewhere. Second highest levels came from the point where a smaller bayou drained into a larger bayou. The copper level there was 54 parts per million, and the silver level was 13 parts per million. The larger bayou coursed between the plating plant and Gulf Coast Bible College, coursing north to south. The smaller bayou, I was informed, drains rainwater from the region where the plating plant is situated. It runs into the larger bayou from the west, draining toward the east.

These early investigative successes seemed to astound Buddy and Phil. From the very start, Buddy established his own pet word for the entire situation: incredible. Before long the two attorneys decided to enlist reinforcements. They arranged for me to meet with Mr. Rusk and Brenda Jenkins of the Werner & Rusk Law Firm. Buddy appraised the law firm very highly.

I met Buddy at his office and he drove me to the Werner & Rusk Law Firm. Brenda was in court when we first arrived, so we met with

Mr. Rusk. This was the only time I spoke directly to Mr. Rusk. Thereafter, Brenda served as negotiator. Brenda's younger age, along with the more secluded posture of Mr. Rusk, seemed a similitude of Nero Wolfe and his associate, except that Brenda was a woman rather than a man.

Mr. Rusk stood and shook our hands after Buddy and I entered his office. Once we were seated, Buddy verbally outlined the purpose of our meeting. I think the facts and evidence concerning the cyanide contamination were presented to Mr. Rusk prior to the meeting. What I remember best are the questions Mr. Rusk posed directly to me. He sat discreetly behind his desk, speaking slowly and deliberately.

"The question now, Doctor Oesch, is what you wish to accomplish," presented Mr. Rusk.

The broadness of such a question was startling, but I had little trouble delivering a response. "Well, eventually I'd like the cyanide polluting to be stopped."

Mr. Rusk threw a quizzical glance at Buddy and leaned contemplatively in his chair.

"I think we would all like to see an end to the poisoning," conferred Mr. Rusk. "I have an interest in humanitarian undertakings. One of my more memorable accomplishments pertains to the legal implementation of a safety device on a particular type of handgun. I imagine there are a few people still living today as a result of that implementation."

Mr. Rusk looked toward me as he completed his statement. I nodded my condoning.

"As a legal firm," resumed Mr. Rusk, "we deal in certain practicalities. The humanitarian aspect definitely plays a part, but there is the matter of financial restitution."

Mr. Rusk's careful wording tipped me off. He was apparently wondering whether or not I would be willing to file a suit against the polluting offenders. Someone, I figured, must have really stressed my religiousness when telling him about me. It is true I believe the Bible, and it is true that the Bible says to love your enemies, but the Bible also says to cooperate with authorities in punishing evildoers, and to take up your arms in time of war. Loving one's enemies does not mean that one should allow evil forces to reign.

"You mean, am I willing to sue?" I asked plainly.

"That's generally a fairly essential component to our active participation in solving problems such as this one," affirmed Mr. Rusk.

Perhaps I would have had qualms about suing if the offenders had ceased their polluting and attempted to right their wrongs. Such was not the case, however, and the continued polluting of the environment could hardly be blamed on ignorance.

"Yes, I'll sue. As long as you work toward getting evidence to solve this problem, you can sue for whatever you decide," I stated. National, state, and city health organizations had all failed to relieve the community of a seriously injurious contaminant. Even if I had detested suing, which under the circumstances I did not, there were no other agencies offering help.

"All right, I think we will be able to work out an agreement," pronounced Mr. Rusk.

Brenda Jenkins arrived before the meeting ended: a very professionally dressed, business-mannered lady, exuding the definite impression that her work was taken seriously. An agreement was drawn up sometime later that my wife and I both signed in Brenda's office. Brenda told us that the suit might take years to materialize, but for the sake of many ailing victims, I hoped some informative evidence would be released long before that.

Chapter 7

```
                    3730 DACOMA                    H.E.W. Clinical Laboratory License # 42-1037
                    HOUSTON, TEXAS 77002           Medicare Identification # 45 6267
                    PHONE 713-681-8477             Medicaid Identification # 204562873

 DATE REPORTED    DATE RECEIVED    PATIENT NAME (D)                        ACCESSION NO
 9-Apr-82         22-Mar-82        CALEB, LABRADOR DOG                     271012-5

 SPRING BRANCH MED. CLINIC   CLIENT NO.    TEST REQUESTED           AGE
 1721 PECH                   84250-02      MISCELLANEOUS TEST
 HOUSTON, TEXAS 77055                      9-37                     SEX

 PHYSICIAN                        REMARKS
                                  DECEASED DOG          SERUM THIOCYANATE

 *** MISCELLANEOUS TEST ***
 RESULT NAME          RESULT              UNITS              NORMALS

 MISC-REFERRAL TEST   NOTE
    THIOCYANATE:      19 UG/ML BLOOD
    CYANIDE:          NOT DETECTED
    DETECTION LIMIT,  0.1 UG/ML BLOOD
    THIOCYANATE AND CYANIDE ARE BELOW THE TOXIC THRESHOLD (100 UG/ML
    AND 0.5 UG/ML RESPECTIVELY).
```

1) Prior Test (dog ill) .27 mg/dl } Same level as given to dogs killed with cyanide)
2) This Test (dog dead) 1.9 mg/dl } in JAMA for
3) Test taken Two days Following death — no cyanide would be expected.   FINAL LAB REPORT (The Td thiocyanate was)
Conclusion: Death from cyanide poisoning. (formed from cyanide)

Clandestine Killer

Sometime in January [*1982*], I flew my wife back to Houston from her parents' home. We spent the night at the Mexicana Motel near the airport. My wife was feeling much better, and we had a very happy reunion. After that, I returned with my wife to the Daniels' home. There we abode until I acquired a new job in Spring Branch, about seven miles west of Gulf Coast Bible College.

I still remember my interview with David Thompson. My involvement with the cyanide problem did not seem to bother him. He owned his own industrial medicine clinic and performed X-rays, electrocardiograms, and other lab tests right in his own facility. His wife, a registered nurse, worked in the clinic as did his daughter who served as receptionist. Only one physician was employed to serve the clinic at that time, and I applied to fill that position.

Before going on, let me explain why I was looking for a full-time job outside of the Heights. Most people seemed to assume that I abandoned the Heights due to the poisonous contamination and my poor health, but this was not the case. It is true that I stopped living and sleeping in the Heights due to cyanide intoxication, but I still worked there for some time. I hoped to find a part-time job in the Heights, and continue serving in my prior office at Gulf Coast Bible College. That way I could continue aiding patients in the Heights who were afflicted with cyanide intoxication. Mr. Saul, however, had other plans for me.

Sometime after Mr. Saul threatened me with blackmail, I made an appointment to meet with Mr. Chandler. Mr. Chandler impressed me as a wise and honest man. Besides teaching classes, I suspect he spent significant time counseling individuals who sought sincere and helpful advice. The actions of Mr. Saul began impressing me as a type of poison. If there are poisons that cause physical problems, then why not poisons that cause social, mental, and spiritual affliction. To be quite honest, I did not believe God wanted me serving under Mr. Saul any longer.

Mr. Chandler welcomed me into his office and directed me to a chair before his desk. There I shared everything that had happened regarding Mr. Saul, and explained why I could no longer serve under Mr. Saul's jurisdiction. I was not sure how Mr. Chandler would react, but I felt certain he was the right man to consult. He advised that I make these happenings known to Mr. Oxten, Board Director for Gulf Coast Bible College. I did as Mr. Chandler advised.

Not long after meeting with Mr. Chandler, I was approached by college officials regarding my willingness to carry on medical practice a couple of days a week at Gulf Coast Bible College. This I agreed to. The idea was short-lived, though, due to decisions made in a subsequent meeting including Mr. Saul. In this meeting it was decided that I would not be allotted further use of the medical office, and that a full-time nurse would be hired to my exclusion.

Several people confided with me, disclosing their unwillingness to remain at Gulf Coast Bible College unless Mr. Saul was dismissed from the staff. These people included teachers as well as students. I could hardly blame them. At the same time, though, I could not help feeling sorry for Mr. Saul. I suspected he was suffering mental effects of cyanide intoxication. My wife and I prayed for him.

Months later I received a letter from Mr. Oxten that read as follows:

Dear Dr. Oesch:

I received your paper on cyanide. It was interesting and very well done. I guess the next step is to find out where it is coming from. This is such an uphill battle.

I sent a copy of your letter to the college. I am no longer chairman of the board because of the vote at the ministerial assembly in Saxton [*may have been Anderson, as in Anderson, Indiana*]. The Chairman of the Board of Wellington was also defeated. A new chairman will be elected at the next meeting.

Thanks for your help,

J.O.

P.S. I am sure you know that Mr. Saul is no longer with the college.

With the option of continuing part-time work at Gulf Coast Bible College expunged, I sought employment through a medical employment agency. Soon I found myself sitting in David Thompson's office. The interview was short. David claimed that I was exactly what he wanted, and the clinic suited my desires perfectly. David was more than glad to permit my private practice into his clinic in addition to the industrial practice already established. He even changed the name of the clinic from Industrial Health Center to Spring Branch Medical Clinic. We soon became devoted friends.

I began working in Spring Branch around the first of February. My wife and I found a two-bedroom apartment near the clinic. We rented some furniture and lived in comparative luxury to our prior abode. The apartment had an outdoor swimming pool and a heated Jacuzzi. By sitting in the hot Jacuzzi before plunging into the pool, we managed to swim on forbiddingly cool nights. We often had the whole pool to ourselves.

It did not take long for my wife and me to discover that Spring Branch was also affected by cyanide contamination. As early summer winds blew more and more consistently from the southeast, and as temperatures grew warmer, our symptoms worsened. It was heartbreaking. Nonetheless, determined to stay together and make the best of it, my wife and I remained at the apartment for two months. My wife took a part-time job as nursery director at church.

A Breath of Cyanide

Work at the medical clinic in Spring Branch went well. I arrived in the office at about 9:30 a.m. and remained until around 4:30 or 5:00 p.m., Monday through Friday. Besides David's wife and daughter, two paramedics were also employed at the clinic.

On the morning of February 22, 1982, a Monday, I received a call from the clinic just minutes before my normal departure time. It was David. David did not need to identify himself; his gruff country accent and friendly, outgoing manner distinctly characterized his voice.

"Doctor Oesch, I think you'd better get down here right away," stated David.

"What's wrong?" I responded.

"I can't stand to see a full-grown man cry. There's a Jimmy Partridge here who claims he's one of your cyanide patients. He can't walk straight, and he breaks out crying like a baby."

"I'm on my way."

The name Jimmy Partridge was familiar to me even though I had never seen the man. He was one of the patients tested positively for cyanide intoxication by a physician besides myself. The doctor who performed the test, Lawrence Billings, M.D., was an allergist in Spring Branch. Doctor Billings had a blood cyanide test performed on Mr. Partridge at BioScience Laboratories. The test yielded a blood cyanide level of 27 mcg/dl.

After entering the clinic, I was quickly ushered to an examining room where Mr. Partridge lay dismally on the examination table. His wife, Rhonda Partridge, greeted me as I stepped into the room. They were a young couple, about thirty years of age.

"Doctor Oesch?" evoked Rhonda.

I nodded. "Yes."

Jimmy turned his head to view me, but made no attempt to rise. He held one hand to his forehead.

"I hate to barge in here like this, I know you're supposed to have an appointment, but Jimmy's so sick, I've never seen him like this," Rhonda explained apologetically.

"No problem, I'm glad to finally meet you," I returned. Rhonda was the one who actually called and informed me about Jimmy's positive cyanide test. I sometimes wondered how many other positive tests in the region went unmentioned. I have no doubt that many individuals with chronic cyanide intoxication received negative tests since blood cyanide may only be elevated for brief periods of time.

"We should really have seen you before," continued Rhonda.

"Well, I'm glad you're here now, anyway."

"Can you do anything for me, doc? I'm dying!" Jimmy interjected with a tone of slapstick humor. It was his way of politely directing our attention to the real issue at hand.

"You do look like you don't feel very well," I acknowledged. Jimmy was a wry comedian, and as I learned later, a very talented musical composer. We struck a mutual friendship almost immediately.

"Don't feel well, ha! I feel like I've been rolled up in a Chinese fortune cookie and chewed alive by a sumo wrestler."

For someone who had just been crying from the mentally-oppressive effects of cyanide intoxication, Jimmy Partridge certainly maintained an impressive measure of wit.

"You'll have to excuse Jimmy, he's that way with everybody," mitigated Rhonda. She seemed to have her hands full managing her husband, but she seemed to enjoy it. "He is sick though, he can't even walk straight, and I had to drive him here."

"It's obvious I'm sick. The question is, what can we do about it?" resolved Jimmy.

It was apparent that Jimmy wanted me to get right down to business. I began checking vital signs.

"How long have you been ill?" I questioned.

"Oh, about three days this time. It never seems to go away completely," answered Jimmy.

"It's gotten a whole lot worse lately though," added Rhonda. "Jimmy's been taking a lot of sick days to avoid going back to where he works. He works right across the street from the electroplating plant. Lately he's been sick at home too. Do you suppose he could be getting exposed to cyanide here in Spring Branch?"

"Maybe, but probably not as much as where he works," I replied.

Time would cause me to reconsider my reply to Rhonda. Weather conditions could definitely affect which direction the contamination spread, and unauthorized dumping of cyanide compounds might disseminate the contamination most any direction.

Jimmy's symptoms and vital signs were consistent with cyanide intoxication. He was first identified with the poisoning after reading a list of symptoms in the newspaper and having his doctor test him. Actually, Rhonda was the one who requested the test; she served in a secretarial pool for several physicians, including Doctor Billings. She told me that Doctor Billings was rather surprised when the test came back positive.

Despite his verbal jesting, Jimmy was in a great deal of distress. He was, in fact, poisoned to the extent that he could not walk and maintain his balance well. His condition also put his wife in a lot of distress.

"He's not dying is he doctor? I mean, he keeps saying he's dying—and I never know whether to believe him or not."

"I think he will feel better with some sodium thiosulfate. It will probably take about thirty minutes to help though…"

"Thirty minutes! I don't know if I can take thirty more minutes of this!" exclaimed Jimmy. "Don't you have anything that will work faster? I'll even take a shot."

"That is serious if he'll take a shot," proclaimed Rhonda.

I almost never used amyl nitrite due to its side effects. It causes an immediate drop in blood pressure and may result in a migraine headache. On occasion, however, I considered the use of amyl nitrite to be warranted by the extent of acute symptoms a patient experienced.

"Well, I do have something he can inhale," I mentioned to Rhonda.

"I'll take it!" blurted Jimmy.

Jimmy drank some sodium thiosulfate and inhaled six breaths of crushed amyl nitrite pearls. I monitored his blood pressure very closely while administering the amyl nitrite, but there was no drastic change. Six more breaths of amyl nitrite were given; this time a significant change was noted in Jimmy's blood pressure, so further administration was withheld. Notable improvement soon occurred, much to the relief of both Jimmy and Rhonda.

"Thanks," said Jimmy. He was able to stand and walk without vertigo. "Now, what happens the next time I get sick? Am I going to have to come in here and faint on your table in order to get any help?"

"No, you can take sodium thiosulfate yourself," I replied. "I'll send some home with you, and if you need more, you can get it from Northwest Pharmacy. The pharmacist there is named Henry Armstrong."

Jimmy looked dismayed. "How come you can treat me and do all this for me, and no other doctor would even tell me what's going on?" he posed.

"Well, most doctors aren't aware of this yet," I returned.

"Aren't aware of it! I read about it in the newspaper, and since my wife happens to work for a doctor, I managed to get tested for it. It's been on television, the radio, and you're saying that doctors aren't aware of it!"

By taking up for my comrades in medicine, I somehow hoped to attract their cooperation in confronting the problem of cyanide intoxication. For the most part I was sadly disappointed, but there were a couple of startling exceptions.

"Well," I stammered, "I didn't know anything about chronic cyanide poisoning myself, at first. I had to search out information all the way from here to California."

Jimmy was ponderously silent. It was apparent that he would digest my comments and derive his own conclusions. With his headache alleviated, his mind seemed shifted to high gear.

"Did my wife mention that she's had some of the same symptoms that I have," inquired Jimmy, embarking upon a new line of investigation.

Rhonda smiled sheepishly as I looked toward her following Jimmy's question. "I haven't told many people about it. I mentioned it to one doctor, and he looked at me like I was having psychological problems," conceded Rhonda.

"She doesn't work near the plating plant, either. She works right here in Spring Branch," added Jimmy.

By this time my wife and I had lived in Spring Branch about three weeks. My wife was just beginning to relapse into illness after her recovery at her parents' home. Although I was suspecting, much to my bereavement, that cyanide contamination was present in Spring Branch, there was not yet objective proof of it. Jimmy had a positive blood test for cyanide, and would soon have a positive urine test for thiocyanate, but he worked near the plating plant.

"It sounds like we should test you too," I suggested, looking toward Rhonda.

"Well, yea, I suppose we should, but I haven't really been sick lately. The next time I get sick I'll come by."

Four days later Rhonda returned. She was ill. I did not feel too well that day either. We both had urine specimens tested by Metpath Laboratories, located several states to the northeast. Both tests were positive for elevated levels of urine thiocyanate; Rhonda's level was slightly higher than mine. [*My urine thiocyanate level was 8.7 mg/L, and Rhonda's level was 10 mg/L. Both of these urines were collected on 2/26/82 and the thiocyanate measurements were performed by Metpath Laboratories, Inc. I also had a urine thiocyanate test done per National Medical Services while working in Spring Branch, with a "date received" by the lab reported as 3/9/82, and with the urine thiocyanate level reported as 6 mcg/ml, which is equal to 6 mg/L. Rhonda and Jimmy are both fictitious names.*] Thus, environmental cyanide poisoning was not just limited to the area of the plating plant and the Heights, it was a very real entity in Spring Branch.

After Rhonda and Jimmy were found to have cyanide poisoning, I started taking notice when patients presented to Spring Branch Medical Clinic with symptoms of cyanide intoxication. Week by week, the number of individuals living in the area who were identified with cyanide poisoning increased. Just five days after Rhonda came to the clinic for testing, one of the physicians she worked for submitted a urine sample to be tested himself. The physician had experienced headaches and malaise for some time. The urine sample was found positive for elevated thiocyanate, with a level over twice that found in Rhonda's urine. Interestingly, given that many cyanide patients were referred for psychiatric evaluation before discovering that they suffered from cyanide intoxication, this physician was himself a psychiatrist.

Some days later, at about 7:00 p.m. one evening, I received a call from Jimmy.

"Hello, Doctor Oesch," I answered over the telephone.

"Doctor Oesch, this is Jimmy Partridge."

"Hello Jimmy. How are you doing?"

"Oh, so so…that medicine you gave me helps—but Rhonda won't take it."

"She won't?"

"No, she doesn't like taking any kind of medicine."

"Tell her it's just a type of salt with sulfur in it," I suggested.

"I'll have to try that, but for right now we've got a more immediate problem."

"What's that?"

"Rhonda's about to come unglued. She says she feels like she's dying, and it's getting worse."

I could tell from the tone of Jimmy's voice that he was not jiving. "And she still won't take the medicine?"

"No, she says she doesn't know what will happen. She says it might make her worse. I'd take her to the emergency room, but we're kind of low on money right now, and they probably wouldn't know what was wrong with her anyway. I was wondering if I could bring her over to your apartment?"

"Sure, bring her on over. Do you know how to get here?"

"I think so, but you'd better give me directions."

I told Jimmy how to find our apartment, then hung up the phone.

"We're going to have some company. Rhonda Partridge is sick and Jimmy's bringing her over," I informed my wife, who was washing supper dishes.

"What's wrong with her, cyanide?" inquired Melody.

"Sounds like it."

"I'm not surprised. I've been pretty sick the last couple of days," noted Melody. "Who talked to you, Jimmy or Rhonda?"

"Jimmy."

"Did he say how bad she is?"

"She sounds pretty sick."

Melody quickly finished the dishes and straightened up the living room. Jimmy and Rhonda lived only about three miles from our apartment. I helped Melody straighten things up.

"Tap, tap, tap…"

Melody stood with me to greet our guests as I opened the door.

"We found it!" remarked Jimmy. "We usually get lost and have to call."

Rhonda followed close behind Jimmy. I shut the door as she greeted my wife.

"You must be Melody," said Rhonda, taking both of my wife's hands as women do. "I'm so glad to meet you."

"Thank you," returned Melody, "come in and have a seat."

Jimmy and Rhonda sat on the sofa. Melody and I sat in two armchairs facing them.

"We don't know how to thank you for letting us come over here like this," said Rhonda as she sat down.

"No problem, we enjoy having company," I returned.

"That's right. We don't have company that often," concurred Melody.

Jimmy and Rhonda seemed to appreciate the friendly reception. They obviously felt uneasy about inviting themselves as patients into a doctor's home, but my wife and I were quite sincerely thankful for their company. The visit, though, was certainly more than a social call. Rhonda was visibly distressed; her hands quivered as she held them folded upon her lap.

"Well, the reason we're here," began Jimmy, "is because Rhonda is about to spaz out on me."

"I can't help it," spoke up Rhonda, "I just feel weird inside. It's like I'm falling to pieces—like I'm about to die. It feels like something is attacking me from the inside."

Rhonda's agitation became very evident as she opened up to us. "Go get the pressure cuff and my stethoscope," I asked Melody.

We tried to reassure Rhonda while taking her vital signs and talking to her about her symptoms. Her rapid pulse, shortness of breath, confused thinking, and extreme apprehension indicated significant effects of cyanide intoxication. As with many patients experiencing cyanide intoxication, Rhonda exhibited decreased ability to comprehend her own condition.

"What do you think it is? Do you think I'm dying?" posed Rhonda.

It seemed rather strange for Rhonda to ask me what was wrong with her. Besides the fact that she recently had a positive test for cyanide exposure, her symptoms were very similar to what her husband's symptoms were when she brought him to the clinic. "Considering the urine test you had done, and the symptoms you're experiencing, I think it appears that you're having symptoms of cyanide poisoning," I explained.

"Are you sure? Couldn't it just be the flu or something?" asked Rhonda.

"She's been like this all evening," stated Jimmy, "you can't talk any sense with her."

"Whatever it is, can you give me something for it? I can't go on like this," pleaded Rhonda.

"I think we should try some sodium thiosulfate," I expressed.

"You mean those salt crystals like Jimmy takes?" inquired Rhonda.

"Right."

"But will those do any good? I'm so sick. I've got to have some relief."

"If that doesn't help, I think we'll have to take you to an emergency room," I confided.

"Emergency room, we can't afford an emergency room," replied Rhonda. "How much of that stuff do I take?"

I measured out three quarters of one cubic centimeter of sodium thiosulfate crystals. Rhonda drank them down with water. I told her the crystals usually provided relief in about twenty to thirty minutes. Rhonda was desperately apprehensive. She repeated over and over that it felt like she was going to die.

When thirty minutes passed and Rhonda experienced no significant relief, she panicked. "I don't feel any different," she said. "Honest, it feels like I'm dying, we've got to do something."

I was not used to seeing such poor response to sodium thiosulfate, it worried me. I spoke to Jimmy: "Listen, maybe we should go ahead and get her to an emergency room. If you can't afford it, maybe I…"

"Oh, I can afford it if we have too," interjected Jimmy. "I'm more concerned about Rhonda. Can you take care of her in an emergency room?"

"No, I'm not on staff at any hospital," I pointed out. "We will have to get another doctor to care for her."

"That's what worries me. Most doctors act like you're crazy if you mention cyanide poisoning," returned Jimmy.

"Dr. Grant believes it's real," inserted Rhonda. She was not missing a word that was spoken.

"Yea, but he's a psychiatrist," replied Jimmy.

"That's all right," I intervened. "As long as he has staff privileges at a hospital…"

"He's on staff at Spring Branch Memorial," informed Rhonda.

"That's fine. Do you know his phone number?" I asked.

"I think it's in my purse."

Rhonda gave me Doctor Grant's phone number and I called him at his home. We had two phones in our apartment, so I called from our bedroom and let Jimmy join in on the other phone in the dining room.

Doctor Grant seemed genuinely concerned:

"Hello, Doctor Grant," he answered.

"Hello Doctor Grant, this is Doctor Oesch. I'm calling in regard to Rhonda Partridge…"

"Is she sick?" inquired Doctor Grant. Rhonda was a secretary where he practiced medicine, so he knew her quite well.

"Yes she is. She seems, in my opinion, to have cyanide intoxication. I tested her for it before, and…"

"Right, I know about that," asserted Doctor Grant. "Is she in the hospital?"

"No, she and her husband are at my apartment right now. Her husband brought her over for me to evaluate, and I gave her some oral sodium thiosulfate, but she hasn't responded like most patients I've treated. She seems pretty shaken up. She says she feels like she's dying. The reason I called is because I don't have staff privileges at a hospital, and I think we had better take Rhonda to an emergency room."

Doctor Grant hesitated. "Okay, I'm on staff at Spring Branch Memorial. There may be some problem with my treating her directly, since I'm a psychiatrist, but I can call a friend of mine to admit her to the hospital. Will you be there?"

The thought had not crossed my mind. "I can come if you would like me to."

"Good. Your advice may be needed. Most physicians aren't too familiar with this problem. Do you know what kind of medical insurance Rhonda has?"

"Hello, Doctor Grant, this is Jimmy Partridge, Rhonda's husband, I'm on the other line," Jimmy broke in. "Don't worry about the finances, I'll just write a check."

"Well, I was just concerned about admitting her to the hospital. Sometimes they want some kind of guaranteed financing ahead of time," construed Doctor Grant.

"No problem," maintained Jimmy.

"All right then, I'll get ahold of Doctor Shelby and have him meet us there right away. How far are you from the hospital?"

"We're very close. It's only about a mile away," I answered.

Arrangements were shaping up effectually. We were just about ready to hang up the phones and put our plans into action when a surprising, but pleasant happening transpired.

"Hello, Doctor Grant," Rhonda's voice sounded in place of Jimmy's voice. She had taken the phone away from her husband. "Listen, I dearly appreciate your willingness to help me like this…but I don't know what to say…I'm better now. This is terribly embarrassing…"

"You're better?" I queried.

"Yes. I'm fine now. That medicine must have finally worked."

"You're sure?" pried Doctor Grant.

"I know it sounds incredible, but I was sitting there when I noticed that I was improving," affirmed Rhonda. "I'm just fine now."

"Well, I guess it just took a little longer than usual for the medicine to work," I surmised. "Thank you very much for your willingness to help, Doctor Grant."

"Certainly. Let me know if anything develops where you need my assistance."

"All right. Thank you. Goodbye."

"Goodbye."

I walked back into the living room. The atmosphere was laden with a gracious sense of relief. Rhonda was smiling.

"I just can't believe how much difference those salt crystals make," Rhonda remarked.

"Actually, she never was sick," jested Jimmy. "This is just her way of livening up an evening. She does things like this when she gets bored."

"Jimmy, cut it out!" admonished Rhonda. "This is the first time Melody has met us. She's liable to think we're a couple of looney birds."

"Well, we might as well not try and hide it. They'll find out sooner or later."

Rhonda laughed and shook her head. "Can you imagine living with someone like that?" she posed, pointing a thumb at Jimmy.

"It must make life interesting," I commented.

Jimmy and Rhonda departed from our apartment in much higher spirits than when they arrived. My wife and I invited them to stay longer, but they said they would rather visit under different circumstances. Rhonda admitted that using sodium thiosulfate might not be such a bad idea.

I never did meet Doctor Grant in person, but he did refer one his patients to my clinic. The lady had been under psychiatric care off and on for twenty years. During the preceding weeks, however, she developed some new symptoms. She complained of heart palpitations, labored breathing, decreased energy, increased depression, and scratchy eyes. There were also times when her hands got very shaky and she became *heavy-headed*. Sometimes her legs grew weak, and once she even fell down from weakness.

Doctor Grant wanted me to evaluate this lady for cyanide intoxication. Her symptoms were definitely suggestive of the diagnosis, and I ordered a urine thiocyanate test. The result was highly positive with a urine thiocyanate level of 41 mg/L. I thought it was interesting that Doctor Grant, a psychiatrist, was able to recognize symptoms of cyanide intoxication in a psychiatric patient. Perhaps it was partly because he had experienced such symptoms himself; his office was near my clinic in Spring Branch.

During the first part of March, I received a phone call from Mr. Chandler, the professor at Gulf Coast Bible College whom I previously consulted for advice. He gave me some alarming news. The news did not involve Gulf Coast Bible College, but rather an incident that occurred in his neighborhood.

"Hello, Dr. Oesch," I answered the phone.

"Dr. Oesch, this is Mr. Chandler. How are you getting along?"

"All right. How about yourself?"

"Trusting the Lord. Listen, I've got some information I thought you might want to know. Last Friday one of my neighbors died and the man across the street from her was taken to the hospital. I live in the Timbergrove area, you know. I think it may have been from the cyanide."

Timbergrove was the heartland of the General Electric plating plant, with the Heights to the east and Spring Branch to the west.

"Did the woman have an autopsy?" I inquired.

"Yes. They decided she died from a heart attack."

"How old was she?"

"She was still pretty young, in her fifties. She was an active, healthy woman too. Her death was a real shock to her family."

A variety of thoughts and tactics were running through my mind. It was too late to test for cyanide, since the woman died three days before Mr. Chandler called. If any blood specimens remained, they could be checked for thiocyanate. I was not sure if the coroners would cooperate though, especially if they were connected in any way with the Houston Health Department. I also disliked the idea of putting the woman's family through any additional stress. Then another approach entered my mind:

"Where is the sick man now?" I posed.

"He's at the Heights Hospital," replied Mr. Chandler. [*I assume this was the Memorial Hermann Greater Heights Hospital.*]
"What have they said was wrong with him?"
"I think they're saying he had a stroke or something. I'm not sure."
"Do you know his name?"
"Yes, his name is Frank Marsh."
"All right, I'll see about looking into this. Thanks for calling."
"Okay, be careful. Goodbye."
"Goodbye."
Since both Frank Marsh and the lady who died became ill on a Wednesday and grew much worse the following Friday, and since they lived in close proximity, it was likely that they both suffered from the same ailment. I remembered that a man was taken to the hospital who lived across the street from Marsha Cheshire when she became ill several weeks before. I acquired Frank Marsh's phone number and called his wife. She agreed to bring home a urine sample from the hospital. This was accomplished the following day.

I drove to the Marsh's residence to pick up Frank Marsh's urine sample. After arriving, I noticed a teenager wearing dark sunglasses drive up to a house across the street. He got out of his car and walked to the front door without looking up or about him. I surmised that this was the house where death had recently stricken. Mrs. Marsh verified my assumption.

Frank Marsh was still at the hospital when I picked up the urine from this wife. Even though four days had passed since he was taken to the hospital, Mr. Marsh's urine still tested positive for elevated thiocyanate at 15.40 mg/L. [*In retrospect, there would almost certainly have been some cyanide in the atmosphere at the Heights Hospital, and likely enough to show at least a small amount of thiocyanate in a urine sample. The level of cyanide in the atmosphere at the Marsh's home, however, was likely much higher than the level of cyanide in the air at the Heights Hospital. Frank's real first name is James.*] This level was several times higher than the upper limit of normal for a nonsmoker, and Frank Marsh was a nonsmoker. He was on no medication while in the hospital, but he improved with time. Considering the location of his house, the nature of his illness, and the result of his urine test, I had no trouble deducing what caused his neighbor's death. Nonetheless, the Houston Health Department still seemed to dominate control of the press and public opinion. It was fearsome to realize how powerful and heartless such an agency could be. It was also fearsome to see how tragically manipulated a poisoned society could be, even in the face of conclusive evidence.

Somewhere along this period of time, I acquired an additional agent for treating chronic cyanide intoxication. It was hydroxocobalamin, commercially available as alphaREDISOL. This vitamin preparation, actually a type of vitamin B12, gave fast and noticeable relief to cyanide symptoms such as headaches and depression. It was the treatment of choice for chronic cyanide intoxication mentioned in foreign literature. The concentration of hydroxocobalamin in alphaREDISOL was much less than desirable for treating cyanide intoxication, but it still proved highly beneficial as an adjunctive treatment to sodium thiosulfate.

As far as my wife was concerned, the major drawback with alphaREDISOL was that it only came in injectable form. There was no oral preparation available for purchase. [*One can now acquire sublingual hydroxocobalamin, as well as sublingual methylcobalamin, through Amazon.*] In actuality, even the injectable preparation could be taken orally, but this did not occur to me until after months of rather painful, intramuscular injections.

Sunday, March 20, 1982, is a day imprinted vividly in my mind. It began normally enough: my wife and I went to church as usual where she was nursery director and I sang in the choir. [*Houston First Church of God, 14400 Northwest Fwy.*] Sometimes my wife recruited me to help babysit two-year-olds, about ten or fifteen of them, which generally left me sprawled out on the floor after emptying the toy box and working to keep the merchandise peaceably distributed. This Sunday would become uniquely unusual as the afternoon sun coursed lazily across the sky, and the novelty began when Bob Hastings approached me after church.

"Doctor Oesch," said Bob, "can I talk with you a minute?"

"Bob was a very composed, unemotional gentleman outwardly, and at first I did not detect the involuntary shakiness in his voice.

"Sure, what is it?" I replied.

"It's Caleb. He's dead," stated Bob. He stood sedately and invoked my reaction with still, serene eyes. I knew that Bob was attached to Caleb. He took the dog for walks quite regularly, and had raised him from a puppy to maturity. "He was only one year and three months old."

"I'm sorry to hear that," I returned, then suddenly I suspected that there was more to Bob's confrontation than a simple announcement. "Was he hit by a car?"

"No, he died right in the backyard. When I found him, he was lying in the middle of the yard with his tongue hanging out of his mouth. If he died from that cyanide, do you suppose he suffered much?"

I had read about agonizing deaths resulting from cyanide exposure, but it did not seem appropriate to mention that fact to Bob. "Well, if he died from cyanide poisoning, the poison may have dulled his senses so much that he really did not perceive the amount of pain he was in," I responded. It was a truthful answer, and about the best one I could conjure. "When did he die?"

"A couple days ago," replied Bob.

"Did you bury him?"

"No, he's in a plastic bag in the trash can."

It was too late to check for cyanide; far more than twenty hours had elapsed without freezing any tissue. Thiocyanate, however, is more stable. Since we had a previous serum thiocyanate level taken when Caleb was ill, the prospect of obtaining a postmortem serum thiocyanate level seemed like a sound investigatory procedure.

"Would you like me to come over and get some serum to test and see if Caleb died from cyanide poisoning?" I inquired.

"He probably smells by now," responded Bob, "but I would like to know. If you'll come over and get the blood, I'll be glad to pay for the test."

"All right, I'll come over this afternoon. How do you get to your house?"

"It's my parents' old house on Pine Street. I bought it from them. You've been there before, haven't you?"

Once Bob mentioned it, I remembered visiting his parent's old home about fourteen years before. There used to be a large, abandoned mill behind the house which I explored with Bob's younger brother, Chad. Chad, like me, also went into medicine, and was a senior at UTMB Galveston when I was a freshman.

"Oh yes, I've been there before," I replied, "but it's been a while. You'd better go ahead and give me directions."

After church I had Sunday dinner with my wife, and then departed for Bob's house with a large syringe, some blood collection tubes, and a couple of needles. My wife declined coming with me on this particular adventure. She did not like returning to the Heights, except perhaps to visit old friends. Drawing blood from a dead dog did not appeal to her.

Bob's directions were easy to follow, especially since they took me through some of my old stomping grounds. At the time of Caleb's death, Kevin Bradley still lived at the house with Bob. Kevin was out of town, however, the day that Caleb died. Kevin traveled quite a bit in order to get away from the Heights. Not long after my visit, he moved away from the area due to the severity of his illness. Bob still did not have, or at least did not admit having any significant symptoms of cyanide intoxication. [*Sensitivity to airborne cyanide varies greatly between individuals. Higher levels of airborne cyanide affect a higher percentage of the exposed population, as would be expected.*]

Bob and Kevin were both at home when I arrived. I remember knocking on the door:

"Come on in," said Kevin, opening the door. "Bob, Doctor Oesch is here!" he hollered, then he turned back toward me. "Can you believe it? I knew that stuff was making Caleb sick. I was sick last week too, that's one reason why I went out of town."

"Yes. I'm going to try and get some blood to test. We can compare it to the blood drawn last time when Caleb was sick."

Bob walked into the living room from a hallway. "Hello Dr. Oesch. Are you ready?"

"I guess so. Where's the body?"

"I'm so sorry I have to rush off, but I've got a meeting," inserted Kevin. "Good luck."

Kevin shook my hand and then quickly departed wearing a sharp-looking suit. I was still wearing the suit I wore to church that morning. Choir practice started at 5:30 pm back at church, several miles northwest of Bob's house, so I planned to drive straight from Bob's house to choir practice. The evening church services came right after choir practice, which did not leave me much time to change clothes. Therefore, I just kept my suit on.

"Caleb's in the trash can outside the back door," directed Bob. "If it's all right with you, I think I'll just stay in here. If you need my help…"

"I think I can handle it," I asserted. Bob apparently did not want to see Caleb's body, and I did not want him to see it either. It was bad enough having to unbag the body myself, without having to watch expressions of lamentation emerge on Bob's face.

The lid was on the trash can. I removed the lid and spied the top of a thick, plastic garbage bag. The bag was tied shut. Caleb was a registered Labrador; the bag was quite heavy. After toting the bag to the center of the yard, I untied it and uncovered the deceased dog's head and neck.

The grossly protruding tongue gave a desperate appearance of agony to the dog's head. No wonder Bob had asked me if I thought the dog had suffered. I remember noting a startling, reddish coloration to the dog's tongue and mouth. There was some malodor as I opened the bag, but not much. The dog seemed less stiff than I would have expected. I took a needle and syringe from my pocket, removed the needle from its cover, and fixed the needle to the syringe.

The carotid artery or jugular vein seemed like reasonable sites to probe for blood or serum. Time after time I gouged the needle through the dog's tough hide and pulled back on the syringe plunger, but to no avail. I tried a different-sized needle, but still no luck.

From time to time Bob appeared behind the back, screen door. After a while he probably surmised that I was having some difficulty.

"How's it coming?" posed Bob from within the house. The back door was open, so only the screen door separated us.

"Not so good," I admitted. It was frustrating. After pulling a large, dead canine from a trash can while wearing my Sunday suit, I certainly did not wish to leave empty-handed. Besides that, the evidence the dog's blood potentially contained could, I thought, help bring solution to the cyanide pollution.

I walked pensively to the screen door and confronted Bob with a grueling proposition: "I can only think of one way I might get any blood serum to test. I guess I'd have to cut through the chest to the heart."

"Do whatever you have to," Bob stated resolutely.

"Do you have a knife?" I asked.

Bob decided to pass up the kitchen knives and loan me a well-sharpened pocketknife. I accepted the knife and returned to my gruesome task. The hide was tough. Once I got through, I pierced inward and twisted the blade until the knife was buried halfway up the handle. At one point the blade burst into a pocket of gas. The smell was caustically repelling. I nearly gagged.

"What's going on?" a new voice called from behind the screen door. I was standing a short distance away from the carcass, waiting for the gaseous stench to disperse. Behind the screen stood Chad Hastings and his young daughter, Sherry.

"Oh, hi!" I returned. It was surprising to see Chad. He was doing a residency in oncology a couple hundred miles north.

"I hear you've got yourself involved in a cyanide case. How's it coming?" asked Chad.

"Well, hopefully I'll come up with some more evidence here. I'm trying to get some serum for a thiocyanate test."

"Is that Caleb?" Sherry asked boldly.

"Caleb's dead. Doctor Oesch is trying to find out what killed him," Chad explained to his daughter.

I looked at the girl standing before Chad. When she was three weeks old, Chad asked me to babysit her while he and his wife went out. [*To the best of my memory, this occurred in Galveston, while we were both in medical school.*] She sure had changed. I hated for her to see the morbid operation transpiring in her uncle's backyard.

"I'm on my way to my mother-in-law's. I just stopped by to say hello to Bob," spoke Chad. "Good luck."

"Thanks, goodbye."

"Bye," said Sherry.

"Goodbye," I repeated.

My observers departed and I knelt back down to my undertaking. The knife tip finally tapped sanguineous fluid. It was deep within the animal's breast. I drew up several milliliters of the non-coagulated blood and transferred it into a special laboratory tube. Success at last.

"Did you get some?" posed Bob.

"Yes," I answered.

Bob came back out and helped me get the bag back into the trash can. It was almost time for choir practice, so I went straight to church from Bob's house. Needless to say, I washed my hands first.

Several days later, back in my clinic in Spring Branch, I received the results from Caleb's blood test. The result was conclusive with a serum thiocyanate level of 19 mcg/ml or 1.9 mg/dl. Caleb's blood had been tested once before when he was ill, yielding a serum thiocyanate level of 0.27 mg/dl. The level after his death was more than seven times higher. Furthermore, in an article published in the Journal of the American Medical Association, the average serum thiocyanate level in three dogs sacrificed by cyanide poisoning was exactly 1.9 mg/dl. I thought that was quite a coincidence.

Chapter 8

Underground

Barbara Preskin became quite enthusiastic in her studies of cyanide effects on cheek cells. It was uniquely unusual to have a group of people knowingly exposed to low doses of cyanide day after day. Once such a discovery was made, one would expect the exposure to stop. Due to the politics in Houston, however, the exposure continued.

Besides her own studies on living cells, Barbara arranged for hair analyses to be done by a doctor in Chicago. She interested him in the study so much that he agreed to do quite a number of the tests free. Furthermore, she brought me into contact with Doctor William Hitt, an outstanding micro-allergist who trained at Johns Hopkins. Dr. Hitt worked at a large medical complex located in the center of Houston. He demonstrated two qualities I was very thankful to see in a medical professional: compassion and courage. [*Dr. William M. Hitt had a Ph.D. in Microbiology and Applied Biology from a number of schools. He finished at Johns Hopkins*.]

Before long Doctor Hitt came up with some very pertinent data. He discovered that many individuals suffering from cyanide intoxication had developed an allergy to cyanide. Cyanide can cause illness easily enough without an individual being allergic or immunologically sensitive to it. Many ill patients, including me, did not show any allergy to cyanide; but some of the more serious cases did demonstrate allergy. Doctor Hitt performed allergy tests on freshly drawn blood; he did not actually expose patients to cyanide. [*I have been able to conclude that cyanide, like beryllium, may act as a hapten, or partial antigen. This means that an individual is immunologically reactive to one or more of their own types of bodily proteins when cyanide attaches to that protein, causing the body to interpret the protein as being foreign to the body*.]

One of the patients most extremely allergic to cyanide was Marie Black. Marie was referred to me after seeking help elsewhere for a prolonged illness which turned out to be chronic cyanide intoxication. The first time she visited the clinic in Spring Branch was toward the end of March. She was a well-mannered, cultured lady from a respectably established neighborhood near Timbergrove. Her home was not far from the General Electric plating company.

"You've got a new cyanide patient here," informed Kristy, our clinic secretary. [*Kristy is a fictitious name, and I cannot recall her real name*.] "Mom's getting a history and vital signs right now."

"Okay, let me know when she's ready."

Kristy's mom, who was also David's wife, was senior nurse at the clinic. I appreciated having someone else to give shots to toddlers. I was willing to do it when necessary, but Mrs. Kay Thompson took over some of the more trying and unpopular tasks that I faced in my earlier solo practice.

"She's ready, Doctor Oesch," called Kristy.

I walked from my office and Kay met me with Mrs. Black's chart."

"Another typical cyanide patient," commented Kay.

I looked over Mrs. Black's chart and soon saw that Kay was right. Fatigue, tiredness, headaches, forgetfulness, and shortness of breath were all common symptoms among cyanide victims. As I interviewed Mrs. Black, the probability that she suffered from cyanide intoxication became almost a certainty.

"Have you noticed any difference in your symptoms when you leave the area where you live for a couple days?" I inquired.

"Well, it's been so long since I've gone anywhere, I'm not sure I remember. I'm leaving next week for a vacation in Hawaii, though," replied Mrs. Black.

"That should be far enough away," I commented. "Pay special attention to how you feel the first couple of days after you leave, and to how you feel the first couple of days after you get back."

"I'll do that. Now, should I get some kind of test done? Is there a way you can test for this cyanide?"

"Yes, we're mainly doing urine thiocyanate tests. It's best to collect the urine about a day after you've noticed significant symptoms of illness. Just drop by the next time you're ill and Kay will order the test for you."

"Well, I've been sick," expressed Mrs. Black, "how about getting a test now, before I leave for Hawaii?"

"Fine."

When the result from Mrs. Black's test returned several days later, I had no trouble concluding why she was ill. She was a nonsmoker, and her urine thiocyanate level was 51.8 mg/L. This was and would remain the highest urine thiocyanate level of any patient tested, including smokers who normally have much higher thiocyanate levels than nonsmokers. Notably, Mrs. Black did not live far from the woman who mysteriously died earlier the same month. She improved dramatically after leaving for Hawaii, and became ill soon after returning to her home near Timbergrove.

As time went by, more and more patients were diagnosed with cyanide intoxication. Quite a number of cyanide patients came to the clinic just by chance, without being specifically referred for evaluation of cyanide intoxication. This convinced me that sizeable portions of the human populace in areas such as the Heights, Timbergrove, and Spring

Branch were suffering from varying degrees of cyanide intoxication. One food store on the north side of Timbergrove seemed utterly plagued with cyanide intoxication among employees. I was the company physician for that store.

During her winter visit to her parents' home, my wife basically recovered from the cyanide intoxication she experienced in the Heights. [*My wife's parents lived in South Carolina, and then later moved to Iowa.*] After returning to Houston, this time in Spring Branch, she seemed okay for a while, but then redeveloped cyanide symptoms. Her condition gradually worsened, as it had in the Heights, until about the second week in April. She woke up one morning crying; the relentless poison racked her body and mind. Melody made no request to escape the environment, but I would not watch her suffer so severely when there was a simple cure. I flew her back to her parents' home.

During the remainder of April, I made arrangements to vacate the apartment in Spring Branch and move west to Katy, Texas. [*I understand that Katy, Texas has really grown since 1982.*] Katy was several miles from Spring Branch, west of the Houston city limits. By this time, the Navy had called me to active duty beginning in July. The actual date of my orders was February 4, 1982, for duty to begin on July 5, 1982. [*Note: although my orders for active duty were dated February 4th, I cannot remember when I actually received those orders.*] My financial situation was tight, and I did not want to lose another deposit on an apartment. Fortunately, James Marshall and Ben McHanly offered to let my wife and me rent an extra bedroom in their house. I moved the first part of May, then flew my wife back to me.

As before, my wife basically recovered from illness after leaving Houston. She did better after returning to Katy than she did in the Heights or Spring Branch. Surprisingly, she still experienced illness, however, when prevailing winds came consistently from the southeast. There was a major bayou flowing out of Houston which passed about a mile south of our Katy home. Whether cyanide was generated from contamination in that bayou, or came from some nearby industrial plant, or traveled several miles on the wind, I did not know. Whatever the case, my wife was anxious to leave Houston for good.

My own health improved a little after moving to Katy, even though I still worked in Spring Branch. James and Ben were both prior residents of Spring Branch, and both suffered from verified cyanide intoxication. Like me, both James and Ben returned to Houston to work. Ben drove a school bus for the Spring Branch School District, and James taught at a community college. Melody quickly adapted to cooking supper for four, rather than two.

The number of patients diagnosed with cyanide intoxication continued increasing. One lady moved to Houston from Utah and went to work at a diet center in Timbergrove. Soon she became very ill, and her illness progressed to the point of attempting suicide. She was a smoker, but her urine thiocyanate was still more than twice the upper limit of normal for smokers. It was the second highest urine thiocyanate of any patient I tested, with a level of 49.9 mg/L. Interestingly, the woman who previously held her job had experienced similar symptoms of illness. This woman also developed thyroid abnormalities; thyroid abnormalities are associated with chronic cyanide intoxication in medical literature.

Meanwhile, my wife and I were hoping, along with many others, that the law firm investigating the poisoning would soon do something to alleviate the problem. As the time of my active military duty drew closer, I became concerned about the public ignorance of the poisonous assailant that frequented the atmosphere in regions of Houston. One day in the office, Mrs. Thompson informed me that a community meeting would be held near the Heights. She thought the cyanide situation might be a topic of discussion and suggested that I attend. Dr. Judith Craven was the scheduled speaker.

I attended the meeting incognito, wearing western boots, blue jeans, and a long-sleeved shirt. My attorney told me to avoid public disputes or comments. I objected to such advice, but it was hard to argue the point when she reminded me about the fiasco that resulted when the problem was previously brought to public attention. The longer that silence persisted, though, the harder it was for me to keep quiet. There were people being poisoned; someone needed to do something about it.

There were not very many people at the community meeting, but Dr. Craven gave no indication that she recognized me. During her entire speech, however, she never mentioned the topic of cyanide contamination. At the end of her discourse she answered a few questions, and then departed. After Dr. Craven's departure, quite a discussion arose among the remaining community representatives. I think they were primarily embroiled over designating funds to repair drainage ditches.

Somewhere in the midst of the community debate a middle-aged, black gentleman made a comment that heightened my attentiveness. I do not remember exactly where or how his comment fit in, but I remember his statement as something like: *Yes, well, remember what happened last fall with the cyanide poisoning in the Heights. They crucified the young doctor who had enough nerve to say something about it.* It was a brief diversion; the discussion quickly returned to the previous topic. I still remember being impressed with the image of a young, crucified doctor—someone who dared take a stand for right and was shot down. Fortunately, being Christian, I knew that crucifixion was not necessarily a permanent condition.

When the meeting ended, I decided to obtain someone's phone number who I could contact and inform about the developments in the cyanide investigation. I approached a man who appeared to be a community leader; he was busy talking with someone.

"Excuse me," I said when there was a break in the conversation, "I was wondering if there is someone who I could contact regarding the cyanide contamination in the Heights?"

"Grace Ledrew," the man replied quickly, pointing to a blonde-haired lady several feet across the room, "that's the lady to talk to. She's been quite involved with that situation."

"Thank you," I returned.

Grace Ledrew was already somewhat familiar to me just from attending the meeting. She was outspoken, opinionated, adroit, diplomatic, and seemingly intelligent. I waited some time for her to finish conversing with someone else, then was dismayed when she quickly exited the room. Determined not to lose an opportunity to establish further communications with the Heights community, I followed her down a hallway to two large, glass doors. Miss Ledrew was unlocking one of the doors; she turned and faced me when she heard my footsteps.

"I'll have to let you out if you want to go out this way," she said without asking any questions. "I have to lock this door back."

"Well, actually, I was just wondering if I could get your phone number," I inquired, planning to phone her later about the cyanide problem.

"No, you can't," Miss Ledrew answered bluntly. She turned back around and resumed her exit.

"I want to talk with you about the cyanide problem in the Heights," I spoke rapidly.

Miss Ledrew suddenly halted and again turned around. She stared at me harshly, then inquisitively. "Who are you?"

"I'm Doctor Oesch. I'm the doctor who…"

"Doctor Oesch!" exclaimed Miss Ledrew. "Why didn't you say so?" She seemed rather embarrassed. "I had no idea it was you, I just thought that some man was after my phone number." There was a short pause: "Can you come over to my place for a while? I'd love to talk with you. My brother would like to meet you too, we share a house together."

"All right."

Miss Ledrew gave me instructions, and I arrived at her house a few minutes later. It was an interesting house, full of bookshelves and books, typewriting paraphernalia, and other signs of literary enterprise. There were two dogs that she shut up in the kitchen. Her brother Rick seemed as placid as she did forcible. They were both very friendly.

"Do you like hot tea?" asked Grace.

"Sure, I'll take some," I answered. Tea was something I never drank at home but usually always accepted when visiting someone. Rick and I sat at the dining room table and talked while Grace fixed some tea and hors d'oeuvres, including crackers, cheese, and crisp vegetables. It was a substantial snack.

"So, what have you been doing the last couple of months?" inquired Grace, seating herself across the table from me.

I told Grace about my practice in Spring Branch, and learned that she was an aspiring writer. We touched upon a number of subjects during our conversation, but the major point of interest, of course, was the cyanide problem. Grace and her brother had both experienced symptoms of cyanide intoxication, and Grace had gone so far as to obtain a special report on cyanide compiled by a physician friend of hers. The report read as follows:

FACT SHEET ON CYANIDE

WHAT IS CYANIDE? Cyanide is a chemical compound made of carbon and nitrogen. It comes in different forms and can be a gas, liquid, or solid.

WHAT DOES IT DO? It prevents the body from using oxygen, and can lead to death from asphyxiation.

WHERE IS IT FOUND? Cyanide is used to fumigate ships, workshops, and dwellings, to spray plants, and is found in chemical labs, in blast furnace gas, in the manufacture of illuminating gas, and in gas from burning nitrocellulose. Nut meats, beans, peas, and seeds are fumigated with cyanide. Cyanides are used to extract gold and silver from ores, and in electroplating and case hardening steel and iron. It is also used to polish, clean, and coat silver, and in photography.

HOW DO YOU GET EXPOSED? Exposure can occur from breathing cyanide fumes, from absorbing the material through the skin, or from eating or drinking it.

WHAT ARE THE HEALTH EFFECTS? Skin rashes and itching can result from skin exposure to cyanide solutions. Respiratory irritation can occur after breathing in the fumes and this produces symptoms of running nose, congestion and nosebleeds. Mild poisoning can produce sudden faintness, drowsiness, weakness, trembling of the muscles, dizziness, and headache. The warning signs of exposure include itching of the throat and nose; burning and redness of the eyes; a metallic taste in the mouth; burning of the tongue; pressure in the head; and a feeling of apprehension.

At high doses, cyanide is highly lethal and will produce flushing, shortness of breath, coma and death.

WHAT DO THE TESTS MEAN AND WHY IS THERE SO MUCH CONFUSION? Cyanide is absorbed quickly and carried to all parts of the body. Part of the cyanide is then breathed out unchanged. Most of the cyanide is broken down in the body to thiocyanate, a much less dangerous and toxic material. The cyanide level is reduced to half in about one half hour to one hour after exposure, and returns to normal range about 4 to 8 hours after exposure. Thiocyanate is then excreted in the urine. Thiocyanate levels take longer to go down: the level is reduced by half in the blood and urine after about two days. Both cyanide and thiocyanate can be found in normal people without any exposure to cyanide. Smoking cigarettes and eating cabbage, almonds, and mustard can all produce measurable cyanide and thiocyanate levels in the urine and blood. Reported normal levels of cyanide in blood range from 0 to 10.7 micrograms per 100 milliliters with an average of 4.8 micrograms per 100 milliliters. (These levels are found in people without any symptoms and without any known history of exposure. The average levels in workers who had been exposed to *cyanide and who had symptoms was higher, but the two groups overlap in the range of levels. That is, the highest of the normal levels was higher than the lowest of the exposed symptomatic worker levels.) Tests for cyanide in the blood are not very accurate at low levels (less than 20 micrograms per deciliter.) Thiocyanate is a better test for checking on a problem.*

It encouraged me to discover some additional individuals who were concerned about the cyanide problem, and who were working to get something done about it. Due to manipulation of the news media, we were forced to work and communicate by phone, letter, and personal contact, but the battle had not been abandoned. Grace expressed her appreciation for my continuing efforts, and I was certainly glad to learn of her efforts. The trip to the community meeting was worthwhile after all.

The Thompson family seemed pleased with the addition of general medical practice to their industrial clinic. Most of our patients seemed to come from the Spring Branch area, but a few of my prior patients from the Heights came from time to time. This gave me an opportunity to inquire about the cyanide situation in the Heights. One of these patients was Kevin Bradley. Kevin was a close friend; I was always glad when he came by.

"There's a student here from Gulf Coast Bible College," informed Kristy, "Kevin Bradley. He says he wants to talk with you."

"Kevin, sure, have him come in," I responded.

As usual, Kevin was dressed immaculately. Even when not wearing a suit, his clothes seemed those of a Sunday preacher. Perhaps knowing he was a preacher influenced my perception.

"Hello Doctor Oesch," greeted Kevin, shaking my hand, "I appreciate your seeing me like this. I hope you're not too busy."

"No, it's good to see you. What's up?"

"Well, I've still been sick with cyanide, though I do some better since I've moved."

"You've moved?"

"Yes. I hated to leave Bob there with all the house payments, but I just couldn't take it anymore. Sometimes I felt like I couldn't breathe, like I was dying. Now, I do a lot better, but I have to go back in there for school, and when I do I get sick."

I had wondered whether or not the cyanide contamination would decrease in the Heights after all the news coverage, and sometimes it seemed that it had, but it apparently persisted. "Are many others sick?" I inquired.

"Yes, but nobody talks about it. You don't know what's going on over there now. If you mention being ill with cyanide, people just look at you like you're crazy. Some of them are saying pretty nasty things about you, too."

"Well, some people get their priorities a little messed up—their pocketbooks seem to take precedence over other people's lives and health," I responded. I do not think I was quite as ignorant of the situation as Kevin thought, though I appreciated his input.

"Well, I'll be glad when this semester's over. I just hope I can make it through my exams. That's one reason I came by—that alphaREDISOL helps, but I have a lot of trouble getting to sleep. Do you think you could give me something to help me sleep at night? This cyanide makes me so jittery and shaky, I just can't sleep."

I had not prescribed tranquilizers to any of my cyanide patients; in fact, I very rarely prescribed tranquilizers at all. Having taken a college course myself while suffering from cyanide intoxication, however, I knew that the illness could affect both sleep and studies.

"Well, I do have some mild tranquilizers here. I'll give you some to use for now during your finals, but only take one per night, and only when you need it."

"Don't worry, I hate taking any kind of drugs," said Kevin. "I'll let you know if these help."

Tranquilizers are a symptomatic treatment. Whatever problem causes an individual to be nervous, jittery, or apprehensive, a tranquilizer may alleviate these feelings. Physicians may treat symptoms with tranquilizers without ever getting to the root of an underlying problem. I was curious to see whether or not a tranquilizer would alleviate apprehension or anxiety that I knew was caused by cyanide intoxication. Somewhat to my surprise, the tranquilizers helped significantly. Perhaps a number of physicians in the Heights were using tranquilizers to treat patients with cyanide intoxication. Perhaps these patients were being diagnosed as having nervous disorders while the underlying cause was escaping notice.

Chapter 9

```
                                    25 February 1988
                    University of California, San Francisco...A Health Sciences Campus

Occupational Health Clinic
San Francisco General Hospital
Building 9, Room 109
San Francisco, CA 94110
(415) 821-5391            Tim Oesch, MD
                          1   Golfcrest
James E. Cone, M.D, M.P.H.
Medical Director          Oak Ridge, TN 37830
John Balmes, M.D., F.C.C.P.
Attending Physician       Dear Dr. Oesch,
Judith Quemfeld, R.N., M.P.H.
Clinic Coordinator        Thank you for your letter of 2/24/88 requesting that I review
Patricia Quinlan, M.P.H., C.I.H.   the blood and urine tests which you kindly provided.
Industrial Hygienist
                          These levels are certainly consistent with the history of
                          exposure to excessive environmental sources of cyanide.

                                              Sincerely yours,

                                              [signature]

                                              James E. Cone, MD, MPH
                                              Assistant Clinical Professor and
                                              Chief, Occupational Health Clinic
```

Repressed Disclosure

My departure date for active duty in the United States Navy drew nearer, and there was still a critical, unrecognized problem of environmental cyanide contamination. After months of silence on the issue, a couple of major newspaper articles readdressed the topic. An article appeared in The Houston Post entitled: *What ever happened to… …victims of 'cyanide poisoning' at city Bible college?* The article was quite interesting, it compared the cyanide problem to the plot for a late, late television show. As the title reveals, it also redirected public focus to Gulf Coast Bible College. I did not mind Gulf Coast Bible College getting publicity, but the article did not mention that a considerably large number of patients were diagnosed with the poisoning who did not attend Gulf Coast Bible College.

The article also gave several statements by Chancellor Fields, Chancellor of Gulf Coast Bible College. [*I am using a fictitious name and title, namely Chancellor Fields, for the President of Gulf Coast*

Bible College. His real name was President John W. Conley. President Conley had many great and admirable accomplishments as are listed in his obituary. He reportedly "spearheaded" the relocation of Gulf Coast Bible College from Houston to Oklahoma City, and it is publicized that the decision to make the move was determined in 1983. The college was renamed Mid-America Bible College, and is now Mid-America Christian University. To the best of my memory, President Conley confided with me that he had a notably high blood cyanide level, reported by the Harris County Medical Examiners Toxicology Laboratory, in regard to persons tested on December 2nd when the Houston Health Department collected blood samples in the college administration building. I only received written reports from the Houston Health Department in regard to in my own patients, and President Conley was not my patient, though I did acquire other results later. The highest blood cyanide level reported by the Harris County Medical Examiners Toxicology Laboratory, at least that I ever received, was 36 mcg/dl, and I think this was the blood result for President Conley. In regard to 36 mcg/dl blood cyanide, this is a notably high level—I only recall finding two blood cyanide levels higher than 36 mcg/dl while in Houston, and they were both from blood collected on December 2nd in my small medical clinic—a clinic that did not have central air conditioning. The wind was blowing from due west that day. In regard to Gulf Coast Bible College, it was founded in Houston in 1953 under the leadership of Dr. Max R. Gaulke and was called the South Texas Bible Institute, and the name was changed to Gulf Coast Bible College in 1955. I am privileged and honored to have studied New Testament Greek at this outstanding institution prior to its relocation to Oklahoma City.] I found the statements [*in the newspaper article*] hard to believe, but they were printed nonetheless. He [*reportedly*] attributed the complaints of ill patients to psychological suggestibility, and claimed that after I left the college the symptoms disappeared. He also [*reportedly*] claimed that I refused to return to Gulf Coast Bible College after my findings were *discredited*. This rather annoyed me. For one thing, the laboratory findings of cyanide poisoning were not exclusively my findings, and they had not been legitimately discredited. For another thing, it was hardly my choice to not return to the college; that decision arose from a staff meeting attended by Mr. Saul. [*What may have been said by Chancellor Fields,* *and what was written in the newspaper, could have been very different. I know this from personal experience.*]

Another newspaper article was entitled: *Health director ends cyanide study review*. In this article the Houston Health Department director, Dr. Craven, officially refuted that some Heights residents had suffered from cyanide poisoning. [*Note: the newspaper clippings that I possess of these two reports, namely* **What ever happened to … … victims of 'cyanide poisoning' at city Bible college?** *and* **Health director ends cyanide study review**, *do not have any dates on them that I can find, and it appears that they were cut out and given to me. My wife and I were not too fond of collecting newspaper reports at this point, especially considering what was being written. The two reports may have been published near the time of another report entitled* **Probers find no cyanide link,** *and this report began on the front page of The Houston Post on July 13, 1982. This July 13th article states that I claimed that residents were probably being exposed to cyanide from water; when, in fact, I had always plainly stated that the cyanide came from air pollution. I would like to mention that Chancellor Fields was quoted in this article as saying that he* "**believed Doctor Oesch was honest and meant well…**", *even though he went on to downplay the existence of cyanide intoxication in the college students. Two more things to mention from this article are that sixteen residents were reportedly examined by a team from the Baylor College of Medicine that found no common link to explain their symptoms, and that the head of the panel from the University of Texas School of Public Health said that the cyanide I found* **may have come from cigarette smoking or other sources**. *The highest blood cyanide levels found came from nonsmokers, and of course the cyanide came from other sources, such as air pollution with hydrogen cyanide and cyanogen chloride.*] The article [*Health director ends cyanide study review*] went on to say that several people from Gulf Coast Bible College were examined by doctors at hospitals. Dr. Craven said that cyanide levels were within normal limits in these patients, and another doctor said that ailments that the patients presented could be attributed to such common problems as stress, diabetes, pneumonia, and urinary tract infections. I spoke to one of these patients later, and she told me that the doctor who examined her said that he doubted they would obtain positive tests for cyanide poisoning even if the patients had actually experienced cyanide poisoning. He said this was due to shortcomings in the type of testing done.

Interestingly, the problems assigned to the above patients, namely stress, diabetes, pneumonia, and urinary tract infections, are all problems that have been associated with chronic cyanide poisoning either by me or by other investigators. In the prior news article, the writer mentioned that I planned to release a report on cyanide poisoning by late June or early July. He knew this because he spoke to me on the telephone before writing the article. My attorney discouraged further attempts to productively utilize the news media, but I did not want to leave Houston in such blighting ignorance. Toward the end of June, my wife and I won a cruise from Los Angeles to Ensenada, Mexico—provided we pay to travel to Los Angeles and back. By this time I was out of debt and we decided to take the trip. I released my news article just before we left. The article reads as follows:

METROPOLITAN EFFECTS OF ENVIRONMENTAL CYANIDE

On Sunday, January 3, 1982, I was contacted by an ex-paramedic who urgently requested help for a close friend. Her friend was demonstrating symptoms of acute cyanide poisoning. I drove to my office and observed two adults carefully transport the patient to a chair inside. She was unable to walk unassisted. Upon questioning, the patient complained of symptoms persisting since the preceding Thursday. These symptoms included burning eyes, shortness of breath, badly decreased appetite, trouble with memory, and an itchy rash. She also mentioned blurring vision which developed over several preceding months.

The woman was perspiring, her pulse and temperature were both mildly elevated. Her pulse was 100 beats per minute and her temperature 99.8 degrees Fahrenheit. A venous blood sample drawn initially was rose red, like arterial blood. This is noted in cyanide poisoning due to decreased ability of body tissue to extract oxygen from blood. She was treated with an oral dose of sodium thiosulfate, which is an antidote for cyanide poisoning, and dramatically recovered within thirty minutes to an hour.

Following the woman's recovery, more venous blood was drawn. This time the blood appeared normal in venous coloration. The woman expressed great relief, including relief from a severe headache with hallucinations and relief from tightness in her chest. She was able to walk from the office without assistance.

The blood taken from this woman was tested and found positive for both blood cyanide and serum thiocyanate, which is a metabolite of cyanide. Notably, the day preceding this woman's treatment her pet bird died. Her brother, who lived nearby, also had a bird which died that day, and he himself became ill and was admitted to a hospital. Another man, who lived across the street from the woman, was also taken to the hospital where he was diagnosed as a stroke victim. To my knowledge, although all these events transpired on the same day, only the woman treated in my office was evaluated for cyanide poisoning.

Among the eighty patients I have recorded with positive laboratory tests for cyanide or thiocyanate as of June 10, 1982, there are many intriguing and sometimes alarming stories. The severity of symptoms range from irksome lethargy to suicidal desperation. There are now at least one hundred positive, objective laboratory tests derived from patients since September 1981. Among laboratories having performed positive tests for cyanide are Bio-Science, Severance, SmithKline, and Mayo Medical laboratories. Laboratories having performed positive tests for urine thiocyanate include Bio-Science, Metpath, and National Medical Services. The evidence for cyanide poisoning in Houston, most notable in Spring Branch and Heights thus far, is enormous both quantitatively and qualitatively. Hopefully the following information will prove useful in identifying and aiding ill cyanide victims, and help to free the Houston environment from a direly potent poison.

To begin with, cyanide is an elusive, destructive agent with a wide variety of toxic capabilities. An article by NIOSH (1) reveals the half-life of cyanide in the blood to be quite brief, between 20 minutes and 1 hour. This makes detection of cyanide in blood a challenging proposal, but does not mean the bodily effect of cyanide is only transient. The actual poisoning by cyanide is caused from intracellular levels of cyanide and cellular damage, rather than by blood levels of cyanide.

An article from Clinical Toxicology (2) by Vogel, Sultan, and Eyck, discloses that moderate blood levels of cyanide may reflect severe poisoning since cyanide is tightly bound inside cells of the body. In the same article, Berlin (3) points out that toxicity from cyanide is due to intracellular concentration, and that blood levels can be misleading. He further relates that any blood level greater than 20 mcg/dl (micrograms per deciliter) suggests a toxic reaction, and that the clinical condition of the patient is a better indicator of cyanide intoxication than the blood cyanide level.

To be specific, literature from the EPA (4) explains that the ferric iron-porphyrin molecule, which is responsible for the catalytic action of cytochrome oxidase inside cells, is where cyanide combines with ferric (+++) iron. A reversible complex is formed which blocks the normal use of oxygen by the cells. As a result, affected individuals may essentially suffocate, not from lack of oxygen in the blood, but from inability to use it in tissues (2). The reason cyanide does not usually combine with iron in the hemoglobin of blood cells is because this iron is mostly divalent (++), or ferrous (4). Cyanide does combine with a trivalent form of hemoglobin called methemoglobin but methemoglobin cannot carry oxygen and normally represents only a small fraction of the total hemoglobin in blood cells (4).

What happens, then, when an individual is exposed to cyanide which binds to cytochrome oxidase within his cells? This depends on several factors. As Baumeister, Schievelbein, and Zickgraf-Rüdel explain in a writing from the Institut für Klinishe Chemie (5), symptoms of cyanide poisoning depend upon the velocity of the increase of cyanide in tissues. This is affected by the form of cyanide contacted, the manner of contact, the amount taken in, and the ability of an individual to detoxify cyanide (5).

To simplify a complicated issue, three categories of poisoning will be considered. First, a single poisoning of significant amount. Second, long-term exposure to low levels of cyanide which do not cause acute or immediate symptoms. Then third, chronic exposure to repeated doses of cyanide which are sufficiently high to cause acute symptoms.

Breathing hydrogen cyanide molecules in the air may cause death within one minute, and as Spencer and Schaumburg further expound (6), those who survive an acute episode may be left with residual damage to the central nervous system resulting from anoxic or hypotensive injury to the brain. When initially poisoned, an individual experiences flushing, a quickened heart rate, breathlessness, headache, and dizziness (2). This may progress to a stuporous, combative phase, then finally to ceased respiration, generalized convulsions, and death. Sometimes a cyanide victim may first be noted with fluid in his lungs. If blood tests are taken, such patients will often demonstrate lactic acidosis, which means increased acidity of blood and tissue fluids (2). In addition, according to Harrison's Principles of Internal Medicine (7), characteristic electrocardiographic changes are noted.

Still on the topic of serious, single-dose intoxication with cyanide, one problem in diagnosis is that the symptoms of severe anxiety mimic the early symptoms of toxicity (2). Before becoming aware of the cyanide problem in Houston, I was awakened one night with an emergency call near my practice. A girl argued with a friend, ran a short distance to her dwelling, and then collapsed unconscious outside the door. Her pupils were widely dilated and completely unresponsive to light. In a few minutes, she regained consciousness, her muscles relaxed, her pulse slowed, and her pupils slowly began showing signs of reaction to light. This was inside a centrally air-conditioned building. An emergency team on the scene with me concluded that she suffered an extreme emotional reaction. At the time, I offered no alternative diagnosis.

Only recently an interesting description of cyanide victims found in coma, by Polson and Tattersall, pricked my memory (8). In it they quoted Reid and Kennedy (9) stating that a cyanide victim may be thought to have had an epileptic fit. Symptoms mentioned included cyanosis, a clammy sweat and froth at the mouth, dilated pupils with sluggish or absent light reflex, labored breathing, rapid and feeble pulse, and tetanic convulsions of the limbs and jaws followed by a period of complete flaccidity. They also included the possibility of incontinence of urine and feces shortly before death, but neither was noted in the patient described above. The patient regained mobility roughly thirty minutes after collapse. No blood samples were taken.

Notably, the depicted patient did not seem to understand or comprehend the bewildering episode she experienced. Like many proven cyanide victims who were diagnosed later, she was primarily encouraged to seek emotional counseling. Also notable in her history were severe symptoms of depression, abdominal cramps, and an attempted or feigned suicide.

Before moving to chronic cyanide poisoning, following is a list of symptoms which may be warning signs of acute cyanide intoxication. These include headache, vertigo, irritation of the mucous membranes of the eyes and throat (5), watering of the eyes, salivation, rapid and noticeable heartbeats, difficulty breathing, weakness of the limbs, and giddiness. Collapse and unconsciousness follow thereafter (8).

Ensuing next is matter concerning subacute, chronic cyanide poisoning. By this is meant prolonged, repeated exposure to cyanide of such low concentration that no acute symptoms are noted. Individuals in this category may be unaware of any exposure to cyanide, and incognizant of any ill effects that they ascribe to poison. Long-term effects of this exposure, however, may be serious and permanent.

Repeated small doses of cyanide have been shown to cause a demyelination in the central nervous system of rats and monkeys (5). In humans, several conditions are assumed to result from the chronic uptake of cyanide in small doses, which as single doses do not cause clinical symptoms. The conditions include tobacco amblyopia, retrobulbar neuritis with pernicious anemia, optic atrophy of Leber, Nigerian nutritional ataxic neuropathy, and sterility in women who are heavy smokers (5). Symptoms associated with Nigerian nutritional neuropathy include painful paresthesia of the feet, numbness in the hands, visual loss, diminished hearing, weakness of the lower extremities, and a broad-based ataxic gait. Visual damage is a prominent feature of the illness (5).

Most patients I have noted with cyanide poisoning in Houston fall into a third category. They have experienced chronic, repeated doses of cyanide and have also suffered various clinical symptoms of both acute and chronic poisoning. There are probably many people in Houston who fall into the second category, that of chronic exposure without acute symptoms, but those individuals would be less likely to seek medical assistance. The following section, then, is most applicable to the majority of patients I have diagnosed and treated, those with immediate symptoms who suffer chronic, and sometimes acute cyanide poisoning.

Tiredness and depression are probably most universal of the symptoms my patients experience. Increased time in bed, restless sleep, lack of motivation, and apathetic withdrawal depict aspects of the depression. Several patients have described extended crying spells which overcame them for no apparent reason. One such crying spell reportedly lasted four hours. Many patients also relate thoughts of suicide which occur during their depression, and most maintain that such thoughts are completely unlike them.

Athletic and mental abilities are also altered in affected patients. Their impairments come and go, but a generalized deterioration occurs during the course of recurring episodes of illness. These episodes last from hours to days, and occur at variable intervals. In a few instances, episodes of relief seem rarer than those of illness. Decreased exercise tolerance, lower grades in school, forgetfulness, and inability to concentrate are also noteworthy features in these patients.

Jacobs (10) mentions several other symptoms of chronic cyanide exposure that are very prevalent in the patients I see, namely weakness, nausea, muscle cramps, loss of appetite, and psychoses. Another author reports pallor, vertigo, indigestion, and breathlessness (8), which are also common among my patients. He further states that in some patients the picture may be that of a mental illness. I have noted that a remarkable number of patients have been advised to see psychologists or psychiatrists prior to their diagnosis of cyanide poisoning. More thorough consideration of the mental and emotional effects of cyanide follows.

Nelson Herwig, a renowned investigator of cyanide poisoning in tropical fish, wrote regarding poisoned fish that atypical behavior is possibly symptom "Number One" (11). An article concerning dog experimentation, printed in the *Journal of the American Medical Association* (12), disclosed notable effects of cyanide poisoning in dogs. It stated that even though recovery from acute cyanide poisoning may seem complete, there are, at times, changes in personality from several days to months later, and at autopsy, degeneration of nerve cells may be found in all portions of the central nervous system. In one case study, a man developed symptoms after one year of exposure to cyanide. Specifically mentioned were severe gastrointestinal symptoms and a generalized disturbance of the nervous system, including behavioral and mental disorders (1). He continued working for 12 years before he was completely disabled and died 2 years after cessation of exposure.

Some time ago I noticed that an alarming number of patients with cyanide poisoning reported either recent divorce or increased irritability with their spouse. Others complained of easily aroused anger and unusual feelings toward other people. One usually friendly couple expressed that times when they were ill with cyanide were times when they would rather not have company. Both this husband and his wife were treated at least once for acute cyanide poisoning and both had positive laboratory tests confirming cyanide poisoning. Many patients are comforted to discover that a mentally-oppressive poison is causing their severe depression and agitation, rather than personal insanity.

A more peculiar symptom that a few of my patients have described is a feeling of detachment from their bodies. Some depict it as passing or floating out of their bodies, and one patient said he felt as though he was one place and his body another. I was intrigued, therefore, by a publication (8) quoting from the *British Medical Journal* (13) that related the same occurrence. An individual denoted as J.B.S., when accidentally poisoned, afterwards said that at the time he felt he had become free and could pass through the bedroom walls. Still another testimony, this time by a medical student, made claim to a sensation of floating while recovering from cyanide poisoning (8, 14).

Another remarkable facet regarding cyanide intoxication is the varying range of tolerance that different individuals display toward equal or similar exposures to cyanide. In one report of chronic cyanide poisoning, a man complained for several years of weight loss, occasional headache, vomiting, and attacks of faintness (8). He then had the symptoms and signs of Parkinsonism. It appeared, however, that his workmates, similarly exposed, were all well.

Many ill cyanide victims question why others about them are not ill or as ill as they are. In one instance, two bachelors were living at the same house where they split costs, one of whom had a young, black Labrador he raised from a puppy. One of the bachelors was very ill with cyanide intoxication while the other, who owned the dog, reported no significant symptoms. The dog owner noted at times, however, that his dog acted sluggish and depressed. Meanwhile, the ill bachelor was definitely diagnosed with cyanide poisoning by a blood test for serum thiocyanate and by allergy testing that revealed sensitivity to cyanide. A considerable proportion of cyanide victims who were tested demonstrated the development of allergy or sensitivity to cyanide.

As time passed, the ill bachelor became so debilitated he was forced to move. Not long thereafter, I received a call from the remaining bachelor requesting that I come investigate the death of his dog. [By ***not long thereafter***, *I suppose I was referring to the preceding paragraph, or perhaps to the ill bachelor becoming debilitated. Kevin did not actually move permanently from the house until after Caleb's death. Also, I presume that Bob called me at home after we spoke at church— I went home and ate a meal with my wife before going to Bob's house.*

In writing this report, I tried to avoid too much identifying information, such as revealing the fact that Bob and I attended the same church.] The 15 month-old Labrador died suddenly in the bachelor's backyard, two days prior to my notification.

Having conversed with animal coroners at Texas A&M University, I knew it was too late to test the dog for cyanide. After death, cyanide may be detected in liver for 5 to 6 hours, and in muscle for up to 20 hours. Formaldehyde will destroy cyanide and should not be used to preserve tissue (8). Freezing will increase the time cyanide is retained, but this dog was not frozen and 20 hours had long elapsed before I was notified.

Once before, when the dog was acting sluggish, his blood was tested for cyanide and thiocyanate. The cyanide was negative, but the thiocyanate level was 0.27 mg/dl (milligrams per deciliter). Thiocyanate, a metabolite of cyanide, is much more stable and will remain in blood for much longer periods of time. It will also remain in expired bodies for longer periods. Knowing this, I decided to check for serum thiocyanate.

In a laboratory study, three dogs which were experimentally sacrificed by cyanide poisoning had resultant serum thiocyanate levels of 0.49, 0.92, and 4.30 mg/dl (12). The average of the three is 1.90 mg/dl. I withdrew some blood, still unclotted, from the expired Labrador and sent it to a laboratory. The level of serum thiocyanate found was exactly 19 ug/ml (micrograms per milliliter), which is 1.9 mg/dl. The obvious verdict was death from cyanide poisoning.

On the subject of thiocyanate, the best laboratory test at present for detecting chronic cyanide poisoning seems to be urine thiocyanate. Serum thiocyanate, that found in blood, has quite a long half-life, but the serum level does not always correlate with clinical toxicity (15). This is consistent with data (16) suggesting that thiocyanate is rapidly distributed into the tissue anion pool (15). The tissue anion pool refers to fluid in the tissues, rather than in the blood. In my own studies, however, serum thiocyanate was at least mildly elevated in the majority of patients tested who had symptoms of cyanide intoxication.

Urine thiocyanate, because it is eliminated irregularly and slowly in the urine (4), may also fail to coincide precisely with the severity of cyanide intoxication a patient experiences. However, it is probably more dependable than blood cyanide or serum thiocyanate in identifying a case of chronic cyanide poisoning. In 1950, Hardy et al observed a group of 25 workers exposed to HCN (hydrogen cyanide) who consistently excreted small amounts of thiocyanate, with average spot urinary thiocyanate concentrations of 6 to 13 mg/L (milligrams per liter) (1). Radojicic in a 1973 study found that smokers always eliminated more thiocyanate in the urine than nonsmokers. His values (n=10) were 4.40±1.40 mg/L for smokers and 0.17±0.136 mg/L for nonsmokers (1). Thus, a relatively firm basis exists for testing cyanide-exposed individuals using urine thiocyanate levels.

One may ask, after reading the above, if there are any ill effects that result from elevated levels of thiocyanate. [*Thiocyanate is considered perhaps fifty times less toxic than cyanide. Chronic elevated levels of thiocyanate may contribute to hypothyroidism.*] The answer is yes, thiocyanate itself has toxic effects, especially inhibition of uptake of inorganic iodide into the thyroid gland for incorporation into thyroxine (1). Therefore, failure to excrete thiocyanate or chronic exposure to elevated concentrations of this ion in the blood may have a deleterious action on the ability and inclination of an employee to perform his work (1). Another source states that thiocyanate poisoning is characterized by severe mental disturbances (8). Bear in mind, however, that thiocyanate is much, much less toxic than cyanide itself.

So then, some patients demonstrate significant symptoms from particular cyanide exposures while others report little effect. Both may eventually suffer permanent damage. The ability of the liver to detoxify cyanide into thiocyanate, the availability of sulfur to facilitate such conversion, and the presence of hydroxocobalamin or cyanocobalamin (vitamin B12) in the liver (5), likely play important roles in an individual's susceptibility to symptoms from cyanide exposure. Furthermore, some persons likely have a hereditary deficiency of enzymes active in the formation of thiocyanate (5). These persons may be extraordinarily vulnerable to repeated doses of cyanide. [*And being hereditary, such extreme vulnerability to airborne cyanide may tend to also occur in blood relatives.*]

There are several other ailments prevalent in patients I am testing for chronic cyanide poisoning that have not been discussed. Cyanide solutions or cyanide aerosols generated in humid atmospheres have been reported to cause irritation to the skin and to the upper respiratory tract and to cause allergic contact dermatitis (1). Burning, itchy rashes are notable features in a few cases. Bronchitis, pneumonia, mouth sores, burning eyes, sore throats, or irritation of genital mucous membranes occur quite frequently. Usually symptoms of local irritation are accompanied by symptoms of cyanide intoxication such as tiredness, depression, and headache. [*Note: I would expect symptoms of burning eyes and throat, skin rashes, bronchitis, and pneumonia to be more prevalent when the major air pollutant is cyanogen chloride as opposed to hydrogen cyanide. I believe hydrogen cyanide is much more prevalent than cyanogen chloride, but I believe airborne cyanogen chloride was a major pollutant affecting my patients in the Heights, Timbergrove, and Spring Branch regions of Houston.*]

A number of patients complained of inguinal pain, and several males have mentioned testicular pain. Females often experience breakthrough bleeding (metrorrhagia) or irregular periods; easy bruising also seems more notable among females than males. There is evidence of increased infection in cyanide victims, apparently from lowered resistance to disease. Outstanding among these infections is glomerulonephritis (kidney infection) that often yields fine, granular casts in the urine. This occurs in males as well as females, and may play a part in the lower back pain commonly reported.

One clue that may suggest chronic cyanide poisoning from a common blood test is hyperchromic anemia. A statistical study of forty consecutive blood tests taken in the fall of 1981 from patients in northwest Houston revealed twenty patients with hematocrits below 38%. The average MCHC (mean corpuscular hemoglobin concentration) among the patients with hematocrits above 38% was 33.5%, with an average hematocrit of 41.76%. For the patients with hematocrits below 38%, the average MCHC was 35.1%, with an average hematocrit which was also 35.1%. The reference range for MCHC given by the laboratory was 32-36, and all the blood tests in this study were done by the same laboratory. [*Elevated MCHC is seen in cases of vitamin B12 deficiency anemia, and low levels of vitamin B12 in the body can result from chronic exposure to cyanide*: see **Nutrition Articles by Richard Kunin, MD, Cyanide Poisoning: A Low Fat Disease, 18 May 2009, OLALOA**. *Of interest, it has been reported that fibromyalgia patients may have lower vitamin B12 levels in their tissues, even with normal serum levels of vitamin B12. I consider airborne cyanide to likely be the world's leading cause of fibromyalgia.*]

Polson and Tattersall, in their book entitled *Clinical Toxicology* (8), tell of a Leeds engineer who was in contact with cyanide in his employment. He died of hyperchromic anemia which, however, was associated with the production of HCl (hydrogen chloride) after the administration of histamine. The book states that this otherwise unexplained illness may have been a manifestation of chronic cyanide poisoning.

Decreased appetite, bloating, nausea, vomiting, diarrhea, and other gastrointestinal complaints common in chronic cyanide poisoning are likely secondary to damage of the mucosal lining of the digestive tract. David Bellwood, in his study on the effects of cyanide upon the digestive tract of fish (17), examined fish exposed to as little as 1 ppm (part per million) cyanide in water for only 2 to 3 minutes. Examination with a scanning electron microscope (SEM) suggested a disruption of the ultrastructural organization of mucosal epithelial (surface) cells of the intestinal mucosa. He went on to explain that the loss of intestinal cells and blood would be debilitating and predispose the fish to bacterial infections. Visible loss of cells (by autolysis) was evident many days after cyanide exposure.

As of June 1, 1982, I had received results on fifty-four individuals tested for blood cyanide since September of 1981. Due to the short half-life of blood cyanide, such tests should be interpreted with regard to probable time-lapse since exposure to cyanide. Smokers may generate low levels of blood cyanide during smoking. In one study which made no distinction between smokers and nonsmokers, blood cyanide levels ranged from zero to 10.7 ug/dl with a mean of 4.8 ug/dl (1). A laboratory specialist conveyed that smokers may have levels as high as 20 ug/dl, whereas nonsmokers should be below 5 ug/dl.

Trace levels of cyanide sometimes occurring in nonsmokers may result from ingesting certain foods. Among foods mentioned as possible contributors are bitter almonds, bitter cassava, fresh leaves of sorghum, unripe bamboo, cherry seeds, apricot seeds, apple seeds, cabbage, broccoli, java beans, and white clover (5). I instructed one of my patients to consume 111.5 grams of fresh broccoli and 33 minutes later drew a blood sample from her arm for cyanide testing. The blood cyanide level was below 5 ug/dl. Another patient who was a smoker and ate fresh broccoli every other day yielded a random blood cyanide level of zero ug/dl.

A Breath of Cyanide

I consider a test abnormally high in nonsmokers if the blood cyanide is 5 ug/dl or above, and high in smokers at levels above 10 ug/dl if at least one hour has passed since that individual smoked. In individuals who smoke immediately before a blood test, one may designate levels above 20 ug/dl as positive for exposure to cyanide other than food or tobacco. In actuality, any amount of cyanide found in blood may be significant. When a laboratory detects any blood cyanide at all in a symptomatic nonsmoker, it is reasonable to consider the test likely positive for cyanide intoxication.

Of the fifty-four persons tested for blood cyanide, twenty-six were positive with levels from 5 ug/dl to 104 ug/dl and averaging 27.14 ug/dl. Thirty-six total blood cyanides were positive, some individuals having more than one test. The average from each individual was used once in calculating the group average. Of the thirty-six positive blood cyanides, two were above 30 ug/dl (both in nonsmokers), and sixteen were above nineteen ug/dl.

Six persons among the fifty-four tested had blood cyanide levels reported only as *less than 10 ug/dl*. These may have been either positive or negative and were not included in the calculated averages. This leaves twenty-two negative blood levels which ranged from 0 ug/dl or *none detected* to 9 ug/dl, with an average of 0.69 ug/dl. [*The level of 9 ug/dl (same as 9 mcg/dl) was in a smoker, and I decided to count this as a negative blood test. In reality, unless a smoker is smoking right at the time blood is drawn, or very shortly before that, any level of cyanide in the blood may be significant.*] Eighteen of the twenty-two negative reports were 0 ug/dl or *none detected*.

Thirty-seven of those tested for blood cyanide are known nonsmokers, and six are known smokers. The average among nonsmokers was 13.5 ug/dl and the average among smokers was 6.1 ug/dl. This does not mean that nonsmokers normally have higher levels of blood cyanide than smokers, in fact just the opposite is probably true. It shows that the environmental poison afflicting these patients is sufficient to override whatever cyanide levels tobacco may normally contribute.

Very obvious in tests for blood cyanide was dependency upon the day and time the tests were taken. On November 24, 1981, six blood cyanides were drawn from 9:50 am to 6:03 pm. The cyanide levels found in these blood samples increased gradually as the day passed, measuring 16, 19, 20, 20, 21, and 24 ug/dl [*ug/dl = mcg/dl*] in that chronological order. On December 3, 1981, six blood cyanides were drawn from 8:55 am until 8:14 pm, with levels of 0, 5, 0, 0, 0, and 8 ug/dl in that chronological order. Each day, tests were performed on six different individuals, demonstrating that environmental cyanide levels primarily determined blood cyanide levels, rather than habits or idiosyncrasies of the particular individuals tested. All twelve tests were performed by the same laboratory [*Severance and Associates Laboratory*]. [*Note: the six cyanide levels stated for November 24, 1981, are all correct. That was the total number of cyanide tests performed on that day, and all of the individuals tested were nonsmokers. I do need to make one correction for that day: two of the tests were performed on the same individual, so there were actually five different individuals tested that day. John Shearin had blood drawn at 2:45 p.m. with a blood cyanide of 20 mcg/dl, and then had blood drawn again at 6:03 p.m. with a blood cyanide level of 24 mcg/dl. The exact times and results of testing for blood cyanide on 11/24/81 were as follows: 16 mcg/dl at 9:50 a.m., 19 mcg/dl at 9:58 a.m., 20 mcg/dl at 10:48 a.m., 20 mcg/dl at 2:45 p.m., 21 mcg/dl at 4:04 p.m., and 24 mcg/dl at 6:03 p.m.*

Then, there are a number of things to point out about the testing on 12/3/81. The first blood cyanide level of zero, obtained from blood drawn at 8:55 a.m., was from a smoker. Also, there was a nonsmoker tested at 2:17 a.m. on that date, with a blood cyanide level of zero, and I did not include him in the reference to six persons tested on that date. Next, there was an individual tested at 4:20 p.m. who may have been a cigar smoker, but I put an "X" over the "C" for "cigars", so I'm not sure about his smoking status. Further regarding this individual, his blood cyanide level was below 10 mcg/dl, and it may have been zero mcg/dl, but I cannot say what his blood cyanide level was for sure because I failed to record a level on his lab report sheet. By this time, I had to obtain any blood cyanide levels less than 10 mcg/dl per phone, because the laboratory was simply printing out levels less than 10 mcg/dl as "less than 10 mcg/dl" on their report sheets, and I failed to call and record an exact blood cyanide level for this person. For these reasons, this individual was not included in the list of six persons tested on 12/3/81.

And then finally, I need to make one more correction in regard to the blood cyanide testing done on 12/3/81. There were seven known nonsmokers, rather than six, tested from 1:00 p.m. to 8:14 p.m. on 12/3/81. The blood cyanide levels for these seven individuals were 5 mcg/dl at 1:00 p.m., zero mcg/dl at 3:14 p.m., zero mcg/dl at 4:00 p.m., zero mcg/dl at 4:15 p.m., zero mcg/dl at 5:25 p.m., zero mcg/dl at 6:30 p.m., and 8 mcg/dl at 8:14 p.m. Note that five of these known nonsmokers were tested from 4:00 p.m. to 6:30 p.m. and that all five of them in a row had blood cyanide levels of zero mcg/dl (none detected). A sixth person, discussed in the preceding paragraph, was also tested during this time period, with his blood drawn at 4:20 p.m.—this person had uncertain smoking status, and his blood cyanide level is simply recorded as "less than 10 mcg/dl". The majority of blood cyanide tests performed in my office that had blood cyanide levels reported as "less than 10 mcg/dl" were found, by calling the laboratory, to have blood cyanide levels of zero mcg/dl, and this person probably also had a level of zero mcg/dl, though I cannot say this for certain. No one was tested more than once on 12/3/81. Thus, there were a total of ten persons tested for blood cyanide on 12/3/81, and seven of them were nonsmokers who were tested during a reasonable time of day to compare to the nonsmokers tested on 11/24/81. These results strongly support the conclusion that the blood cyanide levels, which were obtained from patients who had blood drawn in my office in the Heights, were dependent upon the recent or present levels of airborne cyanide rather than upon the diets or habits of the individuals being tested.]

From results such as stated in the previous paragraph, and from symptoms such as rash, burning mucous membranes, and respiratory problems, I deduced early that hydrogen cyanide gas contaminated the air my patients were breathing. [*I know now that cyanogen chloride was likely a major contributor to the cyanide air pollution in the Heights at that time.*] One patient demonstrated this fact quite dramatically. His blood was drawn in a centrally air-conditioned building, then redrawn about 30 minutes later after walking outdoors. He did not eat or drink anything during this time. The first blood drawn was purple in color (normal for venous blood) and was found to have a blood cyanide level of 21 ug/dl. The next time his blood was drawn it was rose red in color (like arterial blood) and was found to have a blood cyanide level of 104 ug/dl. [*That particular patient, as a matter of fact, was me.*] Both blood samples were tested by the same laboratory [*Severance and Associates Laboratory*]. Interestingly, another patient who was very ill and had bright red venous blood was found to have a blood cyanide level of only

14 ug/dl. [*Remember that cyanide moves from the bloodstream to the tissues, and that rather severe poisoning may not yield very high blood cyanide levels.*]

In another instance, a woman who lived outside Houston returned for one hour after avoiding her job area for two weeks. She complained of illness even after relatively short visits to the location of her job in Houston. During this hour visit she neither ate nor drank, but still contracted a blood cyanide of 55 ug/dl. The blood was drawn at the end of her hour visit. Though considerable effort was made to alleviate her illness, the woman finally had to relinquish her job and avoid the area where she previously worked.

A publication in the *Western Journal of Medicine* stated the range of lethality for blood cyanide as greater than 100 ug/dl (18). In blood specimens from 57 deceased animals, blood cyanide levels ranged from 64.8 ug/dl to 425 ug/dl (18). One man who committed suicide by oral ingestion of cyanide yielded a blood cyanide level of 44 ug/dl (8). A generally stated minimum lethal dose of orally ingested cyanide is about one grain or between 50 mg and 60 mg of anhydrous HCN (8). One boy aged thirteen, who died from drinking a cyanide solution, was estimated to contain 13 mg of HCN within his body (8).

Much less cyanide is required to cause death by inhalation than the levels generally stated for lethality from oral intake. Hydrogen cyanide (HCN) present in the air at 320 ppm (parts per million) is fatal in five minutes (10). Figuring 16 breaths per minute, 500 ml per breath, and 60% absorption of the total cyanide inhaled with each breath, less than eleven milligrams of HCN are fatal in this instance. Within a short period of time 270 ppm are fatal (5), and in less than one hour exposure to 100 ppm is dangerous (8).

Mild symptoms are produced by several hours of exposure to a concentration of HCN in air of only 20 ppm. The upper limit of safety is 10 ppm (8, 19, 20, 21). [*Remember, as previously stated, that at forty hours of exposure per week, industrial workers have been found to develop symptoms of cyanide intoxication at air levels from 0.2 to 0.8 ppm.*] Natural waters do not contain cyanide and its presence normally indicates contamination from an industrial source (22). Cyanide salt may be converted to airborne HCN by treatment with acids, acid salts, or by water (1). The likelihood and rate of HCN release from water is dependent on several factors.

A Breath of Cyanide

The highly variable persistence of cyanide in water is dependent upon the chemical form of cyanide in water, the concentration of cyanide, and the nature of other constituents (4). Cyanide ions combine with numerous heavy metal ions to form metallocyanide complexes. The stability of these anions is highly variable (4). Thus, various proportions of cyanide may be released into the air at particular water conditions depending on the concentrations of different cyanide compounds present in the water.

The boiling point of liquid HCN is 26°C., or 79°F. (10). [*The boiling point of CNCl, namely cyanogen chloride, is 13°C., or 55°F.*] Many of my patients first noticed the onset of symptoms from cyanide poisoning during late spring as temperatures rose. Besides temperature, pH is also important in the generation of HCN from water. A significant fraction of cyanide exists as HCN molecules at a pH of approximately 8, and the fraction increases rapidly as the pH of the solution decreases (4). This means that when a basic solution containing cyanide becomes more acidic, from mixing with rain water or acidic discharge waters, hydrogen cyanide gas may be emitted into the air.

A level of only 1 ppm cyanide in water would be rapidly lethal in an equal volume of air. [*If that quantity of cyanide were present in the same volume of air.*] Since various chemical and physical conditions dictate the form of cyanide in water, the cyanide criterion must be based on the concentration of total cyanide in the water (4). This includes cyanide that is bound to metals as well as free HCN. Less than 18,400 gallons of water with a cyanide concentration of only 0.65 ppm (less than one part per million) could potentially generate enough HCN to form over 63,000 liters of immediately lethal atmosphere, over 315,000 liters of atmosphere dangerous within one hour's exposure, or over one and one-half million liters of atmosphere that could cause acute illness with long exposure.

The only reference value for serum thiocyanate I found in literature, regarding human beings, came from a report entitled *Laetrile Toxicity Studies in Dogs* (12). [*Note that I would later find more extensive reference data for serum thiocyanate levels.*] The reference value given was 0.2 to 0.4 mg/dl, and it was not specified whether this value excluded smokers or not. I have tested fourteen nonsmokers for serum thiocyanate. Five were negative with levels from 0.23 to 0.37 mg/dl, averaging 0.28 mg/dl. When more than one test was performed on one person, his individual average was entered only once in determining the group average.

Interestingly, one patient was positive for blood cyanide with a level of 30 ug/dl, yet at the same time negative for serum thiocyanate with a level of 0.23 mg/dl. The same patient repeated simultaneous testing at a later date that yielded a blood cyanide of 20 ug/dl and a serum thiocyanate of 0.55 mg/dl. This seems to support one observation in which peak thiocyanate concentrations lagged behind peak cyanide concentrations by several days (15). Another observer noted the half-life or decay (half-life) of serum thiocyanate in one patient to be approximately 2 days. The same half-life of 2 days was also noted for the patient's urinary thiocyanate (1).

The three laboratories I use for testing urine thiocyanate levels are Metpath, Bio-Science, and National Medical Services via National Health Laboratories. When using Metpath, a patient cannot have ingested aspirin in any form for at least 48 hours preceding urine collection or the urine thiocyanate test is invalid. Both Metpath and Bio-Science designate the normal urine thiocyanate level for nonsmokers as less than 0.2 mg/100ml or up to 2 mg/L (milligrams per liter). National Health Services gives no reference value for nonsmokers specifically, but lists a single reference value of up to 20 ug/ml, which is equal to the reference value Metpath gives for smokers of up to 20 mg/L. Note that the reference value Metpath gives for smokers is ten times greater than that given for nonsmokers. Bio-Science gives a reference value of up to 3 mg/100ml for smokers, fifteen times greater than that for nonsmokers. The reasoning is that small amounts of cyanide may be emitted from smoking tobacco which gradually build up a significant amount of thiocyanate in urine. Keep in mind that the reference values given are upper limits, and not norms. The norms were listed earlier from a study by Radojicic (1).

I consider a nonsmoker positive for evidence of cyanide poisoning if the urine thiocyanate exceeds 2 mg/L. For smokers, I assume the test positive if the urine thiocyanate exceeds 12 mg/L for every pack of cigarettes smoked daily. Thus, an upper limit of normal for a patient who smoked 1½ packs-per-day would be 18 mg/L. It is still important to remember that patients suffering from chronic cyanide poisoning may yield positive testing at one time and negative testing at another time, depending on varying environmental meteorological conditions.

Wind direction may significantly influence urine thiocyanate levels when HCN contaminates the atmosphere.

Between February 1, 1982, and June 1, 1982, I received laboratory reports on forty-two patients tested for urine thiocyanate. In the case of patients tested more than once, I calculated a single average for each patient to use in calculating group averages. Of the forty-two patients tested, thirty-nine were positive with levels ranging from 3.4 mg/L to 51.8 mg/L; the average positive level was 21.6 mg/L. Only three patients were negative with two levels of zero mg/L, and one of 11.0 mg/L which occurred in a smoker. One of the patients with zero mg/L was also a smoker.

Of the forty-two patients tested for urine thiocyanate, thirty-one were nonsmokers and eleven were smokers. The average level in nonsmokers was 18.21 mg/L, and the average level in smokers was 26.2 mg/L. The highest level occurred in a nonsmoker, and the only two zero levels were evenly divided between one smoker and one nonsmoker. It appears that smoking boosted the average in smokers over that of nonsmokers, but the far greater effect of environmental poisoning makes this observation questionable. Other studies, however, yield sufficient evidence relating long-term cyanide effects with smoking (such as tobacco amblyopia) to add still another reason why humans should not smoke.

The highest urine thiocyanate level in a nonsmoker was 51.8 mg/L. Calculating 50% excretion, in 24 hours, of thiocyanate formed from previous exposure to cyanide, and figuring that the random urine collected is representative thereof, and that a normal 1500 ml excretion of urine during 24 hours took place, this level of urine thiocyanate represents an uptake of over sixty-eight milligrams of cyanide. This amount of cyanide is greater than the previously-stated minimal, lethal oral does, and is much greater than a quantity of cyanide that is potentially fatal by inhalation.

Another patient, again a nonsmoker, had a urine thiocyanate level of 15.4 mg/L on the fourth day after hospitalization for an attack of dizziness. He first became ill on a Wednesday and was hospitalized the following Friday. On that same Wednesday, a woman who lived across the street from this man also became ill, and died the following Friday. Her symptoms, from what I was told, included dizziness, shortness of breath, and an elevated temperature. Several patients I have treated for acute cyanide poisoning had mildly elevated temperatures, but his woman's temperature was reportedly around 104°F. Her death was attributed to a heart attack. I am unaware if any testing for cyanide and thiocyanate took place in her case.

One real tip in suspecting chronic cyanide poisoning has been when a patient's illness dramatically improves within a few days of leaving Houston, and then grows worse again shortly after returning to Houston. This pattern has been more the rule than the exception with my patients. The geographical area apparently affected by the environmental cyanide expands as patient testing expands. At present, the east-west diameter of symptomatic patients verified by laboratory testing is greater than ten miles, and the north-south diameter is greater than eight miles. More severe contamination seems centered in the Spring Branch and Heights regions, but the extent and magnitude of contamination across Houston and neighboring communities is unknown. [*I now know that airborne cyanide is ubiquitous in the earth's lower atmosphere, varying in degree from location to location, with a half-life measured in years.*]

Besides the tests for cyanide and thiocyanate, a micro-allergist located in the Houston Medical Center downtown has tested patients for allergy or sensitivity to cyanide. Very few in his control study, only one out of the first two hundred, demonstrated any sensitivity to cyanide. That one exception demonstrated only a +1 sensitivity on a scale of +1 to +4. Among patients proven or suspected of cyanide poisoning, twenty-five of forty-three, or 58% of those tested, had positive tests for sensitivity to cyanide. The tests ranged from +1 to +3 sensitivity.

While sensitivity to cyanide likely increases the ill effects cyanide imposes upon an individual (some patients apparently develop arthritis associated with chronic cyanide intoxication), several severely ill patients were not sensitive to cyanide. Cyanide seems to be a very potent sensitizer, but is very capable of physiological damage to persons who have no sensitivity. One such individual had positive tests for blood cyanide, serum thiocyanate, and urine thiocyanate, yet tested negative for sensitivity to cyanide. When positive, however, the sensitivity test is strongly suggestive of chronic cyanide poisoning. It also may be performed when actual exposure to cyanide has not been so recent as required with other types of testing.

At this point, one may be curious concerning treatment of cyanide intoxication. Emergency treatment of severe, acute cyanide poisoning may be administered at a hospital emergency room. Inhalation of amyl nitrite perles, one every two minutes, may be used during transport unless blood pressure (systolic) drops below 80 mm/Hg. Amyl nitrite changes hemoglobin to methemoglobin which binds cyanide. This is followed with I.V. injection of 3% sodium nitrite, 10 ml over a three minute period (7). Maximal methemoglobin produced by inhalation of amyl nitrite is 5%; that produced by I.V. sodium nitrite should be close to, but under 40%, with lethal results occurring at levels of 85% (2). Norepinephrine may be needed during administration of amyl or sodium nitrite to maintain blood pressure. Next, 50 ml of 25% sodium thiosulfate is administered I.V. over a 10 minute period. This provides sulfur for production of thiocyanate in the liver. Supportive measures should be initiated, especially artificial respiration with 100% oxygen (7). When available, hyperbaric oxygen is favorable. Treatment for children should include adjustment for size and weight in medication dosage.

Mild attacks of acute cyanide poisoning, where adequate respiration and self-locomotion (ability to walk stably without assistance) are present, may be treated with oral sodium thiosulfate crystals and intramuscular Alpha Redisol (hydroxocobalamin) injections. Some inhalation of amyl nitrite may also be used if blood pressure is carefully monitored. The patient pours one cc (cubic centimeter) of sodium thiosulfate crystals on the back of his tongue, and then drinks them down with one-half glass of water. One-half to one cc of hydroxocobalamin may be given I.M. at the same time. Noticeable improvement should occur between 15 minutes and one hour after treatment. Arrangement for intravenous, emergency treatment should be made if the patient's condition worsens. [*I now recommend smaller doses of sodium thiosulfate pentahydrate, taken more often, in order to avoid gas or diarrhea from taking larger doses of sodium thiosulfate pentahydrate.*]

When treating acute bouts of cyanide poisoning, patient observation should take place for up to forty-eight hours after recovery because of possible relapse (8). Apparently the treatment for cyanide poisoning can promote cyanide displacement, from sites of tissue absorption, out into the bloodstream. This may partly be due to the reversible nature of the reaction where cyanide is metabolized into thiocyanate. If excretion of the thiocyanate is not prompt, there may be some reversal of formation with regeneration of cyanide (1). In the case of relapse, treatment should be repeated (8).

Cyanide replaces the hydroxo component of hydroxocobalamin and forms cyanocobalamin which is vitamin B12. [*Hydroxocobalamin is also a type of vitamin B12, as is methylcobalamin, and they are both superior to cyanocobalamin.*] For patients ill with chronic cyanide poisoning, I recommend ½ to 1 cc Alpha Redisol I.M. daily, and ½ cc sodium thiosulfate by mouth every four hours as needed for headaches and mental depression. Too liberal use of sodium thiosulfate may cause diarrhea, so limitation to symptomatic treatment is advisable. Intake of sodium thiosulfate with food seems to aid tolerance. Children may use half-doses.

In one study, animals were chronically exposed to cyanide with simultaneous administration of hydroxocobalamin. These animals did not show demyelination in the central nervous system on histological examination. Animals that did not receive hydroxocobalamin, or that were given cyanocobalamin instead, did show central nervous system demyelination after chronic exposure to cyanide (5).

The majority of cyanide patients I am treating report significant relief from headaches using sodium thiosulfate alone. Alpha Redisol, though, is probably better for overall maintenance and preventing permanent neurological damage. It is best to use both. To my knowledge, the only place in Houston where both sodium thiosulfate and Alpha Redisol are readily available is Northwest Pharmacy, 15th and Yale, phone 861-3161. The pharmacist acquired these agents specifically to supply patients suffering from chronic cyanide poisoning.

The primary step in treating diseases caused by chronic application of cyanide is stopping further application of cyanide. [*Good luck on that one. I have not missed a single day in taking sodium thiosulfate pentahydrate in over twenty years. I also take alpha-ketoglutaric acid with meals, and 5,000 mcg sublingual methylcobalamin tablets a.m. and p.m., which are less expensive than 5,000 mcg sublingual hydroxocobalamin tablets.*] Thereafter, hydroxocobalamin may be required up to six months to aid recovery (8). At present, Houstonians are still being subjected to various daily doses of cyanide. As knowledgeable citizens, I do not believe we can rightfully allow this to continue.

Bibliography

1.) *Recommendations for Cyanide Standards by The National Institute for Occupational Safety and Health*, pp. 1-2, 45-52, 93-95.

2.) Stephen N. Vogel, M.D., Thomas R. Sultan, M.D., and Raymond P. Ten Eyck, M.D. *Clinical Toxicology*, 18(3), pp. 367-383 (1981)

3.) C. Berlin, Editorial: *Cyanide poisoning: A challenge, Arch. Intern Med.*, 137 (8), 993-994 (1977).

4.) U.S. Environmental Protection Agency, Washington, D.C., 20460. *Quality Criteria for Water*, July 1976.

5.) R.G.H. Baumeister, H. Schievelbein, and G. Zickgraf-Rüdel. *Toxicological and Clinical Aspects of Cyanide Metabolism*, from the Institut für Klinishe Chemie, Deutsches Herzentrum München; Vorstand: Prof. Dr. H. Schievelbein.

6.) Peter S. Spencer, Ph.D., and Herbert H. Schaumburg, M.D. *Experimental and Clinical Neurotoxicology*, pp. 617-618.

7.) Thorn, Adams, Braunwalk, Isselbacher, Petersdorf. *Harrison's Principles of Internal Medicine*, Eighth Edition; McGraw-Hill Book Company, p. 695 (1977).

8.) C.J. Polson and R.N. Tattersall. *Clinical Toxicology*, published by J.B. Lippincott Company in North America, and by Pitman Medical Publishing Company Ltd in Great Britain, pp. 132-155 (1975).

9.) J. Reid and K. Kennedy. *Brit. Med. J.*, i, 56. (1925)

10.) M.B. Jacobs. *Analytical Toxicology of Industrial Inorganic Poisons*, Wiley Interscience Mag: 721-741 (1967).

11.) Nelson Herwig. *Symptoms and Diagnosis of Cyanide Poisoning. Marine Aquarist*, 8(2): 34-40 (1977)

12.) Eric S. Schmidt, George W. Newton, Steven M. Sanders, Jerry P. Lewis, M.D., Eric E. Conn, Ph.D. *Laetrile Toxicity Studies in Dogs, Journal of the American Medical Association*, March 6, 1978, Volume 239, pp. 944-947.

13.) J.B.S. *Brit. Med. J.*, i, 144, (1925)

14.) J.C. Geiger. *J. Amer. Med. Ass.*, 99, 1944-5 (1932)

15.) Matthew M. Ames, Thomas P. Moyer, John S. Kovach, Charles G. Moertel, and Joseph Rubin. *Pharmacology of Amygdalin (Laetrile) in Cancer Patients, Cancer Chemother Pharmocol* (1981) 6: 51-57.

16.) C.J. Vassey, P.V. Cole, P.J. Simpson. *Cyanide and thiocyanate concentrations following sodium nitroprusside infusion in man*. Br J. Anest. 48: 651-660 (1976).

17.) David R. Bellwood. *Cyanide, Freshwater and Marine Aquarium*, Nov. 1981, Vol. 4, no. 11, pp. 31-35, 75-76.

18.) G.W. Newton, E.S. Schmidt, J.P. Lewis, et al: *Amygdalin toxicity studies in rats predict chronic cyanide poisoning in humans, West. J. Med.* 134:97-103, Feb. 1981.

19.) Department of Scientific and Industrial Research, *Hydrogen Cyanide Vapour*. Leaflet No. 2. London: H.M.S.O. (1951).

20.) D. Hunter. *The Diseases of Occupations*, 2nd ed., pp. 597, 600. London: English Universities Press. (1957).

21.) T.A. Gonzales, M. Vance, M. Helpern, and C.J. Umberger. *Legal Medicine*, 2nd ed., pp. 802, 805. New York: Appleton-Century-Crofts. (1954).

22.) *Cyanide, APHA Standard Methods*, 13th ed., 404 (1971).

The preceding report was mailed to major newspapers, minor newspapers, radio stations, television stations, magazines, medical laboratories, and other health professionals. Considering all the news coverage of earlier findings from a single laboratory, I certainly felt that a documented study utilizing six major laboratories and scores of tests would be important, newsworthy information. Since people's lives and health were at stake, I did not imagine that such findings would be ignored. Silence prevailed. I called a local newspaper in the Heights and Timbergrove areas, pleading for them to inform local residents about the further findings. The reply: "I don't want to get sued."

Given the fact that I made no mention in my report of where I thought the cyanide contamination was coming from, why would a newspaper reporter fear being sued for printing objective laboratory findings? Furthermore, isn't there an amendment in our Constitution guaranteeing freedom of the press? There were a large number of American citizens being exposed to poison, and many were ill, yet I was unable to deliver vital information through public communicative channels.

Chapter 10

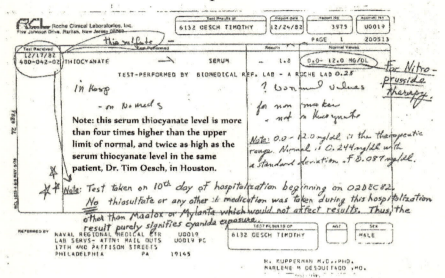

Astounding Rediscovery

With our furniture on the way to Philadelphia, Pennsylvania, my wife and I drove to a nearby naval base in Corpus Christi, Texas. I was assigned to Corpus Christi for about ten days of military indoctrination, then had about a week to reach my permanent duty assignment in Philadelphia. Both my wife and I were looking forward to some cyanide-free air. In Corpus Christi, we were not disappointed.

Having already attended Officer's Indoctrination School in Newport, Rhode Island, my ten days in Corpus Christi were basically a vacation. Only a couple days after leaving Houston, I began working out again. It was the first athletic training I was able to undertake since I began suffering from cyanide intoxication the preceding fall. My wife also began feeling better and joined an aerobics class on the base. By the completion of ten days in Corpus Christi, we were largely recovered from the acute effects of cyanide exposure and we looked forward to resuming normal, healthy lives.

Between Corpus Christi and Philadelphia my wife and I made several stops to visit relatives. We arrived in Philadelphia at about 11:00 pm on July 22, 1982. The naval hospital was enclosed in a tall, chain link fence with barbed wire above. There were no quarters available for my wife and me to stay in, so we asked a guard where the nearest motel was. The motel had pink walls along the hallway, and someone threw a pop bottle that burst not far from us on the parking lot; we only stayed one night.

Thereafter my wife and I stayed at a Quality Inn until invited to stay with friends in Turnersville, New Jersey, the Chapmans. We met the Chapmans at church. My wife hoped to attend school at Glassboro State College, and we found a house in Pitman, NJ, located near the college.

Several weeks passed before settlement came through on our house. We decided to purchase a house rather than rent since I was assigned to work in Philadelphia for three years. My wife registered at Glassboro State College and began classes in early September. We moved to our house in Pitman toward the end of September and found a lovely, local church to attend. Our lives seemed settled and situated at last.

My wife began experiencing symptoms of cyanide intoxication while we lived with the Chapmans, but they were fairly mild and I attributed them to fall allergies. My weight was increasing rapidly [*I had lost a lot of weight with cyanide poisoning in Houston*], and although I too experienced mild symptoms of illness, I was used to feeling somewhat tired during August and early September due to ragweed allergies. It was not until early October that my illness increased to the point that I missed workouts and sought medical attention. The fact that both my wife and I were ill, and that some of my new patients at the naval base had the same symptoms that we did, made me suspect some infectious agent as the cause of our illness. I did not know that there were electroplating plants both where I worked in Philadelphia and within about one and one-half miles of our house in Pitman. [*I also had a lot to learn about other sources of airborne cyanide, as well as the prevalence of cyanide in the atmosphere, and the persistence of cyanide in the atmosphere.*]

After reporting for active duty to the hospital in Philadelphia, I was assigned to work at a dispensary in the naval shipyard about a mile from the hospital. There was a shortage of civilian physicians at the dispensary which were needed to attend to civilian shipyard workers, and I was primarily assigned to work with civilian patients. The dispensary was divided into two separate sections, one for military patients and one for civilian patients. Most of the work was exactly what I was used to, and I quickly made friends with the civilian staff.

Each day after work I visited a workout facility on the base before going home. My weight was back to 157½ pounds, and I enjoyed feeling strength in my arms and legs again. As before in Houston, the first effect of cyanide intoxication I noticed was decreased exercise ability. I became short of breath with only moderate exertion, and my strength began dwindling. At the time, however, I did not know why. My illness was puzzling.

Ragweed season ended, but my illness did not improve; I continued growing worse. Exercise became intolerable. It was all I could do to last through a day's work. One of my patients with similar symptoms was released from work after six weeks of illness. Several others had similarly lingering sickness, and my wife missed several days of school. She lost weight, hair, and energy. One of her teachers guessed her at thirty-four years of age; she was only nineteen. [*Of note, it is not normal for my wife to appear older than her age. Years later, living in Tennessee, my wife was stopped in the hallway of an elementary school and asked for her hall pass. She had to explain that she was a mother, not a student. I think the oldest students in that school were 6th graders.*]

Due to the persisting nature of the illness affecting my wife, my patients, and myself, I suspected a severe viral disease. Coxsacchie virus, the same agent I suspected in several patients in Houston [*before learning that the patients suffered from cyanide intoxication*], was one virus I considered. Other viruses I thought even more likely were those commonly associated with hepatitis. I tested about five of my patients for hepatitis, in addition to tests on my wife and myself, but the tests did not indicate viral hepatitis. Our illnesses persisted.

My wife adapted to her illness by resting and sleeping almost constantly when not studying, cooking, washing dishes, or attending classes. She had to stop exercising completely. I continued working as long as possible, but now and then I missed a day or two as my condition depreciated. I kept hoping and expecting to improve, but my health faltered progressively and relentlessly. Meanwhile, another young doctor I worked with was hospitalized with heart failure. It was decided that he suffered from a viral infection of the heart, though I never heard that any causative agent was ever isolated.

Besides my work at the shipyard dispensary, I was selected as a member of a special medical team known as MMART. This team was designated to aid marines and naval personnel in military emergencies overseas. After becoming ill, I notified my MMART coordinator and asked if my illness needed reported—just in case an emergency should arise and a replacement was needed. He told me not to worry about it since there was little chance of our being called upon. Not long afterwards, the MMART was placed on alert, and I was advised to get several shots.

By this time I was very ill. Besides fatigue, headaches, dizziness, weakness, tachycardia, slight fever, and decreased appetite, I also began experiencing chest pains. Once after a shower I nearly dropped to the floor with a gripping pain in my chest, and I often awoke in the early morning with shortness of breath and chest pain. Being a physician, I knew that the chest pains were comparable to those resulting from coronary insufficiency, a condition generally noted in men considerably older than me. Multiple diagnostic tests continued yielding negative results, yet my illness worsened.

There was a reason why I failed to suspect cyanide poisoning. The illness was so widespread that an environmental etiology seemed unfeasible. My wife was ill in Pitman, my patients were ill in Philadelphia, and at least one of my patients had family members who were likewise ill. Knowing this, I concluded that an infectious agent must have caused the epidemic affliction. With time, I learned differently: there is enough cyanide produced annually in the United States to kill every human being in the United States hundreds of times over. Widespread chronic cyanide intoxication is not unfeasible, it is evident.

My military physician, an internal medicine specialist named Doctor Wendle, was quite frustrated by my condition. He finally told me that he could not find anything wrong and suggested that I was feigning illness in order to get out of possible MMART duty. I found this rather disconcerting. I reported to my Commanding Officer, a lady captain, and told her that I would sign a release that gave me sole responsibility for not taking immunization shots, and that I would serve on my

MMART team despite my illness. With the severity of my condition, I was afraid the immunization shots might kill me.

The lady captain, Captain Martinson, ordered that I be hospitalized and diagnosed. The chief physician in the internal medicine department, a lady physician named Doctor Gilmore, was assigned to my case. On November 1, 1982, I was admitted to the naval hospital in Philadelphia. The following day I became very ill. Chest pain developed before lunch and lasted the rest of the day; when the pain first hit me I became short of breath and was unable to sit up for thirty minutes. My doctor assessed me with questionable esophageal or pyloric spasm and related my symptoms to eating. As I found out later, winds that day were coming from the south.

Winds were not usually from the south during my November hospitalization in Philadelphia. Although I continued having periods of chest pain during my hospitalization, none were as alarming as that on November second. A large number of diagnostic tests were performed, including a heart scan following injection of a radioactive dye into a vein. Still, no etiology was confirmed to explain my illness. I was discharged on November 12, 1982, with the assessment of viral syndrome and possible stress reaction. Doctor Gilmore advised that I have a psychiatric evaluation if my symptoms escalated.

November twelfth was the first date that any mention of a stress reaction or psychiatric evaluation appeared in my hospital record. Notably, on November eleventh I gave Doctor Gilmore a copy of the report I wrote in Houston, entitled: *Metropolitan Effects of Environmental Cyanide*. This occurred at her request; she started asking me questions about my previous cyanide poisoning after extensive testing failed to disclose the cause of my illness. My wife brought me a copy of the report on the eleventh, and I reviewed the report before giving it to Doctor Gilmore the same day.

As I read over my report on the eleventh, it was strikingly apparent that the symptoms I experienced were precisely consistent with those of cyanide intoxication. Despite my prior judgment that cyanide intoxication was unlikely due to the distance between ill patients, cyanide intoxication certainly fit the description of my condition. I pointed this out to Doctor Gilmore as she received the report. Doctor Gilmore seemed interested. She probably took the report straight to the head of the naval environmental department, Captain Galasyn.

When Doctor Gilmore spoke to me on the twelfth, she made no inquiry about how to check for cyanide intoxication. Judging from later events, she probably received misleading counsel about cyanide contamination; she was probably told that my suffering from cyanide intoxication was an impossibility. As I learned later, the naval base in Philadelphia definitely made contact with the Houston Health Department. If this contact was initiated on the eleventh, then my treatment on the twelfth may have resulted from political concerns that stemmed from communication between the naval base and the Houston Health Department. This was only the start. [*And as a note of interest, there was not only a connection between GE and the Houston Health Department, in that GE was permitted to release cyanide into the public sewer system; there was also a connection between GE—specifically the GE plant at 3530 W 12th Street in Houston—and the U.S. Navy. To see this connection, go to the following internet site*: https://books.google.com/books?id=tuBHAQAAIAAJ&pg=PP1&lpg=PP1&dq=Selling+to+Navy+Prime+Contractors+(12/58)&source=bl&ots=9TukNdoiND&sig=ACfU3U1W1sieqXUEcAtIBBQLrfBiknb-gw&hl=en&sa=X&ved=2ahUKEwj37aKGoZroAhXMl-AKHX5EAc8Q6AEwAHoECAkQAQ#v=onepage&q=Selling%20to%20Navy%20Prime%20Contractors%20(12%2F58)&f=false *and there, you will find a book entitled* **SELLING TO NAVY PRIME CONTRACTORS**. *Scroll down in this book to page 121; and there, under the word* **Houston**, *you will find the following:* **General Electric Co., Distribution Assembly Department, 3530 West 12th St. W. A. Pugh**.]

When Doctor Gilmore asked me if I would be willing to talk to a psychiatrist, I knew the implications. To resist such a request may have invited the hazard of confinement. I agreed to a psychiatric interview at any time. It was intriguing to receive the same treatment as several of my prior patients in Houston, but somehow I never imagined it would happen to me. One thing was certain, as soon as I got home I would take some antidote for cyanide poisoning.

My wife received a great deal of support from our next-door neighbors, Lee and Leighann Deere. Their two children were also anxious to help: a boy and girl ages eleven and eight. While I was hospitalized, they often invited my wife over for supper and offered to let her sleep at their home. My wife was already quite ill during this time, and the help we received from the Deere family was deeply appreciated. My wife was consulting a local physician in Pitman, an internal medicine specialist named Dr. DeEugenio.

A grateful embrace followed my entrance into our home after driving myself back from the hospital. It was November twelfth.

"Well, did they figure out what you have?" inquired Melody. She came with me to see Dr. Wendle on a couple of occasions before I was hospitalized, which was before she went to see Dr. DeEugenio. Neither specialist was able to diagnose her illness, but at least Dr. DeEugenio acknowledged that a problem existed, even if he could not identify it. Dr. Wendle, on the other hand, seemed to accuse my wife of feigning illness just as he accused me. My wife was direly ill, and she was not at all impressed by Dr. Wendle's insinuation.

"I don't know about them, but I think I know what it is," I replied.

"What?"

"I think we're getting cyanide exposure again."

Melody looked lividly stricken. "No, I mean, how could we? Are you sure?"

"I intend to find out."

Melody watched as I unpacked some sodium thiosulfate and alphaREDISOL. I took the antidote and soon improved remarkably. Melody followed suit, and also experienced significant improvement. After that, we began noting wind direction when we felt acutely ill. It did not take long to decipher that winds from the north and west brought suffering to our household. Southeast winds came only too rarely; we felt sick more often than well.

The next time Melody visited Dr. DeEugenio, I accompanied her to his office. Dr. DeEugenio congratulated me for diagnosing Melody's illness, and ordered a laboratory test that confirmed that she experienced cyanide intoxication. He also expressed concern about the community, and said he might contact a physician who he knew in the state environmental department. This was encouraging at the time, especially compared to the treatment my wife and I received from physicians associated with the Houston Health Department. There were some future surprises, however, that we did not foresee.

The following Monday, I returned to work at the shipyard dispensary. Knowing that my wife was even more sensitive to cyanide exposure than me, I figured that the cyanide contamination at the base in Philadelphia was worse than in Pitman. This seemed logical since my illness was as severe as my wife's illness, even though I usually withstood equal exposures to cyanide better than her. When I returned to work I soon experienced acute symptoms of cyanide intoxication. These were relieved by doses of antidote. I took sodium thiosulfate orally, and alphaREDISOL by intramuscular injection.

November twenty-second began my second week back at work. Having made acquaintance primarily with civilian personnel, I asked a couple of civilian nurses who I should call if I suspected an environmental problem at the base. One of them informed me that I should call Randy Cobb; she even got me his phone extension. Since I was on a military base, working at a military dispensary, I figured that Randy Cobb was associated with the military environmental department. This was a mistake, but in the long run it was probably a good mistake.

I dialed Randy Cobb's extension:

"Hello, Randy Cobb speaking," answered Mr. Cobb. He did not mention that he worked for OSHA, the Occupational Safety and Health Administration.

"Hello, this is Doctor Oesch. I work at the dispensary here on the base."

"Yes, can I help you?"

"Hopefully so, the nurses here gave me your name to report a possible environmental problem."

With all the evidence of cyanide intoxication, the existence of cyanide contamination was more than just a possibility. Nonetheless, remembering my past experience with health agencies, I knew that acquiring any cooperation toward solving the problem might require careful diplomacy.

"Really, what is it?" asked Mr. Cobb.

"Well, in a prior practice I had in another state, I had quite a bit of experience with a contaminant associated with electroplating. Do they have any electroplating plants on the base here?"

"Perhaps…what kind of contaminant were you dealing with?"

"I was working with patients who were ill from long-term, repeated exposure to low doses of hydrogen cyanide gas. [*I was not informed of the finding of cyanogen chloride in the industrial effluent from the plating plant in Houston until years later, despite the fact that cyanogen chloride was found in the industrial effluent as early as May 12, 1982, prior to my departure from Houston for service in the navy. And to my knowledge, the citizens of Houston were never informed of this finding.*] An industrial plant was apparently discharging cyanide compounds into the sewer system, and with increased acidity from rainwater or other discharge waters, hydrogen cyanide gas was generated into the atmosphere."

"We don't have a problem with cyanide here. I think the sewers were checked for cyanide a couple years ago."

For whatever reason, I've noticed that health officials often seem quite defensive regarding the existence of environmental pollution. It's like going fox hunting with hounds that look the other way when a fox runs by.

"I've had quite a number of patients with symptoms of cyanide intoxication, and there are laboratory tests to screen individuals for cyanide exposure," I persisted.

"Have you received any positive tests for cyanide?"

"No, not yet. I just found out that cyanide was used on the base."

"Well, let me know if anyone tests positive for cyanide," stated Mr. Cobb.

As I hung up the phone, I was left with the unmistakable impression that if anything would be done, I would have to do it myself—with God's help. Furthermore, I was beginning to detect that the cyanide problem in Philadelphia might be handled by health authorities in like manner to the cyanide problem in Houston. In time, the truth would prove far more alarming than any of my premonitions.

By noontime on the twenty-second, I learned the number to one building on the base where cyanide was utilized. When my lunch break came, I went straight to the security office and obtained a pass to visit building forty-one. The building was located in a restricted portion of the base known as the *industrial area*. While walking there, I received quite a few looks from civilian workers [*I recall wearing my U.S. Navy Officer Service Dress White Uniform to visit building 41*]; I recognized a couple of them as patients I had seen in the dispensary. Building forty-one turned out to be about seven blocks south of the dispensary. It was an electroplating shop. [*A copy of my pass to building 41 follows:*]

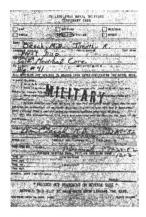

I was a little nervous as I knocked on the door to building forty-one. When it opened, a civilian employee greeted me:

"Hello Lieutenant, can I help you?"

"I'm investigating a possible environmental contaminant," I replied casually. "Could I speak with someone in charge of electroplating?"

"That's all we do in this section, but I'm the only one here right now."

"Do you think you could show me around? I'd like to see what kind of setup you have here."

The gentleman did not appear disturbed by my request; if anything, he seemed almost pleased. "Well, sure, I may not be able to answer too many questions."

"That's all right."

"Okay, come on in."

What I saw inside the electroplating shop was stunning. In Houston, an employee from the plating plant tried to explain the involved process by which discharged cyanide was presumably destroyed. An industrial agent later told me that perhaps fifty million dollars would be required to improve the treatment of cyanide at the plating plant so that cyanide would no longer be released into the environment. As I observed the electroplating process in building forty-one, it became evident that discharged cyanide was released directly into the sewage system without any treatment whatsoever.

"Are there any treatment tanks for discharged cyanide?" I questioned, not satisfied to rely merely upon visual examination.

"No, this place is really behind times."

"Are these the actual electroplating tanks?" I asked, pointing to several large, concrete vats.

"Yes."

We walked upon a raised wooden floor composed of narrow, evenly-spaced planks. Below this lay a solid concrete floor over which ran constantly flowing water. One or two of the electroplating tanks were overflowing as I stood watching. The overflow dropped to the concrete floor below and washed briskly away into the sewage system.

"So you put cyanide compounds directly into these same tanks that are spilling over into the drain?" I posed.

"Right. We have to run them over sometimes because they get too alkaline."

One thing I remembered from experiences in Houston was that electroplating plants keep their electroplating solutions alkaline. Alkaline fluids hold cyanide in solution. More neutral or acidic solutions, such as rainwater, allow cyanide to be generated into the atmosphere as hydrogen cyanide gas.

"What pH do you keep the solutions at?" I asked.

"Well, we don't measure the pH very often. When the tanks get too alkaline to work properly, then we run them over until the pH comes down some."

"You keep them pretty alkaline though, don't you?"

"Oh yea, we keep the solutions alkaline."

"Do you measure the amount of cyanide in the discharge water that runs out of the tanks?"

"No. Like I said, this place is like working in the Dark Ages."

The shortcomings of the electroplating process in building forty-one were plainly obvious. As I surveyed the setup, I regretted that no measurement was made of the cyanide in the overflow water from the electroplating tanks. Then a different idea popped into my mind:

"Do you ever change the solution in these tanks?" I asked.

"No. When they get low on stuff, we just add more. They can get too alkaline after a while, but like I said, we can fix that by running them over."

"How often to you run them over?"

"It depends how often we use them. Some of them are kept running over almost all the time."

Since electroplating itself does not destroy cyanide, but simply releases it from a metal such as copper or silver, then the amount of cyanide released from building forty-one was probably calculable from the amount used. In other words, the cyanide used in electroplating is not used up, it is extracted from a metal that is plated upon another metal. This extracted cyanide, in the case of building forty-one, was simply turned loose into the environment.

I had seen enough. There was one thing left to attempt before departing: "Do you keep records of how much cyanide you add to these tanks?"

"Yes, we keep records of the new added compounds to the tanks."

"Would you mind if I looked at some of those records?"

"No. Do you think there might be a problem here? Come on with me and I'll show you the records."

I followed the gentleman, who appeared to be about thirty-five years of age, to a small office with a desk and file cabinets. There was a single chair beside the desk where I sat down, and the gentleman sat at the desk. He started going through the desk drawers.

"That's why I'm here. I've been seeing a number of patients with symptoms I think may be from chronic cyanide poisoning. In fact, I've been sick myself," I said, responding to the gentleman's prior question.

"Can it give you headaches?" inquired the gentleman, looking ardently into my eyes.

"Yes, that's one of the main symptoms."

"The last couple of months I've had headaches so bad I could hardly stand it. I've been taking Extra-Strength Tylenol like candy. Sometimes I take three or four at a time. I've also been getting chest pains. About two weeks ago I got chest pains so bad that I nearly cried. My wife wanted to take me to the hospital."

"Have you had shortness of breath?"

"I get short of breath just walking up stairs."

The gentleman's symptoms were practically identical to those I was hospitalized with. I noted that he wore rather thick glasses: "Have you had any trouble with your vision lately?"

"Yea, is that from this stuff too? I've just gotten new glasses. My vision is worse now than it was six months ago."

"It sounds like you definitely have symptoms of chronic cyanide poisoning. Hopefully we'll be able to get something done about the problem. Can you find those records?"

"They're in here somewhere."

Before long the gentleman produced some records showing quantities of cyanide compounds added to electroplating tanks during a two-month period the preceding summer. These records showed twenty-three pounds of copper cyanide, eighteen pounds of silver cyanide, nine pounds of sodium cyanide, and ninety-two pounds of potassium cyanide that had been added to the tanks to replace used substances. This represented sufficient cyanide to produce about two billion liters of air at 10 ppm cyanide. Furthermore, there may have been other industrial plants at the shipyard that also utilized cyanide; and to the south, across the river [*Delaware River*], were several additional electroplating plants.

Chapter 11

AFFIDAVIT

I, LTJG Maryjane B. Kelley, JAGC, USN-R, on 14-15 June 1983, checked the medical files of the Philadelphia Navay Shipyard Medical Dispensary, of the following persons to determine if the request and results of urine throcyanate tests ordered by Dr. Timothy Oesch, MC, USN were noted in the files:

```
Norval  ▓▓▓▓▓       ▓▓▓▓▓▓ 5
Gaylord ▓▓▓▓▓       ▓▓▓▓▓▓ 4
Robert  ▓▓▓▓▓       ▓▓▓▓▓▓ 6
Robert  ▓▓▓▓▓       ▓▓▓▓▓▓ 4
Frank   ▓▓▓▓▓ Jr.   ▓▓▓▓▓▓ 7
John    ▓▓▓▓▓       ▓▓▓▓▓▓ 3
Robert  ▓▓▓▓▓       ▓▓▓▓▓▓ 6
H. W.   ▓▓▓▓▓       ▓▓▓▓▓▓ 3
Frank   ▓▓▓▓▓       ▓▓▓▓▓▓ 1
Leonard ▓▓▓▓▓ Jr.   ▓▓▓▓▓▓ 1
Samuel  ▓▓▓▓▓       ▓▓▓▓▓▓ 1
```

There was no indication in the files that such tests had been given. Ann Bettinger, R.N., Occupational Health Nurse Director at the dispensary could not explain why the files did not note the tests. All test are to be recorded in the files. Laura Booth, Administrative Clerk of Record also indicated that test results should be in the file and no where else. She stated that the test results are never kept in CDR DeJesus's office.

I was referred to CDR DeJesus, MC, USN, Senior Medical Officer, who stated that she had the original tests requested and results in her desk office because she did not want them to get lost. She admitted that no notation was in the file and she did not explain why copies of the tests requested and results were not placed in the file in place of the original.

I also questioned CDR DeJesus why Dr. Oesch's lecture in cyanide poisoning was abruptly cancelled. She stated that she did not remember the reason for its cancellation.

_____   _____
WITNESS   MARYJANE B. KELLEY
                                  LTJG, JAGC, USN-R

LT. JAGC, USNR
NLSO, Phil. PA.
19112

Threat After Threat

My visit to building forty-one took a little longer than I anticipated; I returned to the dispensary about thirty minutes late.

"There you are, Doctor Oesch. We've got some patients for you," said a nurse as I entered the dispensary.

"All right," I obliged.

For the remainder of that day, all of the next day, and half of the second day following, I questioned patients who came to my office concerning symptoms of cyanide intoxication. I also mentioned my suspicions of cyanide contamination to the Senior Medical Officer at the dispensary, Commander DeJesus. It so happened that she was attempting to arrange biweekly lectures at the dispensary, and I was assigned to deliver the first lecture on the subject of *chronic cyanide poisoning*. This was encouraging. Urine thiocyanate tests were ordered on several civilian employees, myself, and on an enlisted sailor seen the previous week. The sailor also received a serum thiocyanate test.

I ordered the urine thiocyanate tests carefully, recording whether or not the patients smoked, and if they did, how much they smoked during the preceding two weeks. In addition, just in case Metpath Laboratories, Inc. would be utilized by the military laboratory technicians, I inquired about the use of aspirin. Only one patient had taken aspirin. With positive symptomatic histories and carefully conducted thiocyanate tests, I expected to soon obtain statistically significant data verifying the presence of cyanide intoxication among workers at the base. The data was finally obtained, but not so quickly or easily as I expected.

There was an ominous tinge to my rapidly developing cyanide investigation. After ordering the first urine thiocyanate test, I was transferred to an office where only physicals and prescribed industrial screening took place. Rather than stinting my investigation, this actually boosted it. Practically all the workers who participated in the industrial screening were candidates to cyanide exposure, and a significant proportion complained of symptoms suggesting cyanide intoxication. This enabled me to collect a pertinent quantity of thiocyanate tests in only two and a half days.

Adding a thiocyanate test to the prescribed tests in the industrial screening program was really quite simple. The shipyard workers had so many tests performed on them that one more test was no big deal. If any of them asked why I was ordering this test, I just said that I was testing for possible industrial cyanide exposure. I did not know of any reason why I should not say what I was doing. If someone has been ill from exposure to a poison, then who has more right to know about it than that person himself?

There was someone in the military establishment who apparently did not share my view regarding individual rights. At about noontime on

November twenty-fourth, a knock sounded on my office door. I do not remember who answered the door, but whoever it was instructed me to go immediately upstairs to Commander DeJesus's office. I was also informed that Captain Galasyn was waiting to see me there. I was already aware that Captain Galasyn was in charge of the Naval Environmental Department in Philadelphia.

As I walked through the door to Commander DeJesus's office, I quickly sensed an atmosphere saturated with berating tension. Commander DeJesus looked petrified. Both she and Captain Galasyn stood facing me as I entered. Captain Galasyn was tall and lean; his face looked outwardly amiable in contract to coldly calculating eyes.

"Hello Lieutenant Oesch, Commander DeJesus and I have just been discussing you," stated Captain Galasyn. "Have a seat."

Captain Galasyn and Commander DeJesus seated themselves across the room from me. There were several chairs in the office to accommodate small group meetings.

"I received word that you've been ordering cyanide tests on civilian employees," said Captain Galasyn.

"That's correct," I replied.

Captain Galasyn shook his head slowly from side to side and looked downward. "That's bad. Very, very bad."

I said nothing.

"What made you order these tests?" Captain Galasyn questioned, looking upward interrogatively.

"I found out about the use of cyanide on the base, and I've seen a lot of patients with symptoms of chronic cyanide poisoning," I responded.

"Don't you think you should have contacted my department before ordering these tests?"

"I called Randy Cobb, and he told me to let him know if any of the patients tested positive for cyanide."

"Randy Cobb is not with my department, he's with OSHA," the captain asserted blisteringly.

It was more than obvious that Captain Galasyn was opposed to any sort of cyanide investigation on my part. He surprised me by pointing out that I called OSHA rather than his department, and left me little choice except to apologize.

"OSHA," I evoked, "I'm sorry. I thought he was with your department."

"No, he wasn't, and you won't call Randy Cobb back. Is that clear?"
"Yes sir."
By this point I was beginning to dislike Captain Galasyn's attitude toward the problem of cyanide contamination. He did not seem very concerned about the health of my patients.
"Now, why didn't you let Commander DeJesus know about your cyanide concerns?" inquired the captain.
"I told her I suspected a cyanide problem," I replied.
"Yes, but I didn't know he was doing all this testing," interjected Commander DeJesus. She was obviously anxious.
I offered no objection. Captain Galasyn seemed content with Commander DeJesus's response. He dropped the discussion of her role in my activities, and refocused his grueling query toward me.
"I think taking this matter into your own hands was very unwise, Lieutenant Oesch, very unwise."
I tried to keep my face basically expressionless and gave no reply. Captain Galasyn seemed bent on intimidating me, and for the time being, I thought it might be unwise to inform his that he was not succeeding.
"Commander DeJesus tells me that you were preoccupied with hepatitis sometime back, and now it's cyanide," Captain Galasyn stated demeaningly.
"Before I found out there was cyanide around, I was considering some infectious agent as the cause of my illness and the illness of many of my patients. Some type of hepatitis virus seemed most likely. After I found out about the cyanide, I realized that the symptoms my patients and I were experiencing were precisely those of cyanide intoxication."
Captain Galasyn did not appear very pleased with my explanation. "You've stepped out of your capacity by ordering these tests. From now on I'll handle this problem, agreed?"
Now Captain Galasyn was asking me to commit myself. It is not standard practice in the Navy for a Lieutenant to refuse a request from a Captain. On the other hand, I could hardly allow my patients to go on suffering from cyanide intoxication and say nothing about it. Besides that, I was seriously ill with cyanide intoxication myself.
"Yes sir, I'll not do anything more about the problem providing that you take care of it."
"What do you mean by that?" the captain demanded.

"I mean that as long as you take care of the problem there's no need for me to. I don't mind letting you handle this problem at all. I just don't want the problem to continue."

"And if I don't?" taunted the captain.

Captain Galasyn was leaving me no escape. "If you don't do anything about the problem, then I'll have to," I affirmed.

Commander DeJesus looked very nervous. She peered at Captain Galasyn as if she were watching a horror show. The captain seemed to turn pale for a second, then recovered his rigid amiability.

"I'll take care of the problem, but I want you to stop all of your testing right now. Something like this could end up in a congressional investigation, and I certainly don't want that. I don't even want you discussing this with any of the civilian workers."

"I understand, sir."

"I hope you realize that this is for your own good as well as that of the base," concluded Captain Galasyn while rising from his chair. "Commander DeJesus has a few more words for you. I believe she has something to tell you regarding a lecture you were planning to give on cyanide."

"Yes, we'll have to cancel that lecture," Commander DeJesus inserted obsequiously.

I rose when Captain Galasyn did. Rather than exiting immediately from the office, he walked across the room and put one arm around my shoulders. Commander DeJesus was still on the opposite side of the office.

"If you draw a cyanide test on one more patient, I'll have to put you in a psychiatric hospital," Captain Galasyn spoke softly and confidentially into my ear. "We wouldn't want that now, would we?"

I was pressed for an immediate and intimate response: "I know that happens," I replied. What I did not mention, however, was that the only place I had heard of it occurring was in the Union of Soviet Socialist Republics. Captain Galasyn left the room, and Commander DeJesus further admonished me not to involve myself with additional cyanide testing. When I finally returned to my office, it was under a constant cloud of threat. I decided to await the test results from the urine thiocyanate tests already ordered before attempting anything else controversial. Meanwhile, I continued taking daily doses of cyanide antidote which enabled me to continue work.

A Breath of Cyanide

Somehow, Captain Galasyn found out that I was taking antidote for cyanide intoxication. Perhaps the fact that I had suffered a long-term illness which was relieved by cyanide antidote worried or annoyed him. Whatever the case, he soon paid a personal visit to my office. This time he and I were alone.

My office door opened after brief knocking. "Hello Doctor Oesch, I'd like to talk with you a few minutes."

"Yes sir, come on in," I assented, standing as Captain Galasyn entered.

Captain Galasyn shut the door and stepped to a chair before my desk. "Sit down," he said, motioning toward my chair while seating himself. I sat down. The captain paused before speaking again, leaning forward in morose contemplation. His formidable bearing served to tremulously dramatize our interview. I did not tell him that I was more disgusted than frightened.

"I understand that you're taking some sort of crystals," the captain remarked.

"Right, sodium thiosulfate crystals."

He paused and nodded. "What are those crystals for?"

"They're an antidote for cyanide intoxication."

"I see...from what I hear, this medication really shouldn't do much to make you feel better..."

"No, not unless you have cyanide poisoning," I responded. The captain's insinuation that I was abusing a drug was hardly merited in the case of a sulfur salt. "If anything, it might give you a stomach ache or diarrhea if you take too much."

"Yes, that's what I understand. Who prescribed this medication for you?"

"I already had some," I replied.

At the time, I was not yet aware that sodium thiosulfate is nonprescription; anyone can purchase it whether or not he has a medical license. [*I apparently found out that sodium thiosulfate is nonprescription not too long thereafter. To the best of my memory, I also learned that electroplating workers in New Jersey took oral doses of sodium thiosulfate to counteract their exposures to cyanide, and that this was taking place before I ever came to the state.*] Nonetheless, Captain Galasyn acted as though I was smuggling morphine.

"You mean you're treating yourself?" he inquired sedately.

"Yes, there aren't many doctors that know much about this."

The captain looked downward and shook his head in feigned regret. "Oh, that' bad. I think it's very unwise for a physician to treat himself. I think most of the other doctors who work here would agree with me that it's a very bad thing to do. What about your wife, are you treating her too?"

"Yes I am," I admitted, though I suspected that Captain Galasyn knew the answer to his question before he asked it.

"A doctor who treats his own wife," the captain chided, "surely you've heard that a doctor shouldn't treat his own wife."

"I took her to an internal medicine specialist who diagnosed her with cyanide intoxication. He told me to treat her myself because he didn't know anything about it."

"No, I'm not so sure I agree with that," the captain maintained, "and if I were a patient, I don't think I'd want to go to a doctor who treated himself. Did you have a medical practice before coming into the navy?"

"Yes."

"I think if your patients knew what you were doing, they wouldn't want to come back to you. In fact, I don't think anyone would want to go to a doctor who treats himself."

It was not until later that I realized Captain Galasyn was threatening my future medical practice. I continued contending with him: "Several of my patients knew I was treating myself with antidote for cyanide poisoning. They didn't seem to mind."

"Doctor Oesch, let's get serious now," the captain stated firmly. "I want you to stop taking those crystals."

The captain's request was vexingly absurd. I was only able to continue work because I took antidote, and to stop taking it would almost certainly bring debilitating illness.

"I'd like to stop taking it," I replied. "The only reason I take it is because I get sick if I don't."

The captain was not there to discuss issues or listen to reason. "I don't think so Doctor Oesch. If you stop taking the crystals, you'll find out you're just as well without them."

Captain Galasyn was not asking me how I would feel if I stopped taking the antidote, he was telling me how I would feel—but he was wrong. Yielding to his demand would mean relentless destruction of my own body.

"I hear what you're saying, captain, but I just got out of the hospital where I had serious heart pain. I get acutely ill if I don't take this antidote. Sometimes I need to take it."

"When was the last time you became ill and had to take it?" posed the captain.

"This morning," I confided.

Without pausing, Captain Galasyn lowered his voice slightly and coolly accused me of lying—though I do not think he really thought I was: "I don't believe that, Doctor Oesch."

I did not respond. It seemed wisest to continue allowing Captain Galasyn to think he was intimidating me. I looked downward to avoid eye contact; sometimes the eyes disclose more than the tongue.

"I hope you will consider what I've said to you very seriously," he concluded.

"Yes sir."

He left my office, but there were other visits later—mainly to make sure I refrained from further cyanide testing. On one visit the captain warned that involvement in *such an issue*, meaning cyanide contamination at the base, could be *very dangerous*. A few weeks later I learned more than I cared to about the danger. For the time being, though, I continued waiting for test results to arrive. I also continued taking my antidote.

Having determined not to order any more cyanide tests until I acquired some results from those already ordered, I was presented with quite a problem when two nurses sought me out to evaluate Chester Parkins. Chester was working upon an outside platform not far from building forty-one when he became dizzy and ill. His foreman had him climb down and sit for about an hour or two, but his illness only worsened. When I saw Chester, he was ivory white, his pulse was very weak, and his blood pressure was 80 over zero. He sat with his head buried in both hands.

"How do you feel?" I asked.

"To be honest, doc, I feel terrible," replied Chester, hardly looking up as he spoke.

"What kind of pain are you having?"

"I don't know, it's just...it's just a terrible feeling."

"Does you head hurt?"

"Yea, my head's really aching."

"How about your chest?"

"Well, my chest isn't all that bad."

"How about your breathing? Are you having any trouble breathing?"

"Yea, I can't seem to get my breath—I've got that asbestos, you know…"

It seemed that a lot of problems among the shipyard workers were blamed on asbestos. In Chester's case, he probably did have some emphysema which resulted from asbestos exposure and previous smoking. This likely made him more vulnerable to cyanide exposure because he was more sensitive to oxygen starvation, even if the starvation occurred on a cellular level.

"Where were you when you got sick?" I asked.

Chester disclosed his work location, and I was convinced that he suffered from cyanide intoxication. His condition was critical enough that I clearly had to put politics aside. Besides that, I really had no intention of simply abandoning the problem.

"I think I have something that might help you," I said, "it's nothing dangerous, just a vitamin shot."

"I'll take anything, doc, if you can help this headache."

I walked back to my office, then returned with my personal vial of alphaREDISOL. The nurses administered the treatment as I instructed, and Chester was remarkably better within minutes. Next, I instructed the nurses to acquire a venous blood sample and get an electrocardiogram. The electrocardiogram was abnormal with a depressed ST segment, indicating that Chester's heart might not be getting enough oxygen and might be straining. I decided to get Chester evaluated at a nearby hospital. I also hoped to have him tested for cyanide exposure.

It was no problem getting authorization to send Chester to a hospital emergency room, I just showed his abnormal electrocardiogram to Commander DeJesus. Getting Chester to cooperate, though, was a different story. I talked to him alone in my office.

"Thanks doc, I sure feel a lot better. I think I'll be all right now with some rest," said Chester.

"You may get sick again, especially if you try and stay around here," I remonstrated. "What I treated you for was an environmental contaminant."

"An environmental contaminant…what?"

"There's an electroplating plant near where you were working, and I think you were exposed to some cyanide gas in the air."

"Cyanide," voiced Chester, "isn't that the stuff they had in the news with the Tylenol, when all those people were getting poisoned?"

"Yes it was, but this is from an industrial source."

"Oh, well I'm sure glad I came to you, doc. I mean, most doctors probably wouldn't even look for something like that. But I think I'll be all right now," Chester maintained.

"There's something else I haven't told you yet. Have you ever had an abnormal electrocardiogram?"

"You mean where they hook those wires up to your chest?"

"Right."

"No, why?"

"Well, yours was a little abnormal this time. I showed it to Commander DeJesus, and she definitely wants you checked out at the local hospital."

Chester seemed reluctant, but with the mention of his heart, he finally conceded. "Well, I guess I should then. I don't feel bad though, and I've never had anything wrong with my heart."

"It will probably be best for you anyway, just to get away from the pollution here," I explained. Then I added: "There's also a little favor I'd like to ask of you, if you're willing."

Chester looked somewhat surprised that I was asking a favor of him. He probably wondered how he could aid a medical doctor. "Sure doc, what can I do?"

"I'd like you to take a note to the doctor who treats you at the local hospital. The note will tell him how to test the blood sample we drew. It will also instruct him to get a urine thiocyanate test."

"A urine...what?" posed Chester.

"It's a test to check for the metabolite of cyanide. You see, your blood test might be negative for cyanide. Cyanide does not stay in the blood long, and the lab test might not show any, even though you were sick with it. The thiocyanate test is better because the thiocyanate lasts longer."

Chester became notably concerned. "I don't know, doc. I'd really like to help you, but you don't know these people around here. If they find out I got tested for an environmental contaminant, I might lose my job—and I'm supposed to retire before too long."

"Well, it's up to you. But if you continue getting ill from this, you may need some proof that you've had it. Maybe you could explain your predicament to the doctor at the local hospital and see what he can work out."

"All right, doc. I'll give him the note, anyway."

I accompanied Chester back to the waiting room where the nurses made arrangements for his transportation to the local hospital. After about thirty minutes, Chester began having recurrence of his headache and dizziness. I was aware that cyanide intoxication can relapse after treatment, and I was also aware that the concentration of cyanide antidote in alphaREDISOL was really too low. For these reasons, I treated him a second time with sodium thiosulfate crystals which he swallowed with water. The crystals took a little longer to give him relief, but the relief probably lasted longer.

When Chester arrived at the local hospital emergency room he gave my note to Doctor Schmidt. Doctor Schmidt took the blood sample Chester brought with him and sent it to SmithKline Laboratory. Fortunately the laboratory technician at SmithKline Laboratory automatically tested the blood sample for thiocyanate when he saw that the patient was being screened for cyanide exposure. Unfortunately, a whole blood cyanide test was not done; instead, the serum was spun down and tested for cyanide. A serum test for cyanide is less likely to detect cyanide after cyanide exposure than a whole blood cyanide test.

Although Chester's serum test for cyanide was negative, his serum thiocyanate level was highly positive. It was the highest level of serum thiocyanate I had ever seen in anyone, smoker or nonsmoker. Furthermore, it was even higher than the serum thiocyanate found in the dead dog I tested in Houston. Since Chester had not smoked for a couple years, this finding was attributable to a nonsmoker. To my knowledge, this is the highest, legitimate level of serum thiocyanate ever found in a nonsmoker being screened for chronic cyanide intoxication. It definitely indicates exposure to a sufficient quantity of cyanide to threaten fatality.

Chester's urine thiocyanate test was performed on urine collected after he arrived at the local hospital. [*This was not the naval hospital.*] The level found was 9 mcg/ml, which is equivalent to 9 mg/L. Although this level of urine thiocyanate is definitely positive for cyanide exposure in a nonsmoker, it was not much compared to the serum level of 21 mcg/ml. This indicated that Chester was exposed to cyanide fairly recently; not much of the thiocyanate in his serum had passed through his kidneys and into his urine. The tests supported the time, symptoms, and etiology of Chester's illness; he had been poisoned by airborne cyanide.

My wife's low blood pressure and headaches got better when I started giving her alphaREDISOL. Her general health, though, dourly worsened with time. Clumps of hair began collecting beneath the bed and dresser and in various corners of hallways and rooms as her long, thick hair began limply thinning. By regularly taking both alphaREDISOL and sodium thiosulfate, I was able to continue work without absence. My athletic life, though, was nonexistent. I could not tolerate any amount of exercise.

There are certain social customs unique to the military. Captain Martinson was fairly new as Commanding Officer at the Philadelphia Naval Regional Medical Center, so an *At Home* was scheduled for all the medical officers and their spouses to get acquainted with her. This meant the officers would gather at Captain Martinson's home one evening for hors d'oeuvres and conversation. Due to the large number of officers, both November thirtieth and December first were designated for such a gathering. Most of the dispensary physicians elected to attend the November thirtieth get-together, myself included.

I was wary about taking my wife into Philadelphia, but we decided that an hour or two would not be too hazardous if she took some antidote before leaving. Captain Martinson's home was situated near the naval hospital. It was dark when we arrived, but the night was warm. Knowing the general direction of the nearby base where cyanide was discharged into the sewer system, I checked for wind direction. The atmosphere was still and silent; I could not detect any directional movement of air.

We mingled and talked with the other guests. Most of them were only vaguely familiar to me, and we spent most of our time with Mark Whitley and his wife. Mark was a friend of mine from the dispensary; he was a physician's assistant. Captain Galasyn was also present, but I never saw him looking directly at me. At first it seemed the affair would be frivolously uneventful.

Not long after arriving, both my wife and I developed dizziness and headaches. The windows in the room were wide open to outside air. A few minutes later, a considerable commotion developed as Lieutenant

Jones, a doctor serving in family practice at the naval hospital, became acutely ill. He grew dizzy and pale, and had to excuse himself from the group. Interestingly, two days later he and I would be in opposing beds on ward 1-D of the naval hospital.

Some of the guests expressed marked concern over Lieutenant Jones's sudden affliction. "Oh, he'll be all right," remarked Captain Martinson, "it's just the flu that's been going around. I was sick myself last Friday."

I wondered whether or not Captain Martinson really thought Lieutenant Jones just had the flu. She seemed almost too intent on settling everyone else's minds.

Meanwhile, my wife and I grew more ill. I checked my pulse, and it was over one hundred. With Captain Galasyn in our midst, I thought it might be dangerous to disclose our illness. A little later my dizziness increased so severely I lost my balance and nearly fell down before catching myself on the back of a chair. I certainly did not wish to pass out and make a scene.

I leaned confidentially toward my wife. "We'd better leave, I'm afraid I'll pass out pretty soon if we don't."

"Fine with me, I'm getting really nauseated," replied Melody.

I could not think of any way to honestly dismiss ourselves without relating our illness, so my wife and I slipped out quietly and unannounced. We felt a little better by the time we got home, but wasted little time before taking some antidote. Months later, on March 14, 1983, I would check with the National Weather Service and discover that the last movement of air before we arrived at Captain Martinson's house was from the southwest at 5 knots. When we arrived, at about 7:00 pm, winds were calm. The naval base was located south and somewhat southwest of Captain Martinson's home.

Two days later, Thursday, December 2, 1982, I had a follow-up doctor's appointment with Doctor Gilmore. I needed a note from Doctor Gilmore to excuse me from having to run a mile for time, something I feared might seriously endanger my health, so I refrained from taking antidote on December first and second. I knew that without antidote my illness should be plainly obvious upon examination. This proved true. By the time Doctor Gilmore examined me, my resting pulse was nearly 100 when lying down, and about 120 when sitting or standing. To my surprise, Doctor Gilmore responded by having me readmitted to the hospital that very day. [*The naval hospital.*] She also wanted my wife admitted to the hospital.

I called home, but Melody was at school. Then I called Leighann Deere and left word for Melody to pack some bags and get ready to come into the hospital. Before the day ended, however, I reconsidered my wife's admission to the hospital, and decided against it. My antidote was taken from me and I was forbidden to use it. I thought such action might be life-threatening to my wife, and as it turned out, it was even life-threatening to me. I had no choice about my own hospitalization, but they could not take my wife.

Chapter 12

Summary and Conclusions:

Dr. Oesch is a bright 28 year old male who demonstrates good creative and intellectual ability, excellent problem-solving and reasoning skills, and exceptional judgement in both social and practical situations. Some denial and/or suppression of negative feelings is evident, but this along with his control of impulses and external expression of affect may be a reflection of the influence of his Christian ethics upon his life. No significant psychopathology is evident, nor any salient personality features which would impede his social, emotional, or intellectual functioning.

_____ _____
Edward G. Daniels   Aaron Botbyl, Ph.D.
Psychometric Technician   Licensed Clinical Psychologist

Frame-Up

It did not take long after my December second hospital admittance to decipher that I as tagged as a psychiatric patient. Later, I was able to obtain actual hospital records that revealed that my admitting diagnosis was listed as *CONVERSION REACTION*. This was a technical way of saying that all my symptoms were psychological in origin. A discharge objective written on December second read as follows: *Patient will verbalize relief of symptoms. Patient will verbalize decreasing levels of pre-occupation with cyanide*. In other words, someone planned for me to stop talking about cyanide poisoning.

Not long after joining the patients of ward 1-D, I was surprised to see Lieutenant Jones admitted among us also. He was placed in the bed directly across from me, and I soon initiated a conversation.

"Well, Doctor Jones, what bring you in here?" I asked. This was the same Lieutenant Jones who became ill at Captain Martinson's party.

"They think it's an intestinal virus. How about yourself?" posed Lieutenant Jones.

"I think I'm basically in here for political reasons," I answered. Since Lieutenant Jones and I were both of the same rank, it gave us sort of a mutual trust and comradeship. "I'm real sensitive to exposure to hydrogen cyanide gas, and I think it's an air pollutant in this area."

"So why did they put you in here?" inquired Doctor Jones, expressing some concern over my predicament.

I told Lieutenant Jones how I ended up in the hospital, and why I suspected a political basis to my admittance. He seemed to hear every word I spoke.

"You know," he commented, "my wife's been sick with symptoms like you described, and no one's been able to tell us what's wrong with her."

"Really, so has my wife. Where do you live?"

"Across the river."

"Is it anywhere near Pitman?"

"Not far."

I went on to tell Lieutenant Jones about my wife's problem, and more about my difficulties getting anyone to cooperate in dealing with the cyanide problem. When it came to the political aspects of the situation, he had some very specific advice.

"You say it was a captain that told you not to test anyone else?" asked Lieutenant Jones.

"Yes," I acknowledged.

"You'd better be careful then. Whatever a captain says, goes. If I were having a problem with a lieutenant commander, or even a commander, I might speak up for my rights. A commander can't really do that much to hurt you. But a captain, a captain can do anything he or she pleases and no one will say a word about it."

"Well, thanks for the advice. I'll have to be careful," I returned. Despite how the hierarchy of the navy was systematized, it was still wrong to poison people.

Lieutenant Jones apparently sensed my resolution. "If they try to do anything rash, remember that you're an officer. You have the right to call your congressman before they do anything. They have to let you call him."

"Really? Thanks, I didn't know that," I responded. The truth was that I did not know who my congressman was or what he could do if I did call him. Nonetheless, the information sounded like a good tip.

Lieutenant Jones was quite ill and expressed a profound distaste for the hospital food. He told me that he planned to *pull some strings* and get back home to his wife's cooking. Sure enough, he was discharged from the hospital just a couple of days after his admittance. I told him what type of testing his wife would need to check for cyanide intoxication, but I have no idea whether or not he ever followed up with it.

I remained on ward 1-D for about fifteen days. It was long enough to make considerable acquaintance with the other patients and a number of the health personnel caring for us. Colonel Adams was retired from the air force. I played a number of chess games with him, and did quite well when winds were northern. With southern winds, however, I don't think the colonel ever lost a game. At those times I would even forget that certain chess pieces were on the board.

Colonel Adams was in the hospital for treatment of an ulcer on his foot. On certain nights he would sweat so profusely that he would have to change the sheets on his bed. It did not take me long to notice that his sweating occurred on the same nights that I suffered from cyanide intoxication, nights when winds came from the south. My radio had a weather band, so I checked the wind direction when my symptoms noticeably worsened or improved. On every single occasion that my symptoms worsened, winds had come from the south or southwest. Furthermore, every time I noticeably improved, winds had come from the north. Bear in mind that I checked the wind direction after noting a change in my condition, not before.

Another acquaintance on the ward was Lieutenant Latinez, a compassionate nurse from a tropical island. Despite the fact that I was listed as a psychiatric patient, she came to me one day for some counseling. This was not long after I broke up a heated fight between two hospital corpsmen, an act she seemed to admire. I learned that she suffered symptoms similar to mine and was operated on the preceding year for a gallbladder attack. After the surgery she learned that the surgeons removed a normal gallbladder.

The dearest memory of my second hospitalization concerned a young man named Phillip Sanders. He was receiving some sort of drug rehabilitation. It took little time to decipher that Phillip was a very opinionated, cynical fellow who wished he could do something to help improve a messed up world. I wanted to talk with him, but I sensed that he would only rebel against anything I had to say. What I did, therefore, was pray for him.

Sunday morning I went to a small, protestant worship service. Phillip Sanders, a Moslem, came to the service and sat beside me. When we left the service that morning, Phillip was a Christian. I gave him my New Testament, and he devoured the Scriptures with stunning alacrity. He was scheduled for baptism on Christmas Eve.

A Breath of Cyanide

Bill, Jack, and Bernie were three cutups, all hospital corpsmen. They had such laudable tasks as making beds, taking blood pressures, and carrying lunch trays. I was very quickly accepted into their comradeship, despite being an officer, and seemed to gain more trust from them than their supposedly sane military bosses. Thus, from time to time, I received tips on what transpired in medical meetings where I was discussed. At one point, I was advised that there was talk of placing me in an institution.

There were not many patients on our ward, but while I was there, at least two heart attacks and one death occurred. A number of patients appeared to have symptoms of cyanide intoxication, but there was little I could do about it. One man was placed on our ward prior to gastrointestinal surgery, but the surgery had to be cancelled because he began seeping blood from his intestines and became anemic. I wanted to tell his physician that cyanide can affect the clotting system, and that this poor patient was experiencing cyanide exposure. His physician was Doctor Wendle, though, so I exercised some silent discretion instead.

I was permitted to walk down a hospital corridor to a pay telephone and call my wife. Every evening I did so. Suspecting that I might never receive any report of the urine thiocyanate tests that I ordered at the base, I asked my wife to call the laboratory and try to obtain the results by phone. Somehow she managed it, and the results were positive. [*My wife actually obtained a number of the test results, but not all of them. All of the results, along with the order sheets for those tests, would be obtained later.*] Afterwards, I asked my naval physician about the tests at the shipyard, and she said they all were okay. Being poisoned may have been okay with her, but it was not okay with me.

One morning I woke up with bluish fingernails. Later I learned that my lips were blue also, but there was not a mirror at my bed. I think my blood pressure the evening before was 80/40, a seriously low reading. Without access to my antidote, I was at the mercy of the environment. Chest pain came and went, as did shortness of breath, dizziness, altered thinking abilities, muscle aches, and weakness. I knew that my heart was probably failing from cyanide intoxication, but who would listen to me?

"Look at my fingernails," I remarked to Mrs. Bryant, a civilian nurse practitioner who worked for the government. More than any other time during my hospitalization, I just wanted to scream—*I'm being poisoned, come on, can't you see I'm being poisoned?!*—but I did not.

I knew that any such action would probably result in additional psychiatric comments in my hospital record, that it might give my military superiors an excuse to institutionalize me, and that it would probably fail to bring me proper medical treatment anyway.

"Are you cold?" asked Mrs. Bryant. Her eyes were nervously widened.

"No, I'm not cold, but I've never seen my fingernails this color before. Could I get you to take my blood pressure?

"Sure.

Mrs. Bryant quickly obtained a blood pressure cuff and reported my bluish fingernails to the nurses' station. It seems like I can remember hearing a comment sound from the nurses' station: *Tell him he'll be all right*. Mrs. Bryant returned with the pressure cuff and took a reading. I do not remember exactly what the reading was, except that my systolic blood pressure, which is the highest number in a blood pressure, was over 70. Nothing was done about my blue fingernails. Dr. Gilmore had written in my chart that a physician should be contacted if my systolic blood pressure was below 70, but it was not. It should be noted, however, that 70 is an extremely low systolic blood pressure for an adult American male. With a pressure below that, I may not have even been conscious.

Standard Form 508					
CLINICAL RECORD			DOCTOR'S ORDERS (Sign all orders)		
DATE AND TIME START / STOP		℞	DRUG ORDERS (Another brand of a generically equivalent product, identical in dosage form and content of active ingredient(s), may be administered UNLESS checked here)	DOCTOR'S SIGNATURE	NURSE'S SIGNATURE
2/9 1830			MD orders received. ① alpha Redisol 1 vial to be kept on ward Call MD for Syst. BP <70		

There seemed to be hardly any test that was not performed on me. Perhaps someone hoped to find something to blame my illness on besides environmental pollution with cyanide. On one occasion I was taken to the local civilian hospital for a CAT-scan of my brain, both with and without injected iodine dye. I remember vomiting forcefully after the iodine was injected into a vein. While there, I slipped a note for Dr. Schmidt to a nurse. The note disclosed that Chester Parkins' test for cyanide exposure was highly positive. Whether or not the note did any good, I do not know.

On December 11, 1982, I experienced definite and apparent symptoms of cyanide intoxication during the early morning hours. A nurse entered the following note in my hospital record in order to relate my subjective complaints: *I feel kind of bad today—my pulse is up, I have a headache and occasional shortness of breath. The wind is from the south—I even called the weather bureau to verify it. I should be okay this afternoon though as the wind is shifting, from the north.* The note was not entirely correct, I heard the weather report on the radio rather than having called on the telephone, but it still reveals that I was plainly communicating symptoms consistent with cyanide intoxication. I was even able to basically pinpoint the directional source of the pollution. Nonetheless, the nurse assessed my illness as an anxiety reaction.

By December eleventh, I was getting a little aggravated by the stubborn refusal of my military physician to take me seriously regarding cyanide intoxication. Considering my acute symptoms, I figured that a blood test for cyanide just might prove positive—if the blood was handled properly and the selected laboratory knew what they were doing. Adamantly, I requested that someone draw my blood for a cyanide test. Somehow, perhaps because it was Saturday, I managed to succeed. The doctor on call, Doctor Weiss, dictated the following order: *Draw blood cyanide level*. Later that day, Doctor Gilmore also signed the order.

When Nelson Martinez, a corpsman, drew my venous blood into a vacu-tube, it was bright red in color. Since the blood was drawn directly from my vein, through a needle, and into a tube from which the air was previously evacuated, the bright red color was not due to exposure of my blood to oxygen in the air. I made sure Mr. Martinez noted the color of my blood. [*Sometime thereafter, I obtained an affidavit from Mr.*

Martinez, but I got the date wrong on the affidavit. The date I wrote on the affidavit was "December 18, 1982," a week after the actual date when the blood was drawn, namely "December eleventh, 1982." I corrected the error after becoming aware of my mistake, but then I chose to simply cross out the dates since the "18" was changed to "eleventh" <u>*after*</u> *Mr. Martinez signed the note:*

> Nelson Daniel Martinez
>
> When I drew doctor Timothy R. Desch's venous blood ~~on December 18, 1982~~ eleventh it was bright red in color, like arterial blood. I verify this statement by signing upon it.

Following this, I instructed the health personnel on my ward to put the blood on ice and advised them that the test for cyanide should be performed as quickly as possible. The blood sample was not received by a laboratory for testing until six days later. [*This is why the* **Test Received** *date on the scanned copy of my serum thiocyanate level shown at the beginning of chapter ten is given as* **12/17/82**, *when the blood was actually drawn on 12/11/82. December 17, 1982, also happens to be the date when I was discharged from the hospital.*]

In spite of the prolonged transit time, I suspect that my blood sample drawn on December eleventh was positive for cyanide. The test result was later missing from my hospital record, and I had no luck trying to obtain it by phone, which is precisely why I suspect the test was positive. One fact that probably worked to my favor was that most laboratories list therapeutic reference values rather than normal reference values for expected levels of serum thiocyanate. Therapeutic reference values are those values resulting from medical use of a drug which boosts levels of thiocyanate [*most likely nitroprusside*]. These levels are used to adjust drug dosages. Normal reference values are much, much lower.

A serum thiocyanate test, which is often performed in conjunction with a blood cyanide test, was performed on my blood. The test was done by Roche Clinical Laboratories, Inc. located in Raritan, New Jersey. I learned from speaking to a toxicologist at Roche Clinical Laboratories that the normal reference value for serum thiocyanate in adult, nonsmoking males is 0.244 mg/dl with a standard deviation of 0.087 mg/dl. A value over 0.4 mg/dl indicates likely exposure to cyanide, and a value over 0.6 mg/dl indicates a definite exposure to cyanide, but a value less than 0.4 mg/dl does not necessarily rule out exposure to cyanide. My serum thiocyanate level was 1.8 mg/dl, an extremely high level that indicated exposure to a sufficient quantity of cyanide to cause death in some individuals.

The therapeutic reference value listed by Roche Clinical Laboratories for serum thiocyanate was 0 to 12 mg/dl. The lethal level for thiocyanate is about 20 mg/dl. Obviously, thiocyanate is far less toxic than cyanide. Seeing this reference value, my military superiors surmised that they had acquired a negative test for cyanide exposure. This may be the only reason that the test was shown to me. When I told Doctor Gilmore that the test was actually highly positive for cyanide exposure, and attempted to explain why, she basically seemed to ignore me.

Another notable fact regarding my serum thiocyanate test was the result of a prior serum thiocyanate test performed on blood that was drawn on December second, nine days earlier. Although the result of this prior test failed to appear in my hospital record, my wife was able to obtain the result by calling the laboratory. My serum thiocyanate level on December second was 0.3 mg/dl, 1.5 mg/dl less than that on December eleventh. Since my diet in the hospital was controlled and I received no medication, this finding clearly and unmistakably revealed that I received a very significant exposure to cyanide while hospitalized.

After voicing my desire for a blood cyanide test on the eleventh, I was soon visited by the Commanding Officer herself, Captain Martinson. I was sitting on my bed eating lunch when she appeared.

"What seems to be the problem?" voiced Captain Martinson.

"Hello ma'am. I seem to be quite ill. I'm dizzy, I have a headache, I'm short of breath, and I have tachycardia," I responded.

"What do you think's causing it?" she prompted.

"Well, I'm real sensitive to cyanide exposure, and I've noticed that I'm ill when winds come from the south, and better when they come from the north."

Captain Martinson looked rather disgusted. She stepped forward and took my wrist in order to take my pulse. At that particular time my pulse was very rapid, probably over 120 beats per minute. A startled expression momentarily mounted her face.

"You seem to be upset," she said, "you'd better lie down. Just relax."

My pulse rate decreased when I lay down, just as it had when Doctor Gilmore examined me before my hospitalization. Captain Martinson stood at the end of my bed and took my pulse from my ankle after unsuccessfully attempting to find it in my foot.

"There, you're better, now," she said, then she started turning to leave.

I was not going to let her off that easily. "I visited an electroplating plant at the base," I interjected, "building forty-one. They used enough cyanide there to generate fifteen and a half million liters of air a day at twenty parts per million cyanide. I can show you the calculations of how I obtained those figures."

"I'm sure you can," Captain Martinson voiced with careless sarcasm. She turned quickly and left me to my thoughts. I definitely had something to think about. After all, the Americans were supposed to be the good guys.

Later that same day I also received a visit from Doctor Gilmore. She wrote the following note in my chart: *Patient complains of headache and tachycardia and anorexia and mild flank pain this am. Stated he knew this would happen because of a shift in the winds from north to the south. This was verified via weather report. However as day progressed the winds shifted from south back to north and symptoms resolved except for his mild chronic anorexia.*

One evident difference exists between what I actually told Doctor Gilmore and what she wrote down. I did not find out that the wind was coming from the south until after I became ill. Doctor Gilmore, on the other hand, insinuated that I became ill after discovering the direction of the wind. This was more supportive to her psychiatric diagnosis. I did know that winds were supposed to become northerly later that day, but knowing that was not what made me feel better.

Perhaps the most depictive disclosure of my complaints associated with wind direction occurred on December sixteenth. The nurse's note includes the following: *Reports vague complaints that woke him up at 0430 (slight dyspneic, fast pulse) but these resolved now. Still feels 'sick.' Refers to winds blowing from direction of the Philadelphia Naval Shipyard directly into this ward. Physically stable now. Continues to believe cyanide is in environment and causing his symptoms. Accept patient's belief matter-of-factly. Maintain patient's trust in staff.*

This note reveals how the medical personnel were probably directed to manage me. They were to sympathetically listen to what I said, but were not to believe it. As it turned out, some of them believed me anyway. Some of them, in fact, experienced symptoms similar to mine. Not all those who experienced symptoms, though, were courageous enough to confide with me.

Shortly after my discharge from the hospital, I found out that another patient besides myself experienced ill symptoms on December sixteenth. The patient was an infant placed on another ward at the Philadelphia Naval Hospital for a respiratory problem. On the sixteenth, this infant experienced apparent seizures and passed out. The infant was rushed to a children's hospital and placed in intensive care. She was eventually diagnosed with fulminant, toxic hepatitis—cause unknown. Notably, she recovered quite rapidly after removal from the Philadelphia Naval Hospital and transport to a hospital more distant from the naval base. This occurred on the very day that a nurse somewhat sardonically noted my claim that pollution from the direction of the base was affecting the hospital environment.

I was befriended during my hospitalization by Chaplain Baggott, a chaplain who visited our ward from time to time. He listened with concerned interest when I told him my naval physicians were trying to stick me with a psychiatric diagnosis. Before long, he had me taking some prescribed psychiatric tests. The results of these tests, he said, might not carry much weight with naval authorities—but it was worth a try. As it turned out, these test results were strongly opposed to the psychiatric diagnosis finally decided upon by my military superiors.

The military psychiatrist who finally yielded a diagnosis that seemed to please Doctor Gilmore and Captain Galasyn was Commander Mangrum. I spoke to another military psychiatrist first, Captain Jacobs, but he basically deferred my diagnosis. I spoke to Commander Mangrum for about an hour and fifteen minutes on the evening of

December twelfth. Interestingly, Commander Mangrum told me that he experienced symptoms such as mine himself, and that no one had definitely diagnosed his problem. When our interview drew to an end, he told me that there was nothing wrong with me psychologically, and that he was going home. I was shocked to later discover that he gave me the diagnosis of *Chronic Paranoid Disorder*. Perhaps the fact that both Doctor Gilmore and Captain Galasyn discussed my case with him before he wrote my diagnosis on December fourteenth had something to do with his apparent change of mind.

[*From my actual hospital record, one of the pages has the following three notes:*

12Dec82 2250 (10:50 pm) Interviewed patient at length on ward tonight from about 2130 to 2245. Very pleasant, verbal, and cooperative. Will give requested opinion after reading patient info. tonight. J. Mangrum, CDR, MC, USN
12/13/82 Pt to have an EEG tomorrow. Will discuss the case with Dr. Mangrum & Dr. G tomorrow. Gilmore
14Dec82 After reviewing the history with Drs. Gilmore and Galasyn, the probability of the patient's beliefs about cyanide poisoning, although presented with much preparation and detail, being delusional are very high. They would not be expected to yield to persuasion. In my opinion, he manifests as Chronic Paranoid Disorder, as defined in DSM-III.

Note that the record indicates that three naval officers discussed my case, two of them commanders, and one of them a captain. A captain, of course, outranks a commander; and Captain Galasyn happens to be the officer who threatened me at the shipyard dispensary.]

I was more than ready for the announcement of my discharge from the hospital on December 17, 1982. Doctor Gilmore made no mention of the Medical Board I would receive a few days later. A Medical Board, in this case, is a document recommending expulsion from the navy on medical grounds. The medical grounds my Medical Board would claim would be: *Paranoia, Chronic, Severe, Unchanged, EPTE.* EPTE mean *existed prior to entry* and serves to exclude the recipient, in this case myself, from any financial benefits. Doctor Gilmore gave me a thirty-day convalescent leave. The only stipulation in the leave was that I had to return in two weeks for an office visit.

Again, there was jubilant reunion when I returned home to my wife. We packed a couple suitcases and gladly left the industrial nesting grounds behind us, or so we thought. As it turned out, the city where we went to visit my brother had about five electroplating plants, and the town where my folks lived boasted a federally-financed penny plant where zinc slugs were plated with copper. It seemed to be rather difficult to sidestep cyanide in eastern U.S. cities. I was able to play some football at my folks, though, which was the first exercise I was able to perform in two or three months. Discovery of the electroplating plants did not occur until a subsequent vacation.

We returned to Philadelphia for my two-week appointment, planning afterwards to visit my wife's family for a couple of weeks in Iowa. Much to my wife's disappointment, Doctor Gilmore informed me that I would have to remain near Philadelphia to receive a pending Medical Board. This meant staying home in Pitman. To make matters worse, western and northern winds were predominant, and my wife's illness in Pitman continued to worsen. To her devoted credit, she made no request to again flee for refuge with her distant family. In time, though, I would be forced to make that decision for her—to prevent her death.

On about January 10, 1983, I received notification that my Medical Board was complete. Seven pertinent paragraphs from the Medical Board follow:

The impression of the medical staff was that there was no identifiable medical illness. There did, however, appear to be a psychiatric condition characterized by a preoccupation with cyanide poisoning as evidenced by his labile symptoms dependent upon the direction the wind was blowing, and of his having begun evaluation of people in the Shipyard, who had no documented exposure to cyanide, as well as the documented negative workup in Houston of those cases that he identified as having cyanide intoxication. The evaluation in Houston was performed by staff members of Baylor Medical College and were found to be negative for cyanide, but positive for an assortment of other medical complaints including galactorrhea, mild hypertension, and mild diabetes.

The service member was seen in psychiatric consultation on 2 December 1982 while on the Medical Inpatient Service. He gave as his chief complaint cyanide poisoning and reported symptoms of tachycardia, decreased appetite, and mild weakness. He presented a detailed history of having discovered cyanide poisoning in Houston, where in 1981 he was working in civilian General Practice, and related it to an electroplating plant. He increasingly came to the belief that many people were affected and had diagnostic tests for cyanide done on a number of patients with a variety of physical symptoms and somatic problems. His interpretation of the laboratory results allegedly confirmed for him the presence of poisoning. He brought this to public attention. A 'Blue Ribbon panel' was established to investigate his charges, reportedly sampled water and air over a three month period, and submitted negative findings. Lt. Oesch claimed the right tests were not used. The Houston Health Department, believing patients were being misdiagnosed and mistreated, is said to have initiated action at that time toward removal of his state medical license. He states that during that time he experienced intermittent depression with suicidal thoughts and saw a civilian physician. (Note: the preceding sentence was a starkly blatant lie, as opposed to more abundant false insinuations. Besides the fact that I never entertained thoughts of suicide, I never saw a civilian physician during my entire illness in Houston. Doctor Hitt, the micro-allergist who tested my wife and me at my request, was not a physician.) [*Dr. Hitt was a Ph.D.*] *He reports never having seen a civilian or other psychiatrist or mental health professional.*

Psychological testing was recommended. This was done and the results submitted 5 January 1982. In summary, 'psychological testing revealed this patient to be defensive, guarded, using rationalization and intellectualization defense mechanism as well as somatic defenses to deal with anxiety, depression, and stress. Strong evidence of psychosis, thought disorder, or paranoia was not found, although this is difficult to state unequivocally due to defensive posture assumed by the patient. Intellectual level appears high.

The Medical Board reviewed the case and the diagnosis is Paranoia, Chronic, Severe, Unchanged, #29710, EPTE; manifested by preoccupation with cyanide poisoning in different locations, the undertaking of repeated tests on patients to determine and prove the presence of such poisoning, denial of any question about the accuracy of his beliefs or interpretation of results, and self treatment.

Precipitating Stress: Minimal (routine duties of military service). Preservice Predisposition: Severe; held same beliefs as at present when working as a civilian General Practitioner in Houston, subjecting numerous patients to tests for cyanide poisoning. His ideas and work were evaluated there and his allegations were considered without merit. Military Impairment: Severe (Unfit for duty). Social Impairment: Considerable. Industrial Impairment: Severe. Follow-up Care: Psychotherapy and possible use of medication if motivation develops and/or if hospitalization appears indicated. He is not recommended for transfer to a VA Hospital at this time because of organization he shows even in the face of his fixed beliefs.

The Medical Board is further of the opinion that the patient is unfit for further military service as a result of physical disability and that his condition was neither incurred in nor aggravated by a period of active duty. The physical disability existed prior to enlistment and has not progressed at a rate greater than is usual for such disorders. Industrial adaptability is essentially as before enlistment. The service member fails to fulfill the minimal standards for enlistment or induction as set forth in A.R. 40-501, Chapter 2. The Medical Board recommends that the service member be discharged in accordance with BUMEDINST 1910.2G.

The Medical Board is further of the opinion that the service member is competent to be discharged to his own custody and at this time does not appear to constitute a menace to himself. Should more evidence of depression arise, short term hospitalization is indicated to facilitate a suitable transition to civilian life. Should that occur, it is recommended that the service member be transferred to a Veteran's Administration Hospital or another hospital of his choice. He is considered potentially hazardous to the care of patients because of his strong focus on cyanide poisoning and relative disregard of other possible diagnoses or known illnesses. Recommendation is made that states where he holds medical licenses be informed of the findings, opinions, and recommendation of the Medical Board.

In reading the Medical Board, I was amazed at the way an official-appearing document with long sentences could doctor up brazen nonsense. The Medical Board was signed by four individuals: Captain Galasyn, Doctor Gilmore, Captain Martinson, and Captain Jacobs. It was an obvious frame-up. Doctor Gilmore asked me whether I wanted to accept the Medical Board or write a rebuttal. I had no intention of accepting it, but I decided to see what kind of response I would get from Doctor Gilmore by acting undecided.

I looked up at Doctor Gilmore inquiringly. "Well, I certainly don't agree with what's written in there—but I've heard that it usually doesn't do much good to rebut one of these things. They usually just end up doing what they want to anyway. Is that right?"

Doctor Gilmore looked troubled. "You realize we're dealing with your future medical practice here," she stated. Her words seemed to almost astound her, as if she herself were surprised by what she was saying.

"My future medical practice?" I posed.

"Yes. If this Board goes through, you could lose your civilian license to practice medicine. Your whole career may be at stake here."

I sat contemplatively for several seconds. It seemed that Doctor Gilmore did not really have her heart in the Medical Board. Perhaps she had more heart than stripes.

"Well, it's probably the right thing to do anyway, because I sure don't agree with what's written in this Board. I'll write a rebuttal."

Doctor Gilmore seemed relieved.

Chapter 13

```
Mental Status Examination:
Dr. Oesch was neatly and appropriately dressed in a three piece suit.
Initially tense, he relaxed maintaining good eye contact through the
interview. He was friendly, warm, and cooperative. Normal in its
rate rhythm and tone, his speech was spontaneous, coherent and
goal directed. His mood and affect overall was full, expressive and
appropriate. There was no evidence of perceptual disturbances, no
symptoms of depression, no ideas of reference or influence, no
magical thinking or thought incertion or broadcasting. There was no
evidence of derealization or depersonalization. He denied suicidal
idiation. His sensorium was intact, revealing an above average
intelligence and an ability to use abstract thinking and reasoning.
There was no impairment in his judgement.

Summary:
Dr. Oesch is a 28 year old white married male. He presents himself
in a warm friendly manner. There were no abnormalities in his
speech, mood or affect. There was no evidence of a thought disorder
nor of an underlying organic process. He manifested above average
intelligence and an ability to think and reason abstractly. His
judgement ability was intact.

Accessment:
No significant underlying psychopathology detected.

                                   Cheryl L. Sanfacon, M.D.
                                   Psychiatrist
```

Unnerving Apparition

"*That's not true! That's a lie!*" exclaimed my wife. She became rather provoked while reading my Medical Board.

"You've got a point, dear," I agreed. It was somehow refreshing to hear my wife's candid remarks.

"I'm not going to let them get by with this. I'll sit right on President Reagan's front steps if I have to."

That was my wife. Her green eyes sparkled and flashed with determined intensity. On one side was the U.S. Navy, General Electric, and the Houston Health Department; and on the other side sat a five-foot-one-and-a-half-inch female who would not yield an inch of truth. I was thankful to be on her side.

"I've sure got some work to do," I noted. "I only have a few days to write a rebuttal."

"You're going to tell them these are lies, I hope," proposed Melody.

"Yes, but probably not quite in those words."

Melody did not like people denying the existence of an environmental poison that caused her day after day of tortuous illness. She liked it even less when they accused her husband of insanity because he dared to mention the problem. She was definitely an emotional inspiration; there was not an ounce of *give up* in her entire body, despite her ailing physical condition.

I was backed farther and farther into a corner from which there appeared no flight except to fight—or yield to evil, but that was out of the question. Still, I hoped to obtain some cooperation from the military authorities at Philadelphia. Though possibly naïve, I figured that some of my military superiors were perhaps acting in ignorance. After writing a rebuttal that would clearly prove the existence of cyanide intoxication in myself and others, I half-expected to see some objective enlightenment. As things turned out, I learned that my military superiors possessed qualities worse than ignorance.

I purchased a used, electric typewriter from a mall store in Pitman. Fortunately, I took two years of typing while in high school. Utilizing the data I obtained from building forty-one on the base, the information Melody acquired from talking to a medical laboratory in order to obtain laboratory results, and numerous facts that discount several claims in my Medical Board, I soon constructed a seemingly irrefutable rebuttal. I wondered if the rebuttal was too harsh, but my wife thought it was too soft. Perhaps she was right.

My Medical Board rebuttal, dated January 13, 1983, read as follows:

From: LT Timothy Oesch, MC, USNR   *January 13, 1983*
Subj: Medical Board Report; Rebuttal
Saturday morning, December 11, after ten days in ward 1-D of the Philadelphia Naval Hospital, I experienced markedly increased symptoms of cyanide poisoning. These included headache, altered sensorium, shortness of breath, dizziness, weakness in my extremities, and chest pain. Upon request, a corpsman drew a sample of my venous blood. The corpsman noted, as I did, that the venous blood was bright red in color, like arterial blood. This blood was tested by Roche Clinical Laboratories, Inc., and found to contain a serum level of 1.8 mg/dl thiocyanate. Along with my symptoms, I also had verified orthostatic tachycardia that persisted when sitting or standing.

A Breath of Cyanide

Since the normal values listed by Roche Clinical Laboratories, Inc. were for therapeutic management of patients receiving nitroprusside, I called a toxicologist at that laboratory to find out what normal serum levels of thiocyanate are for individuals not on nitroprusside therapy. Normal for adult, male nonsmokers is 0.244 mg/dl. The toxicologist referred me to a report in 'Clinical Toxicology', in case I wished to verify or expound upon the information he gave me. He stated that 79 adult males were tested in obtaining the normal value listed above. The normal level the toxicologist gave me for smokers was 0.837 mg/dl with a standard deviation of 0.279 mg/dl. I am a strict nonsmoker and do not like the smell of cigarette smoke; I avoid breathing smoke from others whenever possible.

I was on absolutely no medication while in the hospital, and my serum thiocyanate level of 1.8 mg/dl was very high. Figuring the serum thiocyanate to have been 1.5 mg/dl higher than normal, and taking into account that thiocyanate is dispersed into the interstitial fluid as well as the serum, this represents 225 mg of thiocyanate in my serum and interstitial fluid. About 100 mg of cyanide are required to generate this quantity of thiocyanate, and 100 mg of cyanide is a very serious dose. The toxicologist at Roche Clinical Laboratories, Inc. also verified that the normal serum thiocyanate level of 0.244 mg/dl would be the proper reference level to use in testing an adult, male nonsmoker for cyanide poisoning.

Besides the symptomatic, objective physical, and laboratory evidence of cyanide poisoning mentioned above, there was also an environment factor consistent with the findings of December eleventh. I had mentioned previously, during my hospitalization, that my symptoms grew much worse when the wind came from the south. There are several electroplating plants that use cyanide located south of the Philadelphia Naval Hospital. Some are reported to be in New Jersey [across the Delaware River]; one is located in the Philadelphia Naval Shipyard. In the early morning of December 11, 1982 the wind in Philadelphia was coming from the southwest at 5 to 7 knots. This persisted from midnight until 0548 am.

There were several occasions in the hospital when my condition grew dramatically worse, and several occasions when my condition very much improved. In every instance, I noted the change in my condition before checking with the weather station to find out the wind direction, not after. Also in each instance, the wind was from the south when I dramatically worsened, and from some other direction when I improved. Thus, the connection of wind direction with my symptoms, since my symptoms came before checking the wind direction, was made on an objective basis, not on a subjective basis.

Two laboratories have found my urine positive for abnormally high levels of urine thiocyanate since I began working at the Philadelphia Naval Shipyard. Though I was taking sodium thiosulfate during the time these tests were taken, an occupational specialist has verified that treatment with sodium thiosulfate does not elevate thiocyanate levels in an individual who is not exposed to cyanide. This makes sense, because free serum cyanide is completely metabolized in the liver of normal individuals, and the availability of additional sulfur could not induce the formation of thiocyanate beyond 100% of the cyanide available for formation of thiocyanate. Only in instances where individuals are significantly affected by cyanide intoxication does sodium thiosulfate prove helpful, and even then, elevated levels are only commensurate to elevated levels of cyanide. Therefore, elevated levels of thiocyanate are not less meaningful nor less pertinent because an individual is taking sodium thiosulfate. [Note: this entire report was notably lengthy and repeated quite a bit of data that is already previously mentioned in this book, so I will partly summarize the content, but I will also include some data that has not been previously mentioned.]

One of the urine thiocyanate tests done on myself was collected at my home in Pitman, New Jersey. It was tested by Bio-Science Laboratories and found to be positive with a urine thiocyanate level of 0.3 mg/100ml. My wife, who does not commute to Philadelphia, was also tested and found positive with a urine thiocyanate level of 0.6 mg/100ml. These tests were both positive according to the reference range of 'NORMAL UNDER 0.2' printed on the report and ascertained by a toxicologist at Bio-Science Laboratories.

The other [on myself] urine thiocyanate test was performed on urine actually collected at the dispensary located on the Philadelphia Naval Shipyard. In fact, I purposely collected the urine a day or two after a visit to the industrial section of the shipyard [the "test received" date on the laboratory report is 11/24/82], following which I experienced increased symptoms of cyanide intoxication. This urine was tested by National Medical Services and found to have a level of

A Breath of Cyanide

21 mcg/ml thiocyanate [this would be 2.1 mg/100ml]. While ill with chronic cyanide poisoning in Houston, my urine was tested by National Medical Services and found to have a level of 6 mcg/ml thiocyanate. Although the level from the Houston test was above normal for a nonsmoker, it was obviously far less than the urine tested from Philadelphia. This level, 21 mcg/ml, is over five times higher than the upper limit of normal for nonsmokers given by the toxicologist at National Medical Services.

[Skipping now to another paragraph of interest.] Urine was collected from nine civilian patients at the shipyard on November 22, 23, and 24. [I would later have results from thirteen civilians at the shipyard; and including me, two military members.] All nine patients suffered from symptoms of chronic cyanide poisoning, varying from mild to moderately severe. Careful history as to the amount of smoking by each patient during the preceding week was taken, but this information has not yet been retrieved for use in reporting. The information was written on the laboratory request slips. Information about recent smoking, therefore, must mostly be estimated from histories given in the patient charts. The majority of these patients, however, were selected for screening because of no significant use of tobacco during the preceding week. This enables much more sensitivity and makes results easier to interpret.

According to patient records, two of the nine patients smoke 10 cigarettes daily, which amounts to one-half-pack of cigarettes. One of these patients yielded a urine thiocyanate of 5 mcg/ml, and the other a urine thiocyanate of 21 mcg/ml. Another patient reportedly smoked cigars only. To the best of my memory, he had smoked only one cigar during the preceding week. His urine thiocyanate level was 19 mcg/ml. Still another patient was reportedly a pipe smoker, his level was 6 mcg/ml urine thiocyanate. Two of the reported nonsmokers had levels less than 5 mcg/ml urine thiocyanate, and the third a level of 13 mcg/ml urine thiocyanate. The eighth patient had no mention of smoking in his chart, and yielded a level of 11 mcg/ml urine thiocyanate. Finally, the ninth patient was confirmed as a nonsmoker before resorting to chart records, and had a level of 6 mcg/ml.

[Next comes extensive details regarding Chester Parkins, the gentleman who had severe symptoms of cyanide intoxication and received positive testing through a civilian hospital, mentioned previously.]

On page seven of the Medical Board Report [not previously mentioned], it is reported that air sampled in the dispensary measured 0.0009 part per million HCN. From what I was told, this was the lowest amount of HCN, found in the air, of several tests taken at the shipyard. The highest level reported, to my knowledge, was about one part per million. Depending on the method of air sampling, this may be significant. Despite the strengths or weaknesses of the air sampling, however, patient testing at the shipyard was definitely positive for cyanide. Wind direction on December 2, incidentally, was from the north and northwest until afternoon, then from the southeast, then the west, and finally steady from the southeast at 1852 until midnight.

[Note: I mentioned the northern winds on the morning of December 2, 1982 in the preceding paragraph because that is the morning that air samples were collected by the naval environmental department at the shipyard to be tested for cyanide. Northern winds may have blown the pollution south of the Delaware River rather than north over the shipyard. Also, the only air level of cyanide recorded in my Medical Board was the lowest level reported by the laboratory that performed the tests.]

[Next comes more about my symptoms and wind direction.]

Also on page one [of the Medical Board] begins information supplied by the Houston Health Department. This department tried very hard to deny the cyanide contamination in Houston, but evidence accumulated against them. At least six, major, medical laboratories reported objective levels of blood cyanide, serum thiocyanate, or urine thiocyanate that are above the upper limits of their own stated normal values. Other doctors identified additional patients suffering from cyanide poisoning, and also acquired additional, positive lab tests. A large law firm employed private, environmental investigation that yielded positive findings, and a class action lawsuit is underway. Considering the lawsuit and the apparently culpable posture of the Houston Health Department, nothing attributed to my present case by the Houston Health Department should be considered veritable or usable. The Director of the Houston Health Department has now resigned. [She apparently resigned in 1983.]

[*Next comes data on my symptoms, including some low blood pressures and low-grade fevers, and my good response and ability to work in regard to taking antidotes to cyanide.*]

On page six [*of the Medical Board*] are a couple rather significant factors. The fact that I did not consider cyanide poisoning until the end of my first hospitalization, and that I searched ardently for some other etiology of illness in myself as well as other similarly afflicted individuals at the shipyard, does not characterize a preoccupation with cyanide poisoning. In actuality, the problem may have been considered sooner, but I was unaware that industrial cyanide compounds were utilized in the vicinity. The fact that my symptoms worsen or improve dependent on wind direction is very much in keeping with the major process of environmental cyanide contamination described in the included article, 'Metropolitan Effects of Environmental Cyanide.'

Regarding the cyanide poisoning in Houston, there are pertinent factors that should not be ignored. Certain committees, including a 'Blue Ribbon panel,' conducted given operations by request of the Houston Health Department. Much of the information interpreted by these committees was supplied by the Houston Health Department. As mentioned previously, the Houston Health Department is now in a precarious position legally, the director has resigned, and information they provide regarding myself would be questionable.

Another statement toward the end of page six, that I saw a civilian physician in Houston, is not true. Furthermore, although my illness with cyanide was at times severe, I never entertained thoughts of suicide. Then finally, it was a patient who brought the cyanide problem in Houston to public attention, not me. I do not say this necessarily to my credit, but it is a fact that was misrepresented by the Houston Health Department and is again misrepresented on page six of my Medical Board Report.

On page eight it is stated that I ran repeated tests on patients to prove the presence of poisoning. The fact is, I never ordered more than one test from any patient at the shipyard [remember that the tests for Chester Parkins were ordered by an outside, civilian doctor] for cyanide testing except for one individual. That person had two tests ordered, a urine thiocyanate and a serum thiocyanate. He claimed to smoke from three to five cigarettes total in a day's time. His urine thiocyanate level was 11 mcg/ml, and I do not know the result of his serum thiocyanate. This particular patient was active duty military. Even regarding myself, I only ordered one test from the shipyard for cyanide testing. That was a test for urine thiocyanate, as mentioned previously.

Toward the center of page eight, it is stated that my ideas and work were evaluated in Houston and considered without merit. None of the attorneys that I know of, including the major law firm that is pursuing a class action lawsuit, demanded any commission from their clients other than on a contingency basis. Considerable expense was involved in obtaining proper environmental evaluation, yet the expense was provided at the cost of the law firm. This exemplifies the fact that the evidence at hand was considered significantly positive. In addition, other health professionals not only acquired additional positive testing for cyanide, but expressed admiration of my willingness to act on behalf of a large number of people suffering from medically substantiated cyanide poisoning.

A last comment regarding page eight addresses the statement that my physical disability was not incurred nor aggravated by a period of active duty. During the month I spent in transit between Houston and Philadelphia, the symptoms I suffered from chronic cyanide poisoning in Houston subsided. As when I moved to Houston in 1981, the symptoms of chronic cyanide poisoning began and progressed very slowly after moving to Philadelphia. Letters written in the early weeks after my arrival in Philadelphia, including one written to my attorney in Houston, clearly state that I was feeling well, had gained up to 157½ lbs., and was working out five days a week athletically. Records at the nautilus workout center sponsored by special services, Naval Support Activity, should evidence when I was working out, when my illness progressed to the point that I began missing workouts, and when workouts ceased. The center is located on the base. Furthermore, employees at the center should be able to verify the extent of strenuous physical exercise I was able to perform during my first weeks in Philadelphia. This is because I worked out regularly, and because my physical abilities, when I am well, are far above average and therefore noticeable to observers. Members are required to sign in before each workout.

[*Next, I reiterate how my symptoms began prior to finding out about the cyanide pollution, and I go on to describe what I found when I inspected building forty-one at the shipyard.*]

[*My rebuttal concluded with the following:*] Most of the above information regarding potential cyanide output [*regarding building forty-one*] was presented to a representative of the Department of Environmental Health, a branch of the Naval Regional Medical Center, on November 24, 1982.

Sincerely,
LT Timothy Oesch, MC, USNR

At the time I wrote the preceding rebuttal, I still did not have copies of the urine thiocyanate test results that I ordered at the dispensary. [*Remember that my wife called the laboratory and obtained some of the results by phone.*] Later events disclosed that the tests were probably kept from me purposely. Not only were the test results withheld from my office, they were not even placed in the charts of the patients for whom they were ordered. Fortunately, I smelled a rat, so to speak, long before writing my rebuttal. I slipped up to the dispensary laboratory and found most of the patients' names. My wife then obtained their test results by calling the laboratory.

Without possession of the laboratory orders for urine thiocyanate, I did not know which of the patients were smokers and which were not. Attempts to reach the patients by public telephone proved futile. Knowing that it was vital to find out whether or not the patients smoked in order to interpret their lab results, I called the dispensary and requested the patients' smoking histories from their charts. I had several friends at the dispensary, and their help provided usable data. More precise information was obtained later.

Besides being the date on my rebuttal, January thirteenth was an important date regarding the cyanide contamination in Pitman. On that date, my wife and I drove north for about two hours to meet with health officials at the New Jersey State Health Department in Trenton, New Jersey. Our appointment was at 2:30 in the afternoon. After we arrived, my wife and I were split up and sent to different offices. I met with a physician named Doctor Chowsky.

Little did I know that the State Health Department was interviewing me to screen for a psychological problem. Someone had spoken to them before my arrival. For over an hour Doctor Chowsky belittled my claims and tried to dissuade my beliefs about cyanide contamination. He displayed his own lack of knowledge on the subject at several points, once even stating that hydroxocobalamin is not a treatment for cyanide intoxication. This was rather disenchanting since hydroxocobalamin is the foremost treatment for chronic cyanide poisoning mentioned in published literature.

After patiently and painstakingly explaining my assertions to Doctor Chowsky, and correcting his math when he accused one of my calculations of error, Doctor Chowsky finally demonstrated a slight change of heart.

"I don't know whether I should tell you this or not," related Doctor Chowsky, "but we talked to Captain Martinson, the Commanding Officer at the naval base, before you arrived."

"Really," I responded. The preceding hour of obstinate resistance suddenly seemed explained.

"Yes, and she assured us there was nothing to your cyanide story. She said you were basically just a troublemaker and had caused nothing but problems since you arrived at the base."

Despite the cyanide ordeal, it was still rather startling to hear that Captain Martinson referred to me as a troublemaker. If anything, I was probably too passive at times.

"It sounds like she didn't want anyone here to listen to me," I commented.

"You may be right. I've had some training in psychiatry, and whatever you are, you're definitely not paranoid," stated Doctor Chowsky.

I was glad to hear Doctor Chowsky grant me a clean bill of health regarding paranoia, but there was still the problem of cyanide contamination. "There's been a lot of attention directed toward me, fussing over whether I'm crazy or not crazy, but how is my mental condition going to affect the objective presence of cyanide?" I posed. "I'm not asking anyone to take my word on this issue, there are objective test results from six or seven major laboratories."

Doctor Chowsky stewed over the matter intently. "Let's say you're right. There is still a lot of work to be done, there need to be several papers written on the subject...how would you feel about me writing those papers?"

A Breath of Cyanide

This was certainly a new approach. First Doctor Chowsky denied the very existence of cyanide contamination, then he turned around and asked how I would feel about him writing papers on the subject. Just in case there was some sincerity to his proposal, I gave him all the encouragement I could.

"I don't mind you writing papers. You can write all the papers you want to. I'll even help you—I'll answer any questions and give you all the information I have," I replied. There was no real certainty in my mind about Doctor Chowsky's motivation. He seemed enthralled with the prospect of publishing scientific articles, maybe more so than with the idea of relieving human suffering. On the other hand, perhaps he was continuing his psychiatric probing. Nonetheless, whatever the case, I welcomed the thought of another physician helping to bring badly needed recognition to a serious health problem.

"Of course you'll be recognized as the first one to discover the problem," added Doctor Chowsky. "That's obvious."

"Fine."

It was two full hours after entering Doctor Chowsky's office before we finished our discussion. Doctor Chowsky agreed to order urine thiocyanate tests on my wife and me, and urine specimens were obtained from both of us before we left. Soon after leaving, my wife let me know that she was very displeased with the treatment she received from the physician who interviewed her. "He acted like I was making the whole thing up, or like I didn't know what I as talking about," she remarked with disgust. I did not doubt her in the least.

Doctor Chowsky told me that we would receive the results of our urine thiocyanate tests in a couple weeks. The urine samples were sent to Metpath Laboratories, Inc. Over a month later I was still waiting to receive the results. I wrote the following note to the New Jersey State Department of Health:

Dear Sir: (or Ma'am)

My wife and I had blood and urine specimens (urine only on myself) taken at your facility on January 13, 1983. Please mail me copies of the results of testing on those specimens to my home at the following address: [I then wrote my address in Pitman.]

I am enclosing $5°° to cover costs of copying and mailing; any excess may be donated to your facility.

Thank You,

Timothy Oesch, M.D.

About one week later the health department sent me the following reply:

> *Dear Dr. Oesch:*
> *I'm sorry but we cannot find any record of your tests.*
> *I am returning your check with this note.*
> *Sorry we couldn't be of any help.*
> *NJSDH*

Needless to say, I got a sick feeling in the pit of my stomach as I read the report. This was a far cry from the cooperation I hoped to receive from the health department. As in Houston, the health department proved more hindering than helpful. I called Metpath Laboratories, Inc. and asked if they would give me the laboratory results directly. The laboratory agreed to do so, but said that they would need a reference number from the health department in order to find the results in their computer. I called the health department three times, but they would not give me the reference number requested by Metpath Laboratories, Inc. to aid in finding my laboratory results. To this date, I still do not know the outcome of those tests.

On January 14, 1983, I decided to expand my own investigation of the cyanide contamination in Pitman. With a considerable amount of encouragement, including paying for the test myself, I finally persuaded Leighann Deere to have a urine thiocyanate test. Since I was not licensed in New Jersey, acquiring the test was more complicated than in Houston. Mrs. Deere was experiencing a few symptoms of cyanide intoxication, but the only way she would agree to have her urine tested was on behalf of my wife's illness. I told Mrs. Deere that a positive test found in our next-door neighbor would help confirm the environmental origin of my wife's illness. On those grounds, Mrs. Deere agreed to be tested.

Doctor Williams, a physician in a nearby town, ordered Mrs. Deere's urine thiocyanate test. A special effort was made to send the urine sample to a laboratory other than National Medical Services since National Medical Services still had no reference value for urine thiocyanate levels in nonsmokers. Furthermore, I suspected some sort of political tie between National Medical Services and the naval base in Philadelphia. In time, these suspicions proved substantial.

Mrs. Deere's urine sample was sent to SmithKline Laboratory. As it turned out, SmithKline Laboratory performed serum thiocyanate tests but not urine thiocyanate tests. The urine specimen was forwarded to National Medical Services. A few days later I received the result. The urine thiocyanate level was significantly positive at 8.0 mcg/ml, but the reference value was listed as *up to 20 mcg/ml* for a nonsmoker.

I was disgusted. After all the work performed in order to obtain a urine thiocyanate test on Mrs. Deere, National Medical Services adjusted their reference value to make the test appear normal. Considering that precisely the same reference value was used previously to include smokers, the application of the value to a nonsmoker was obviously wrong. Furthermore, the value was ten times higher than that listed for nonsmokers by other laboratories. Obviously, the reference value had more political basis than medical basis.

Sometime in January I received a newspaper clipping in the mail. I believe my father-in-law found the article while reading a newspaper at his home in Iowa. Three paragraphs in the clipping related to the State of New Jersey. Those paragraphs, taken from a Cedar Rapids newspaper, read as follows:

The committee report included several tales of bungled law enforcement in New Jersey, which generates more toxic waste than any other state. Testimony cited delays, listless investigation and misrepresentations of progress by the Inter-Agency Hazardous Waste Strike Force, which received $1.5 million in federal funding between 1978 and 1981.

Witnesses also provided evidence that the Istellois, Preivone, and Blastell [fictionalized names] families control toxic waste disposal in the state, the report said.

The panel recommended that the FBI initiate prosecutions without waiting for EPA referrals and that state police do more to help halt trucks that carry the wastes.

In light of the disquieting newspaper article, the deviant behavior of the New Jersey State Department of Health dwindled any hopes of help from them. I called National Medical Services and inquired about the basis of the *up to 20 mcg/ml* reference value that they listed for urine thiocyanate in a nonsmoker. A toxicologist there told me that the reference value was based on an article in *Archives of Biochemistry and*

BioPhysics, Vol. 39, pp. 292-299, printed in 1952. I found the article in a library and noted that no mention whatsoever was made as to whether the subjects tested were smokers or nonsmokers. Furthermore, the method used to measure thiocyanate was an earlier method that tended to give falsely elevated levels in the urine.

To discover that a medical laboratory makes an occasional error is worrisome, but to discover that they purposely forward false information is ominous. No matter how ill a patient may be, correct objective data from a medical laboratory is important in designating a particular etiology. My next-door neighbor looked at her laboratory result and concluded that she had a negative test, when in fact it was notably positive. All the difficulty of ordering the right test on the right person at the right time was foiled by a single stroke of prevarication. National Medical Services presented a threat to the disclosure and solution of a serious problem, perhaps more so than the naval and health departments combined. Objective testing could disprove subjective claims of the health department and naval base, but National Medical Services tampered with the objective data itself. [*Of note, my more recent experience with National Medical Services has definitely been more positive than my experiences in the 1980s. In fact, National Medical Service is now my first choice for having urine thiocyanate testing performed. I was very pleased and encouraged when I recently went onto their internet site and discovered that their "Reporting Limit" for urine thiocyanate is now 0.10 mcg/ml. They give a somewhat high reference range for urine thiocyanate in nonsmokers; namely, "usually less than 3.6 mcg/ml"; but this may simply reflect the fact that it is now "normal" for us to be inhaling some cyanide. The reference range they give for urine thiocyanate in smokers is, "usually less than 15 mcg/ml." A copy of the first page from a sample, positive report from their laboratory, presenting a very high urine thiocyanate level of 50 mcg/ml, follows:*

A Breath of Cyanide

NMS Labs
200 Welsh Road, Horsham, PA 19044-2208
Phone: (215) 657-4900 Fax: (215) 657-2972
e-mail: nms@nmslabs.com
Robert A. Middleberg, PhD, F-ABFT, DABCC-TC, Laboratory Director

CONFIDENTIAL

Demo Report

Report Issued 03/30/2020 13:32
Last Report Issued 03/25/2019 07:14

88888
Clinical Example Report
Attn: Example Reports
200 Welsh Road
Horsham, PA 19044

Patient Name 4440U-POS
Patient ID 4440U-POS
Chain 19000264
Age Not Given   DOB Not Given
Gender Not Given
Workorder 19000264

Received 02/01/2019 08:55

Sample ID 19000264-001
Matrix Urine
Patient Name 4440U-POS
Patient ID 4440U-POS
Container Type Clear vial

Collect Dt/Tm Not Given
Source Not Given

Approx Vol/Weight Not Given

Receipt Notes   None Entered

Analysis and Comments	Result	Units	Reporting Limit	Notes
4440U Thiocyanate, Urine				
Analysis by High Performance Liquid Chromatography/Tandem Mass Spectrometry (LC-MS/MS)				
Thiocyanate	50	mcg/mL	0.10	ELEVATED
CDC/NHANES (2013-2014) U.S. general adult population: Non-smokers: Usually less than 3.6 mcg/mL Smokers: Usually less than 15 mcg/mL				
Thiocyanate (Creatinine corrected)	10	mg/g Creat	0.020	
CDC/NHANES (2013-2014) U.S. general adult population: Non-smokers: Usually less than 3.7 mg/g creatinine Smokers: Usually less than 16 mg/g creatinine				
Analysis by Colorimetry (C)				
Creatinine	5000	mg/L	100	ELEVATED
U.S. Population (10th - 90th percentiles, median) All participants: 335 - 2370 mg/L, median 1180 (n=22,245) Males: 495 - 2540 mg/L, median 1370 (n=10,610) Females: 273 - 2170 mg/L, median 994 (n=11,635)				

This test was developed and its performance characteristics determined by NMS Labs. It has not been cleared or approved by the US Food and Drug Administration.

Results for sample 19000264-001 are continued on next page

Page 1 of 2   NMS v.40.0

As can be seen from the preceding, sample report, great progress has been made by National Medical Services in regard to urine thiocyanate testing.]

I visited a medical library in a neighboring state and researched the matter of urine thiocyanate reference values. Literature on the subject was strongly in support of Metpath Laboratories, Inc. and Bio-Science

Laboratories, which both listed reference values only one-tenth of that listed by National Medical Services. I again called a toxicologist at National Medical Services and told him what I discovered about the article they claimed as the source of their of their urine thiocyanate level. He offered no argument. Then I conveyed more pertinent information which I found at the library and pointed out that other laboratories gave values consistent with the literature—namely a reference value for urine thiocyanate in nonsmokers of *up to 2 mcg/ml*. The toxicologist thanked me for the information and indicated that they would correct the reference value.

Time passed and a bill arrived in Mrs. Deere's mailbox for her urine thiocyanate test. I responded to the bill by sending the following letter to the hospital where she had the test:

Payment for the urine thiocyanate test performed on Leighann Deere, patient number 87325293 [fictitious number], dated 1/14/83, is being withheld at my request pending correction of the reference value for urine thiocyanate in nonsmokers. The reference value printed by National Medical Services was 'up to 20 mcg/ml' for nonsmokers; this is in error. Bio-Science Laboratories and Metpath Laboratories, Inc. both state 2 mcg/ml as the upper limit of normal in nonsmokers, as verified by examples of lab reports from those laboratories. This is only one-tenth of the value given by National Medical Services. An enclosed article discloses the average urine thiocyanate level in nonsmokers as indeed below 2 mcg/ml, and the following article gives average urine thiocyanate levels in smokers. It is obvious from reading the articles that the reference value of up to 20 mcg/ml applies to moderate to heavy smokers, not to nonsmokers.

Two other articles are enclosed that regard chronic cyanide poisoning. As noted in the first article, the levels of thiocyanate generated from smoking may surpass the levels generated by cyanide from an industrial, environmental source that is causing chronic cyanide poisoning in an individual. It is very important, then, that Mrs. Deere have proper reference values for evaluating possible exposure to environmental cyanide. This is true not only from a medical standpoint, but also from a medicolegal standpoint and for community health.

Some time ago I contacted National Medical Services about their listing of 20 mcg/ml as a reference value for urine thiocyanate in nonsmokers. They conceded that the reference value needed to be corrected. I do not believe Mrs. Deere should be held responsible for any payment until a corrected report is received by Doctor Williams and/or myself, and made available to her. I would appreciate notice when such has been accomplished.

Sincerely,
Timothy Oesch, M.D.

The lab reports included with the preceding letter were performed during the spring of 1982, giving an up-to-date reference level for urine thiocyanate of zero to 2 mcg/ml. Accompanying literature included articles from *Clinical Chemistry,* 25(5):678-81, May 1979; *Archives of Environmental Health,* Vol. 5, July, 1962; *Laboratory Diagnosis of Diseases Caused by Toxic Agents,* edited by F. W. Sunderman and F. W. Sunderman, Jr.; and *Industrial Toxicology,* Hamilton and Hardy, Third Edition, Publishing Sciences Group, Inc., 1974. This information clearly established the inadequacy of National Medical Services' falsely elevated reference level for urine thiocyanate in nonsmokers. I anticipated a correction of the reference value, but all Mrs. Deere received was additional bills. Finally, in order to prevent any damage to Mr. and Mrs. Deere's credit rating, I paid the bill despite the failure of the laboratory and hospital to provide a corrected report.

January fourteenth was a gravely momentous day. For weeks my wife's health had worsened, but she remained perseveringly at my side. On this particular evening we sat together on a sofa watching television. Melody was quite ill. She was experiencing sensations she had never known before.

"Oh...it's coming back," lamented Melody, holding a clenched hand to her breast.

"You'd better lie down," I advised.

Melody lay down on the sofa and I sat on the floor.

"Does that help any?" I asked.

"It's not as bad, but it's still there. It feels like someone is pushing down inside my chest. It hurts worse if I try to sit up."

I knew firsthand what uncanny feelings distressed my wife's mind. The pains of a cyanide infested heart are practically identical to those of coronary insufficiency. Memory of blue-tinged fingernails infused my thinking. I lifted Melody's hand and pressed against her nails; the color was still good.

"I'll get you some alphaREDISOL. I'll put it in some juice," I said.
"I don't know if I can drink any right now," remarked Melody.
"Well, just do your best."

After months of living with repeated bouts of cyanide exposure, I was used to seeing my wife endure trying episodes of illness. We lived with the constant hope that the environmental poisoning would somehow be recognized and corrected. This night was different. Melody's chest pain continued relentlessly, keeping her awake in bed until about three o'clock in the morning. I considered taking her to an emergency room. When morning finally came, I lost no time having Melody contact her mother in Iowa.

My mother-in-law arrived in Philadelphia by jet and I drove her to our home in Pitman. The next morning, January sixteenth, my wife's car served as the vehicle to transport her and her mother to Iowa. I did not send her away simply because she was ill, I sent her away because I feared for her physical life. The following letter prepared by my father-in-law on March 16, 1983, describes Melody's condition upon her arrival in Iowa:

TO WHOM IT MAY CONCERN
The purpose of this letter is to express my evaluation of my Daughter's (Mrs. Melody Oesch) physical condition in mid-January 1983...

My wife took a flight to Philadelphia on January 15, 1983 in response to a phone call from our daughter, Melody, describing her illness and physical condition, relating to a positive blood test for Cyanide.

They arrived in Iowa on the 17th of January, by automobile.

Melody's appearance was frightening from the standpoint of the last time I had visited with her in August of 1982 right after her arrival in New Jersey.

Melody had lost a considerable amount of weight and her clothes appeared to be much too large for her, hanging loosely on a gaunt frame.

Her color was very pale and she looked as though she hadn't rested for weeks. She was nauseated and suffering from pains and headaches.

Her hair was almost straight and had a very dull appearance.

When she tried to eat, even the sight of food would make her ill.
She didn't have enough energy to sit up except for very short periods of time.
I sat and cried and prayed for her condition when I was by myself.
We coaxed her to eat, took her to a beautician to attempt to restore her hair, and exposed her to clean air and sunshine along with a lot of Parental love and affection.
Her beautician found a coating on her hair, but was unable to identify the source.
Melody gradually regained some of her lost weight, and her overall appearance was greatly improved.
Her energy level was improved but still needed to come to a higher level to allow her to return to her normal activities.
Melody returned to Philadelphia in late February after spending about six weeks with us in Iowa.
We are still deeply concerned about her overall health and feel that any change in her continued improvement would be an indication of her exposure to Cyanide in the air and would require her to be tested for such.

With my wife about a thousand miles west of me, I set myself about the business of selling our home. Friends of mine where I attended church in Pitman informed me about nearby electroplating plants—so I knew I would have to move before bringing my wife back. The nearest electroplating plant turned out to be about one and one-half miles northwest of our house, which explained why we were ill when winds came from the north or west. Five more plants were located several miles north of us.

One of my friends at church, Terry Flanders, actually served as an engineer at an electroplating plant several miles west of Pitman. He was very interested in the information I had accumulated about chronic cyanide intoxication. I told Terry about the electroplating plant I had inspected at the naval base, and he said they were certainly violating state regulations by expelling cyanide waste directly into the sewer without treatment. One thing that should have concerned Terry was his own health. He had recently started having seizures of unknown etiology and had his driver's license suspended. In addition to this, another young man where Terry worked mysteriously died of a *heart attack* without any previous heart disease. He died in his sleep.

Perhaps the most concerned individual I knew in Pitman was Mrs. Catherine Lawton. There was good reason for her to be concerned—she suffered blatant symptoms of cyanide intoxication. Besides headaches, nervousness, forgetfulness, hair loss, and tiredness, she had episodes of severe muscle weakness. One time the muscles in her legs became so weak that she was unable to walk up a stairway. Her doctor treated her with sedatives.

Mrs. Lawton did not receive a test for serum or urine thiocyanate. I was willing to order the test for her, which I could do so long as I did not charge money or prescribe treatment—not having a medical license in New Jersey. With a lack of support from her husband, though, who did not seem inclined to believe that an invisible substance in the air was causing his wife's illness, Mrs. Lawton was fearful about having a test done. It seemed that the possibility of a negative result threatened her: those who claimed her illness was psychological in origin might use a negative test result to harass her further. I explained that negative test results were not at all conclusive in cyanide intoxication, and that only a portion of the tests performed would turn out positive; and that a positive test, on the other hand, was quite conclusive for cyanide exposure—but she still failed to acquire a test. Nonetheless, it was Mrs. Lawton who first informed me about the electroplating plant on the northwest side of Pitman, and who invited me to a Pitman Township environmental meeting. She was a member of a small group that met together and discussed environmental problems in the area. The primary topic of discussion was a landfill.

Mrs. Lawton hoped to recruit some aid in dealing with the cyanide contamination in Pitman through Mr. Frank Joules. She spoke to Mr. Joules before inviting me to the environmental meeting. Mr. Joules expressed some interest and agreed to talk with me, but he did not want anyone to bring up the subject at the meeting. He was afraid the existence of such a problem might interfere with *superfund* money designated toward work on the landfill by the EPA. Apparently millions of dollars were supposed to come to Pitman for work on the landfill.

The meeting reeked with irony. Argument as to whether the chemicals dumped into the landfill should be toted away, or cemented and fenced in, passed back and forth. Toting the chemicals away was obviously a better idea, but more expensive. Meanwhile, measurement of pollutants in water draining off the landfill revealed diminishing levels. If anything was going to be done to prevent pollution, it should have been done years before. Still, I did not object to cleaning up the dump site. What I did object to was the ignoring of a dire air pollutant that swept through the community. It seemed like inoculating a drowning man for chickenpox.

Not long after the environmental meeting, I met with Mr. Joules at his home. Mr. Joules criticized the state health department harshly and warned me not to associate with them. What he did not warn me about was himself. Just weeks after our meeting it was disclosed that he forged his college diplomas and was acting as some sort of charlatan. There was very little if any political progress made in Pitman. Whether or not the millions of dollars poured into the town for work on the landfill, I do not know.

A record snowfall blanketed Pitman after my wife's departure. Due to failing health, I was obliged to hire two teenagers to shovel snow off my driveway so I could back my car out of the garage. Less than two years before, I competed in collegiate track. [*When I attended Bob Jones University for advanced communications during the spring of 1981, I competed in an intramural track meet for my fraternity.*] Inhaling environmental cyanide, at least in my case, transformed an athlete into an invalid—and I was probably not the only one.

Catherine Lawton informed me that she had never seen so many people die of heart attacks in Pitman, and expressed her concern for a young boy who was disabled by mysteriously weakening muscles. This followed one of the most frightful experiences of my life. Although I was less concerned about my own health than my wife's health, I still suffered significantly in Pitman. Sodium thiosulfate was a regular component of my diet, and I took alphaREDISOL from time to time when my symptoms worsened. Some of the worst spells I experienced came during the early morning. Perhaps this was partially due to several hours passing since taking any antidote to cyanide intoxication.

One morning I awoke at about 3:00 am. My wife was in Iowa. Labored breathing and a swimming sensation imposed themselves upon my consciousness; a heavy, dull feeling of suffocation hung in my chest. I rose and stumbled to the bathroom where a container of sodium thiosulfate sat in the medicine cabinet. The fluorescent light in the bathroom was rather dim, but it still served to disclose an unnerving apparition.

My hand froze in place at the edge of the cabinet mirror. The white of my eyes was not white; the eyes that stared back at me were grossly pink. I looked closer; bright, red blood seeped through the mucous membranes beneath my eyes. Never before had I seen anything like it, not in a patient, not in myself—perhaps I had seen something similar in medical photographs or a late, late show. Horrendous thoughts of anticoagulated blood infiltrating my brain tissue stressed my mind.

Cyanide is known to affect the coagulation system. Animals that die from cyanide poisoning may retain unclotted blood for extended periods, and people with cyanide intoxication may bruise and bleed easily. While in the naval hospital, I recorded symptoms I experienced from December eleventh to December thirteenth on a paper hand towel. The symptoms were recorded as follows: *Saturday morning—acute symptoms (headache, tachycardia, shortness of breath, general achiness); Saturday evening—decreased appetite (ate jello for supper), itchy rash left leg; Sunday morning-joint pain, some lower back pain, muscle twitches, headache, felt weak (much better than Saturday though); Monday morning—nose felt stuffed, left nostril (also had headache), blew nose and blood came out*. Thus, I was acquainted with bleeding tendencies from cyanide intoxication before ever facing the ghastly spectacle in my bathroom mirror.

Somehow, perhaps because cyanide can induce giddiness, I found my terrifying appearance somewhat humorous after recovering from the initial shock. I really did look like someone made up for a Halloween party. It also seemed funny that a modern society of educated citizens could be poisoned day after day, and seemingly preferred slowly dying in consequence more than admitting an ecological error. In actuality, of course, none of these facts were too humorous. The plague of cyanide doubtlessly endowed Pitman with numerous individual tragedies.

I took some sodium thiosulfate, some alphaREDISOL, and even some amyl nitrite. Within thirty minutes to an hour I felt better and my eyes appeared less pinkish. The next day, I called Terry Flanders and inquired about the price of a gas mask to wear while sleeping. He informed me that he could order such a mask for about 125^{\circ\circ}$. Considering the financial burdens facing me with selling our house and my wife's illness, I decided to take my antidote more carefully and put off buying the mask unless I experienced another bleeding episode.

Fortunately, to this point, the episode has been a once-in-a-lifetime experience.

Chapter 14

Congress of the United States
House of Representatives
Washington, D.C. 20515

July 13, 1983

Dear Mr. Secretary:

I have been contacted by my constituent, Timothy R. Oesch, a former resident of Houston now on active duty with the U.S. Navy as a Lieutenant in the Medical Corps.

Inside Help

On January 17, 1983, I reported back to the naval hospital for duty. My medical privileges were taken away from me on the grounds that my illness interfered with my work. Rather than working directly with patients, I was assigned to work in the educational department. It was rather curious that I was given the diagnosis of *paranoia* and then appointed to teach. Teaching is one of the last things someone should be expected to do after being labeled paranoid.

The educational department was located on the eighth deck of the naval hospital. I made friends quickly and thoroughly enjoyed teaching classes to corpsmen, nurses, and physicians. I also sat in on paramedic lectures and learned a few things I never picked up in medical school. My illness still plagued me, but I was able to endure by taking frequent doses of sodium thiosulfate. My work was gratifying.

The legal department was on the sixth deck, two floors below the educational department. I dropped down one day to ask a question about my income tax. The legal officer, Captain Breach, seemed rather surprised to confront a doctor who he did not know. He struck up a conversation with me and discovered that I was working on the eighth deck rather than treating patients. This intrigued him further, and I soon found myself telling Captain Breach all about my situation.

As a result of my conversation with Captain Breach, I learned that legal services were available to me at the naval base. Soon an appointment was set up for me to speak with two military attorneys,

Lieutenant Brooks and Lieutenant Norris. Lieutenant Brooks was leaving the military in April, so Lieutenant Norris followed my case to take over after Lieutenant Brooks departed. There was no problem gaining permission from the educational supervisor to take out time for legal appointments. I sent information about my case to Lieutenant Brooks prior to my first appointment.

Lieutenant Brooks was sharp and energetic, a courageous young man about six feet tall and moderately stalky. Lieutenant Norris stood about five feet and five inches high with a bundle of blond hair pinned tightly upon her head. She was skeptical, shrewd, careful, and eventually very helpful. I was fortunate to obtain legal aid from two individuals who demonstrated qualities of motivation other than a desire for military advancement. One of the first suggestions I received was to immediately begin preparing a second rebuttal—my first rebuttal, they said, would almost certainly be rejected.

The first group to consider my first rebuttal included three of the officers who constituted my Medical Board: Captain Galasyn, Captain Jacobs, and Commander Gilmore. Captain Galasyn made no written comment. Captain Jacobs responded by simply stating, *A review of the case has been made and the findings of the Medical Board stand as written.* Commander Gilmore was much more extensive. Her comments, officially classified as a surrebuttal to my rebuttal, were as follows:

The enclosed letter from Dr. Oesch, regarding the validity of his assertions of cyanide exposure, is most representative of the thought processes and behavior for which his is being Boarded.

I've discussed this rebuttal with Dr. Jason Mills, head toxicologist of National Medical Services Laboratory in Willow Grove, Pennsylvania.

He has a copy of Dr. Oesch's comments and is preparing a statement regarding the validity of his comments. Dr. Mills gave me his permission to state that these assertions are totally absurd and without scientific basis. Dr. Mills' prepared statement will be forwarded upon its receipt by this Command.

A light came on in my head when I discovered that Commander Gilmore acquired backing from a toxicologist at National Medical Services. The bizarre reference value forwarded by the laboratory, the inexcusable source given for evaluating nonsmokers, and the failure to correct an admitted error suddenly became more than coincidence. There was a naval base located in the same town as National Medical Services. [*Note also that the calculated flying distance from Willow Grove to Philadelphia is 13 miles. National Medical Service is now apparently located in Horsham, PA, which is about three miles north and somewhat west of Willow Grove.*] I also recalled having a negative report from National Medical Services for urine thiocyanate just one day after a highly positive test for serum thiocyanate from another laboratory. No wonder the Naval Medical Center permitted the utilization of a laboratory that did not even have a specific reference value for urine thiocyanate in nonsmokers—they were apparently more interested in political manipulation than medical veracity.

To pursue my suspicions further, I suggested that Lieutenant Brooks call National Medical Services and directly question them regarding urine thiocyanate reference values. Lieutenant Brooks called the laboratory and was connected with Dr. Mills. Upon questioning, Dr. Mills stated that the reference value for urine thiocyanate in nonsmokers was *up to 20 mcg/ml* and that the reference value for smokers was *up to 50 mcg/ml*. I was astounded, not only by the astronomically high values given, but also by the political ignorance in stating values so plainly erroneous. Before long, National Medical Services recanted on Dr. Mills' statement and claimed that the value of *up to 20 mcg/ml* was for both smokers and nonsmokers, with no specific value for nonsmokers, and that this had been their reference value for a long time—with no recent changes.

Although Commander Gilmore's surrebuttal was dated February 2, 1983, the final rejection of my first rebuttal did not come until March third. The rejection came from Vice Admiral Leo Crowler, Chief of Naval Personnel. With this rejection, I became firmly aware that reason and objective data were not sufficient. The individuals evaluating my reports did not seem sympathetic to rational logic. I would have to accumulate sufficient evidence to override their adverse claims.

If I thought my first rebuttal was conclusive, my second rebuttal seemed ineluctable. With the help of my attorneys, the resources of two medical school libraries, objective test results, and several personal testimonies, I could not imagine anyone reading it and continuing to belittle cyanide intoxication. Lieutenant Norris was less optimistic; she did not think the *established military powers* would pay much mind to the merits of my rebuttal. As it turned out, Lieutenant Norris was more correct than me. My second rebuttal, dated March 29, 1983, read as follows:

From: LT Timothy Oesch, MC, USNR
Subj: Medical Board Report; Second Rebuttal

Table of Contents

1.) Second Rebuttal ... pp. 1-19
2.) Serum thiocyanate Reference Values ... pp. 20-24
3.) Thiocyanate and Blood Cyanide levels ... pp. 25-28
4.) Positive Testing for Cyanide Exposure Among Shipyard Workers ... pp. 29-31
5.) Airborne Cyanide and Urine Thiocyanate Levels ... pp. 32-37
6.) Blood Cyanide Levels ... 38a-38f
7.) Laboratory Result Sheets ... pp. 39-65
8.) Thiocyanate Testing On Myself In Philadelphia ... pp. 66-68
9.) National Weather Service Verification ... pp. 69-75
10.) Sheet From Medical Record (hypogammaglobulinemia) ... pp. 76-77
11.) Cyanide and Hyperventilation ... pp. 78-83
12.) Cyanide and Tachycardia ... pp. 84-98
13.) Cyanide and Symptoms of Coronary Insufficiency ... pp. 99-108
14.) Advised Use of Precautionary hydroxocobalamin ... pp. 109-113
15.) Health Record Information ... pp. 114-126
16.) Symptoms of Chronic Cyanide Poisoning ... pp. 127-131
17.) Factors Pertaining to Chronic Cyanide Poisoning ... pp. 132-133
18.) Entities Associated With Chronic Cyanide Poisoning ... pp. 134-138
19.) Decreased Vision Within Last Year ... pp. 139-150
20.) Chronic Cyanide, Glucose Catabolism, and Diabetes ... pp. 151-159
21.) Miscellaneous Facts About Chronic Cyanide Intoxication ... pp. 160-171

22.) Report from Iowa … pp. 172-173
23.) First Rebuttal … pp. 176-182
24.) 'Metropolitan Effects of Environmental Cyanide' … pp. 183-210

[*This second rebuttal is a lengthy report, and much of it has already been addressed in this book. The written rebuttal itself, namely pages 1 through 19, ended as follows:*]

If the above requests for revocation of a psychiatric diagnosis and affirmation of chronic cyanide intoxication are not granted, then I hereby exercise my right to request a fair hearing.

Sincerely,
LT Timothy Oesch, MC, USNR

Chapter 15

Honorable John F. Lehman, Jr.
July 13, 1983
Page 2

The provisions for the evaluation of a service member's fitness for duty are set out in the Disability Evaluation Manual (SECNAVINST 1850.4A, 30 March, 1982). Foremost among these is a presumption of fitness for duty which can be overcome only by clear and convincing evidence of the member's unfitness. Based on the definition of this standard in the Manual and from the use elsewhere of the evidentiary standard of a preponderance of the evidence, I must presume that these phrases carry their full legal meaning. I question how the Navy diagnosis of Lt. Oesch was found by the R.P.E.B. to have met this high standard of evidence when so many material points were in conflict.

Lt. Oesch's future, not just as a naval officer but also as a physician, is at stake. The decision is not simply one of fitness or unfitness, the Manual clearly empowers the Boards to delay decisions in order to seek better evaluation or to resolve conflicts or questions. The Manual sets out an objective of evaluation under its provisions as "the equitable consideration of the interests of the Government and the individual service members." Therefore, I strongly urge a most scrupulous review of this case by your office and the Physical Review Council.

Thank you very much, and I look forward to hearing from you at your earliest convenience as to any further action taken on this case.

With best wishes, I am

Sincerely

Bill Archer
Member of Congress

Honorable John F. Lehman, Jr.
Secretary of the Navy
Department of the Navy
The Pentagon
Washington, D. C. 20350

Challenge

On March 29, 1983, I hand-carried the following memorandum to the Commanding Officer's secretary:

From: LT Timothy Oesch, MC, USNR
To: Commanding Officer, NRMC Philadelphia
Subj: Redress of Grievances; Request for
Ref: (a) NAVREGS, ART 1106

  (b) UCMJ, ART 138
 1. Pursuant to ref. (a) the following requests are respectfully submitted:
  (a) Revocation of Medical Board with primary psychiatric diagnosis.
  (b) Affirmation of diagnosis of chronic cyanide intoxication based on symptomatology as substantiated by published literature, and based on objective laboratory testing which is definitely positive for cyanide exposure as substantiated by published literature.
 2. In an attempt to have these matters resolved at the lowest level possible, this request is submitted. A failure to redress the regarded grievances may, within about two weeks' time, result in my pursuance of remedies through reference (b).
 Respectfully,
 LT Timothy Oesch, MC, USNR

 Before my Medical Board was ever presented to me, Captain Martinson had to give it her approval. The preceding request gave Captain Martinson a chance to reconsider that approval. I was not sure what to expect from her, but I soon received a strong hint. On April 1, 1983, she signed a letter asking for the termination of my special pay—meaning that she wanted to stop the payment of money that I received for being a physician. This amounted to several hundred dollars a month.

 It was more than clear that I would receive nothing but stubborn resistance from the Command in Philadelphia. On April 12, 1983, I turned in two additional documents to the Commanding Officer's secretary at the naval hospital. One document was a rebuttal to the termination of my special pay, and the other document was a *Request for Redress of Complaint of Wrong Under Article 138, UCMJ*. Our house in Pitman sold in late March, and the costs of selling our house left my wife and me in a poor position for a reduction in pay. Both documents were written with the advice of my military attorneys.

 The rebuttal to the termination of my special pay read as follows:

From: LT Timothy Oesch, MC, USNR
To: Surgeon General

A Breath of Cyanide

Via: Commanding Officer, Naval Regional Medical Center, Philadelphia and Commander,
   Naval Medical Command
Subj: Termination of Additional Special Pay; Rebuttal to
Encl: Request for Redress of Complaint of Wrong Under Article 138, UCMJ

1. Whereas recent forfeiture of substantial financial investment was incurred from sale and evacuation of a home purchased six months previously, forcing acquisition of funds through temporary loan; and
2. Whereas the sale of the home was necessitated by illness from an environmental contaminant, the susceptibility to which is verified on a navy physical given on 08JUN82 prior to active duty at NRMC Philadelphia; and
3. Whereas the Navy assigned placement not only in a region largely polluted by the designated pollutant, but assigned the concerned subject to duty at a location only a few blocks from an industrial operation utilizing the designated pollutant; and
4. Whereas objective laboratory testing, symptomatology, and response to specific antidote definitely and obviously confirmed illness from the designated pollutant; and
5. Whereas NRMC Philadelphia not only failed to take proper action in treating illness from exposure to the designated pollutant, but attempted discharging the concerned subject on primary, psychiatric grounds without any subsequent disability pay or benefits whatsoever; and
6. Whereas a request for redress of complaint of wrong under article 138, UCMJ, has been forwarded, a copy of which follows;
7. It is hereby requested that additional special pay not be terminated.

   Very Respectfully,
   LT Timothy Oesch, MC, USNR

The Article 138 Complaint, which was also enclosed with the preceding rebuttal, read as follows:

From: LT Timothy Oesch, MC, USNR
To: Commander, Naval Base, Philadelphia, Pennsylvania

Via: Respondent, Commanding Officer, NRMC Philadelphia
Sub: Request for Redress of Complaint of Wrong Under Article 138, UCMJ
Ref: (a) Article 138, UCMJ, MCM 1969 (Rev.)
(b) Article 1106, Navy Regs., 1973
(c) Article 1109, Navy Regs.
Encl: (1) Letter of Complaint to Commanding Officer, NRMC Philadelphia, Dated 29March83.
(2) Complaint of Wrong Under Article 138, UCMJ; Two Page Report Giving Supportive, Published Sources.
(3) Supportive Medical Records.

1. Pursuant to references (a), and (b), I, LT Timothy Oesch, MC, USNR, hereinafter referred to as the Complaintant, lodged a Complaint of Wrong with the Commanding Officer, NRMC Philadelphia, hereinafter referred to as the Respondent.

2. Pursuant to reference (b), Complaintant requested redress, in writing, a copy of said request being attached as enclosure (1) and hereby incorporated by reference. Since no action has been taken, and a reasonable time has passed, the complaint is forwarded directly to Respondent's superior.

3. The specific relief requested is:
   (a) Revocation of Medical Board with primary psychiatric diagnosis.
   (b) Affirmation of diagnosis of chronic cyanide intoxication based on symptomatology as substantiated by published literature.

4. The reasons for the request are as follows and are supported by enclosures (2) through (3):
   a. Attempted subterfuge of industrial cyanide pollution.
   b. Misdiagnosis, mistreatment, and potential, negligent homicide.

5. Pursuant to reference (c), a copy of this request has been provided to Respondent.

Very Respectfully,
Lt Timothy Oesch, MC, USNR

The next page was a copy of the memorandum that I turned in to the Commanding Officer's secretary on March 29, and the two pages thereafter read as follows:

A Breath of Cyanide

With an extensive background in diagnosing and treating chronic cyanide intoxication, I came to recognize the presence of such at the Philadelphia Naval Shipyard during the fall of 1982. After ordering a few screening tests, I was confronted by a captain from the environmental department at NRMC Philadelphia. Even though none of the screening tests were back, the captain threatened me when he discovered the tests had been ordered. He told me that I would be admitted to a psychiatric institution if I tested one more person for cyanide exposure. This was obviously demanding that I violate the physician's sworn responsibility to his patients

I decided, rather than reporting the captain's behavior without supportive evidence, to wait until I received the results from the screening tests. To this date, I have not been allowed to see those results, but I know from calls to the laboratory that they positively indicated exposure to environmental cyanide according to published, industrial literature. One of several articles supporting this claim is 'Br J Ind Med' 32(3):215-9, Aug. '75, which gives the formula $M=0.65C$, where M equals milligrams of thiocyanate in urine in 24 hours, and C equals air concentration of cyanide in ppm (parts per million). Using this formula, and taking factors such as smoking into consideration, some of the shipyard employees were evidently exposed to average, workday air concentrations greater than thirty parts per million cyanide prior to their urine thiocyanate tests.

The propensity to develop symptoms or illness from exposure to atmospheric cyanide varies greatly from one individual to another. Persons with lesser resistance to cyanide exposure can be very seriously affected. One factor that has compelled my extensive research of chronic cyanide intoxication, is my own, critical vulnerability to chronic cyanide exposure. After developing illness at the naval shipyard, I had to take antidote for cyanide several times daily in order to prevent debilitating illness. The environmental captain who threatened me initially, further coerced me to stop taking antidote for cyanide intoxication. This was fully enforced when I was admitted to the naval hospital on 02DEC82.

The naval hospital is roughly one mile north of the shipyard. As objective testing on blood drawn ten days after my admittance to the hospital proved, the atmospheric cyanide contamination, at times, reached at least as far as the naval hospital. This is consistent with prior studies on the extent of cyanide contamination from a source in Houston, Texas. Prior to, and during my hospitalization, I fully informed my physician and the medical personnel attending me that I was suffering from chronic cyanide intoxication. This was of little avail, however, since the health personnel were informed beforehand that I was a psychiatric patient, and that they should treat me as such.

My antidote for cyanide intoxication, hydroxocobalamin, was completely withheld during my entire hospitalization from 02DEC82 to 17DEC82. My hospital records clearly reveal that during that period of time I experienced significant symptoms which were completely consistent with cyanide intoxication. These included tachycardia, as explained in 'J Clin Invest' 52:3115-28, Dec. '73; hyperventilation, as explained in 'J Appl Physiol' 39(2):199-204, Aug. '75; symptoms of coronary insufficiency, as explained in 'Cardiovascular Research' 9(1):38-46, Jan '75; and other symptoms such as weakness, altered mental abilities, and gastrointestinal disturbances, as noted in the book, <u>Industrial Toxicology</u>, *Hamilton and Hardy, Third Edition, Publishing Sciences Group, Inc., pp. 225-228, 1974. Findings consistent with cyanide intoxication included hypotension, noted in* <u>Harrison's Principles of Internal Medicine</u>, *eighth edition, p. 695, 1977; bright red venous blood, explained in* <u>Clinical Toxicology</u>, *Polson and Tattersall, second edition, p. 138, 1969, reprinted in 1975; and hypogammaglobulinemia, a recently identified component of some cases of chronic cyanide intoxication verified by Dr. Hitt, Ph.D., a micro-allergist who practices in Houston. Dr. Hitt may be reached for comment on this finding by calling his office in Houston. [I provided the phone number to Dr. Hitt.]*

Less than ten milligrams of hydroxocobalamin were finally placed on the hospital ward after insistent and ardent requesting on my part, but I was never allowed to have any. The recorded order for alphaREDISOL, a commercial form of hydroxocobalamin, stated that an M.D. was to be called if my systolic blood pressure dropped below 70 mm/Hg. Considering the physiological state of an adult, American male with cyanide intoxication to the extreme that his systolic blood pressure is below 70 mm/Hg, the availability of less than ten milligrams of hydroxocobalamin appears more like travesty than treatment. My blood pressure did drop to recorded levels of 80/40 mm/Hg, 90/42 mm/Hg, 90/54 mm/Hg, 90/70 mm/Hg, 90/52 mm/Hg, 84/60 mm/Hg, and

82/60 mm/Hg, any one of which, along with my symptoms of altered sensorium and chest pain, suggests the possibility of cardiogenic shock. On at least one outstanding occasion, I even complained of bluish coloration appearing beneath my fingernails. Adding to this the fact that hydroxocobalamin is considered harmless in large doses, and that its use is prescribed even in cases where cyanide poisoning is suspected but not confirmed (see 'Anesthesiology' 44(2):157-60, Feb. '76), my medical management amounted to blatant, life-threatening malpractice.

On 11DEC82, my blood was drawn and found to have a serum thiocyanate concentration of 1.8 mg/dl. In a study in which serum thiocyanate was measured in 167 nonsmokers, published in 'Clin Chem' 20(10):1344-8, Oct. '74, the very highest level found was less than 0.6 mg/dl. Considering the difference of 1.2 mg/dl [between the highest level of 0.6 and my level of 1.8] to be evenly dispersed in three liters of serum and nine liters of interstitial fluid, just this increased amount of serum thiocyanate alone represents the conversion of 64.8 milligrams of cyanide. This is more than enough cyanide to cause fatality, and even though it may have been acquired over a considerable period of time, it definitely poses a dangerous threat to a vulnerable individual whose body does not detoxify cyanide as quickly as that of the average person. Persons who detoxify more proficiently, although they experience no acute symptoms, may still suffer neurological damage from long-term cyanide exposure.

My Illness, then, was misdiagnosed and mistreated. This would be more excusable if not for the fact that I clearly stated that I was suffering from chronic cyanide intoxication. My history of chronic cyanide intoxication is plainly stated on the military physical I took prior to active duty, and I made it clear that I was suffering from chronic cyanide intoxication prior to my hospitalization on 02DEC82. Also prior to that hospitalization, I demonstrated dramatic improvement of my symptoms by use of specific antidote for cyanide. Furthermore, the library in the Naval hospital itself has several books and articles pertaining to cyanide intoxication. Thus, confinement in an area where I suffered cyanide intoxication, and denial of treatment which I clearly denoted and requested, substantiates evidence of politically motivated malevolence, much less medical malpractice.

Sincerely,
LT Timothy Oesch, MC, USNR

Also included with the Article 138 Complaint were seven supportive pages from my medical records. An introduction to those pages preceded them as follows:

The following page, a narrative summary of my hospitalization from 02DEC82 to 17DEC82, is quite revealing. First of all, note that the symptoms listed are classic symptoms of cyanide intoxication. Secondly, note that it is plainly stated that several serum thiocyanate levels were obtained, yet my hospital record has only one result for serum thiocyanate. None of the other serum results were made known to me. [My wife was able to obtain the result of a serum thiocyanate test on blood drawn on December 2, 1982, the day I was admitted to the hospital, and the level was 0.3 mg/dl.] These missing thiocyanate tests are in addition to a missing blood cyanide test ordered on 11DEC82. [I was never able to obtain the blood cyanide result.]

The missing serum thiocyanate tests could be very helpful in establishing the nature of cyanide contamination affecting NRMC Philadelphia, especially by comparison to my symptoms and to my serum thiocyanate level of 1.8 mg/dl on 11DEC82. [It may be a note of interest to the reader that the Philadelphia Naval Hospital was slated for closure and disposal in 1988; it was opened in 1935.] It is consistent with other indications of subterfuge, however, that these test results are missing. The one serum thiocyanate result I received, may have only been given to me because the reference values listed were for therapeutic levels of thiocyanate rather than for detecting exposure to cyanide. This made the test result appear negative to an individual inexperienced and unknowledgeable in the field of cyanide intoxication. In actuality, the test result was very high, unmistakably positive for exposure to a significant quantity of cyanide. If this had been known, I may have never been informed of the result. [In retrospect, perhaps Dr. Gilmore had something to do with my receiving the report. I think she may have had some conscientious objection to Captain Galasyn's tactics.]

Finally, in the last paragraph, note the unabashed claim that screening tests for cyanide poisoning were essentially normal, both in myself and in other individuals screened at the Naval shipyard. The fact is, screening tests for cyanide poisoning were highly positive, both on myself and on other individuals tested at the Naval shipyard. Published articles regarding reference values for thiocyanate strongly support the highly positive status of the findings. Only unqualified, personal opinion supports the claim of negative testing; and this opinion, it appears, is based on subterfuge. The former statement applies to the head toxicologist at National Medical Services in Willow Grove, Pennsylvania, as well as to personnel of NRMC Philadelphia.

The second page following is a copied sheet from my medical record demonstrating that both blood thiocyanate and blood thiosulfate levels were ordered on 02DEC82. These are examples of missing tests. [In retrospect, these tests may have been ordered to try and claim that elevated thiocyanate levels were somehow caused by taking sodium thiosulfate as an antidote, which I was taking prior to my hospitalization. Thiosulfate, of course, does not produce thiocyanate in the absence of cyanide. I do not know what the thiosulfate level was, but the serum thiocyanate level was 0.3 mg/dl, which is not very high. My wife was able to obtain the 0.3 mg/dl level from the laboratory. Also of interest, I recently discovered, while reading through a report issued by Lando W. Zech, Jr., Vice Admiral, U.S. Navy Chief of Naval Personnel, dated March 3 1983, the following statement: **Repeat screening for urine Thyiocyanate** *(misspelled in the report)* **was positive on 2 December, at which time the patient was taking Thiosulfate. At this time, the Thiocyanate level in the urine was measured at 21 micrograms per milliliter...** *It is notable that this urine thiocyanate level is exactly the same as the thiocyanate level in my urine that was collected in November at the shipyard dispensary, and it is also notable that there appears to be an attempt to blame the positive finding on the fact that I was taking sodium thiosulfate, and it is further notable that I was not informed of this finding: I have been able to search my hospital records and discover that this test was ordered, but I did not become aware that the result of the test was positive with a urine thiocyanate level of 21 mcg/ml until the year 2020.] The third page following is another sheet from my medical record verifying the presence of hypogammaglobulinemia [of note, I was tested for AIDS, which was, of course, negative; and it is further of note that rather extensive testing was performed, perhaps to try and come up with something to blame my illness on rather than cyanide; in addition to other studies, I received a CAT scan of my brain with contrast, a thallium heart study, and an arterial blood stick], and following this is a copy of my physical* *examination which was performed on 08JUN82 prior to active duty in Philadelphia. The examination consists of four sheets; especially note the remarks given in block seven of the final sheet. These remarks include both a blood cyanide level of 104 mc/dl, which is over a minimal lethal level; and a serum thiocyanate level of 0.9 mg/dl, which is plainly positive for cyanide exposure in a nonsmoker. Bear in mind that NRMC Philadelphia maintains that both the illness I experienced in Houston and the illness I experienced in Philadelphia are psychological in origin, rather than due to cyanide intoxication, which leaves them opposing a blood cyanide level of 104 mcg/dl, a serum thiocyanate level of 1.8 mg/dl, and a urine thiocyanate level of 21 mcg/ml, all in a nonsmoker. This is not knowledgeably feasible, again indicating the presence of politically based subterfuge.*

[As an addendum, one thing I was embarrassed to include when I originally penned this book, and even avoided mentioning when writing my complaint letters, had to do with temperature recordings while confined in the naval hospital. Severe episodes of environmental cyanide intoxication can cause low grade fevers, and I was found to have low grade fevers on several occasions. My military superiors, or at least one of them, apparently did not like this—after all, a fever is difficult to explain when claiming that an illness is psychological in origin. The response was to order that all of my subsequent temperature readings be taken rectally, insinuating that I was somehow making my mouth hot every time a corpsman came to take my temperature. I don't drink coffee, and such an insinuation was absurd. A large poster was fixed to the wall behind my bed with the words, 'Rectal Temperatures Only,' written in large letters; and to the best of my memory, the letters were in red print. The corpsmen were instructed to subtract one degree when recording my temperature in my chart, since rectal temperatures generally measure about one degree higher than oral temperatures; however, they were still instructed to note that the temperature was taken rectally. Obviously, this effectually made my temperature appear one degree lower than my actual temperature, since a degree was being subtracted while still recording that it was a rectal temperature. I was much younger back then, and it was notably embarrassing to have visitors come to the hospital with the 'Rectal Temperatures Only' poster mounted on the wall behind my bed, but at least the corpsmen were

considerate enough to hand me the thermometer and permit me to take my own rectal temperatures.]

[*On a more serious note, there is another issue I decided not to mention in my book or in any of my complaints. A corpsman, who I befriended, suspected that his baby died from airborne cyanide pollution. This corpsman joined me in the research and investigation of cyanide pollution and its effects. But then, one day, this corpsman drew me aside and told me that Captain Martinson threatened him, telling him that his 'ass was grass' if he had anything to do with the cyanide situation. He indicated that Captain Martinson seemed very serious in regard to her threat. I responded by telling him that there was likely little that a corpsman could accomplish in regard to the matter, and I advised him to simply back off. In consideration of his safety, or at least his future military career, I kept our conversation confidential. Over thirty-five years have now passed since the conversation between the corpsman and me, and I do not think that he would mind my disclosing what he told me; in fact, I think that he would want me to do so.*]

With the writing of the preceding complaint, my willingness to resist malfeasance was no longer confidential. Already, after turning in my request to the Commanding Officer on March 29, I was assigned to *home subsistence*. This meant that I would no longer work in the educational department, or anywhere else. I was simply told to stay home. My attorney told me that such an assignment was an administrative accusation that I was unfit for work.

The possibility of a future court case and the need for political assertion grew imposingly evident. Collecting all the available information at hand which might be useful in proving my claims seemed highly advisable. My military attorney, now solely Lieutenant Norris, suggested that I begin considering the requisition of outside help. In turn, I requested that she look into the matter of the missing laboratory results that were ordered on the shipyard employees. I was able to make contact with one of these employees, and the result of his thiocyanate test was withheld from his medical chart.

One suggestion I carried out was to contact the Poison Control Center in Atlanta, Georgia for information on cyanide intoxication. Any information on cyanide intoxication that they gave would carry significant political authority. The Poison Center was very cooperative, and put me in personal contact with Dr. Windell Holmes. Dr. Holmes was sympathetic to my theories of environmental cyanide contamination, and agreed that wind direction might play a role in community illness. Unfortunately, the Poison Center had a paucity of information on chronic cyanide poisoning—I offered to send them information from my research.

The one area where the Poison Control Center in Atlanta did have helpful information was in regard to nitroprusside therapy. Nitroprusside is a hazardous drug used for severe cases of high blood pressure; it has the toxic side effect of partially converting into cyanide inside the body. Dr. Holmes [*I think Holmes is a fictitious name, and that his name may have been Dr. Turk*] told me that at therapeutic doses of nitroprusside, blood cyanide levels would range from 5 to 15 mcg/dl. He also confided that the presence of cyanide at these levels in nonsmokers who were not taking nitroprusside therapy would suggest environmental cyanide exposure. The average blood cyanide level among nonsmokers tested in Houston, including both positive and negative results, was 13.5 mcg/dl. The average positive level [*in nonsmokers*] was over 27 mcg/dl.

Dr. Holmes further stated that a frankly toxic level of blood cyanide, meaning an acutely toxic level, is 50 mcg/dl. This more than qualified my blood cyanide level of 104 mcg/dl as an acutely toxic level. The Poison Center in Atlanta informed me that they would mail the information they had to me, but I never received a letter from them. Later, I called back to check on the information, and was informed that the information had, in fact, been mailed about two weeks earlier. I never found out why I failed to receive the letter from Poison Control in Atlanta.

With the discovery that cyanide contamination is a widespread problem [*there are major sources of airborne cyanide pollution other than electroplating*], and after political resistance to disclosure of the problem from various health authorities, I decided to attempt new means to educate an unknowing society. The obstacle to such education was not medical or scientific, it was moral and political. In searching my mind for individuals who might be courageous enough and concerned enough to undertake such a politically daring task, I decided to confide in five individuals who had little association with the medical field. What they lacked in medical knowledge, I hoped they would more than make up for in moral fortitude.

Four of the persons I notified [*or at least attempted to notify*] were outstanding religious leaders. Each of them received data about the cyanide intoxication, including *Metropolitan Effects of Environmental Cyanide* and my second rebuttal. I also wrote each of them a personal letter. Two were close associates, so I simply put both their names on the same letter. The three personal letters read as follows: [*Note: I am not 100% certain about my memory regarding all of the names of the religious leaders, so I am retaining the fictitious names in the following letters. To the best of my memory, however, the names in the second and third letters were Dr. Jerry Falwell, and Dr. Bob Jones and Dr. Bob Jones, Jr.*]

Dear Pastor Glynn:
Your ministry, which directly confronts the need for moral and political reformation, is certainly relevant to our nation's present, ethological condition. The booklet you circulated reinforces and substantiates an inner conviction which is kindling in the hearts of Christian Americans from one coast of our country to the other. The forces of evil would have us believe that Christianity is a pacifist religion, but it is not, it is a powerful, dynamic reality. If there is any man who should place himself between perpetrators of evil and those crimes they perform, it is the Christian. Surely both the spiritual and physical well-being of this nation are dependent on the working of true Christianity.

My own willingness to stand against socioeconomic corruption has been extensively challenged during the past two years. Medical involvement with a serious environmental problem very quickly ushered me into political and moral battlegrounds. I am ethically compelled to disclose the existence of the problem to an uninformed populace, but such may only be accomplished through non-venal means. Please prayerfully consider what role the Lord will have you take in shedding light on this unscrupulously shrouded issue.
Sincerely,
Your Brother In Christ,
Timothy Oesch, M.D.

Contact Persons:
    LT Norris, Attorney [*Phone number was given.*]
    Timothy Oesch, M.D. [*Phone number was given.*]

Timothy Swiss

Dear Dr. Allen:
For many years I have followed and admired your courageous ministry for truth and right in this nation. Recently, due to my involvement with a widespread environmental problem, I have had occasion to wrestle with various felonious agents myself. These experiences have indicated that solution to the problem may only come through employment of non-venal communicators, such as yourself. Surely both the spiritual and physical well-being of our country are dependent on the working of true Christianity. Please prayerfully consider what role the Lord will have you take in shedding light on this unscrupulously shrouded issue.
Sincerely,
Your Brother In Christ,
Timothy Oesch, M.D.

Contact Persons:
  LT Norris, Attorney [Phone number was given.]
  Timothy Oesch, M.D. [Phone number was given.]

Dear Dr. Wells and Dr. Wells, Jr.:
The semester I spent as a graduate student during the spring of 1981 has been a dynamic inspiration in my life. Little did I know just how applicable and helpful the courses I took would be within the first two years of my departure. Not only the academic instruction I received, but also the courageous, contagious spirit to stand for right and truth without compromise, has been an inner support throughout subsequent political and emotional struggles. My medical involvement with an environmental problem very quickly entered political and moral arenas, as the following literature explains, and I am now seeking to reach an uninformed populace through non-venal channels. I have been thoroughly convinced that both the spiritual and physical well-being of this nation are dependent on the working of true Christianity. Please prayerfully consider what role the Lord will have you take in shedding light on this unscrupulously shrouded issue.
Sincerely,
Your Brother In Christ,
Timothy Oesch, M.D.

Contact Persons:

A Breath of Cyanide

LT Norris, Attorney [*Phone number was given.*]
Timothy Oesch, M.D. [*Phone number was given.*]

The fifth person I entreated for aid was the President [*President Ronald Reagan*]. I sent mostly the same material to him as the preceding four individuals, including the following personal letter that was mailed on April 9, 1983:

Dear Sir:
People are sick and dying from an environmental contaminant which has been disclosed and objectively proven, yet degenerate political subterfuge continues to prevent solution of this grave problem. The problem is chronic cyanide intoxication from environmental dispersion of cyanide refuse, notably occurring in connection with industrial electroplating. It has been over a year since medical testing on human blood and urine has revealed the presence of the contaminant clearly and conclusively. During that year, fiscally preponderant industrial tycoons and collaborating health officials have relentlessly handicapped sincere efforts to educate and help unfortunate individuals who suffer from chronic cyanide intoxication. Evidence now indicates that the problem is likely as widespread as electroplating itself, national in scope, and probably affecting untold masses of humanity. [*I would later consider other sources of airborne cyanide to be greater contributors than electroplating to the overall levels of cyanide in the atmosphere, such as biomass burning in regard to automobile exhaust and coal-burning power plant emissions; iron and steel production; carbon fiber production; and petroleum refineries. Nonetheless, plating industries that utilize cyanide compounds may contribute to significant illness in areas proximal to those industries.*]
*Rather than affronting objective patient studies, recalcitrant opposers to revelation of this problem have staged farce counter studies, and have focalized on individual personalities, thereby drawing attention away from real facts and issues. The objective findings speak for themselves. As one involved citizen, I have been threatened with blackmail, threatened with loss of my medical license, threatened with psychiatric institutionalization, and have been further advised that my involvement in such a matter could be **very dangerous**. Indolence on the part of morally principled and medically aware persons would be dangerous to many, many individuals who are unknowingly afflicted*

with chronic cyanide intoxication. The time has come to put a stop to indiscriminate carnage by lucratively and politically animated criminals, despite their socioeconomic positions or professional pedigrees.

A composition of material follows which conveys both political and scientific facets regarding chronic cyanide contamination. The materials were actually compiled in rebuttal to an attempt by NRMC at Philadelphia to discharge me from the Navy on psychiatric grounds, an attempt which followed my disclosure of environmental cyanide contamination at the Philadelphia Naval Shipyard. Nonetheless, the material is well documented and pertinent to a study and understanding of cyanide contamination in general. It includes many details of my involvement with the problem in two, widely separated geographical locations. Published articles and references are included to verify medical and environmental claims.

Not mentioned in the following presentation is a recent episode involving the State of New Jersey Department of Health in Trenton, New Jersey. My wife and I, while living in Pitman, New Jersey, both submitted urine specimens to be tested for thiocyanate concentration. After several weeks, I inquired about the test results by mail, and was informed that the health department could not find any record of our tests. The laboratory was willing to look for the results, but needed an account number from the health department. Although I called the health department three times, I was not able to acquire their account number with Metpath Laboratories, Inc. I was told a physician would call me, but he never did.

The preceding paragraph is only a sample of the bureaucratic hedging surrounding this issue of industrial cyanide contamination. It is unfortunate that such strong political safeguards rise to harbor culpable polluters, when sufferers of chronic cyanide intoxication remain helplessly and ignorantly vulnerable. The medical proof of chronic cyanide poisoning among American citizens is substantial and definite. Appeals for recognition and solution of the problem have been forwarded earnestly and extensively, but peccant political intervention has stinted efforts to help. On behalf of the health and lives of American citizens in industrial areas [I know now that cyanide is a ubiquitous air pollutant with a half-life measured in years, and may affect vulnerable individuals in areas that are not considered industrial], your implementation of public cognizance regarding chronic cyanide intoxication is respectfully requested.

Sincerely,
Timothy Oesch, M.D.

Copies to:
   Dr. Allen
   Dr. Wells
   Dr. Wells, Jr.
   Pastor Glynn

Contact Persons:
   LT Norris, Attorney [*Phone number was given.*]
   Timothy Oesch, M.D. [*Phone number was given.*]

Toward the end of April, I received the following response from Pastor Glynn:

Dear Dr. Oesch:
Thank you for your recent letter and study on cyanide poisoning. I appreciate the time you have sacrificed to compile this information. Due to my schedule I have not yet had the opportunity to give this subject the attention it deserves. Please be assured of my concern in this area and know that I will seek God's direction regarding His will for my involvement in this issue.

May God richly bless you,
Pastor Glynn

On April 21, 1983, Commander Martinson issued a report refuting my Article 138 Complaint. She did not directly address the topic of my mistreatment while hospitalized, but she did include the following paragraph regarding my claim of politically based subterfuge:

The comments of LT Oesch that a 'politically based subterfuge' exists are unjustified. Following LT Oesch's assertions, air samples were taken from the plating shop identified by LT Oesch as the likely source of cyanide. In addition, air and water samples were taken from various locations, including the shipyard dispensary where LT Oesch worked. The results listed below, are all well within acceptable, safe limits. 10 ppm is the level above which action must be taken to reduce concentration. (American Council on Governmental Industrial Hygienists Threshold Limit Value Committee for 1983 standards) As can readily be ascertained, none of the levels obtained approach either the 'action level' of 10 ppm or the 30 ppm which LT Oesch alleges in his Article 138 complaint.

To test air on a given day for the presence of cyanide means little or nothing unless the tests are positive. This was not the only shortcoming, however, in the testing referred to by Captain Martinson. Not only were the tests performed by a naval laboratory, the samples of air and water were collected by the Naval Environmental Department at Philadelphia—headed by Captain Galasyn. Furthermore, rather than testing discharge water from the electroplating tanks mentioned in my first rebuttal, water from nearby rinse tanks was tested. The water that should have been tested was overflow water from the electroplating tanks themselves.

Eventually, Lieutenant Norris informed me that she confronted a naval officer who had access to urine thiocyanate results from tests I previously ordered on civilian employees. I contacted that naval officer in person, and copies of those test results were soon in my possession. [*The acquisition of all of the copies of urine thiocyanate tests from workers at the shipyard apparently did not occur until later, after my First Hearing.*] This shed entirely new light on the shipyard situation. Copies of the order sheets to the tests revealed more precise smoking histories and other details that enabled better interpretation of the tests. There were also additional test results to those I had already acquired.

Using the newly acquired test results from the shipyard, I composed the following manuscript:

Chronic Cyanide Intoxication At The Philadelphia Naval Shipyard

Since cyanide is very fleeting, both in the environment and in the bloodstream, it may be compared to the actual flame of fire. In cases of fire damage, generally speaking, the more flame present, the longer the flame is present, and the more often the flame is present, the greater will be the damage by fire. Likewise, in the human body, the more cyanide present, the longer it is present, and the more often it is present, the greater will be the ill effects of cyanide intoxication. The damage caused by fire is much longer lasting than the actual presence of flame, and the illness caused by cyanide is much more persevering than the periods when cyanide is actually present in the environment or bloodstream.

The comparison between cyanide and flame is very applicable to understanding environmental testing for cyanide. Imagine that a particular neighborhood is subjected to numerous fires started by a gang of local arsonists, but that the weather is very damp, and daily showers of rain extinguish the fires not long after they are started. The amount of damage caused by the fire depends upon how busily the arsonists keep the neighborhood ignited, and upon the prevalence of rain. A significant decrease in rain can be very harmful without added initiative on the part of the arsonists, and heavy outbursts of rain can practically obliterate all attempts of arson.

Next, consider an environment that experiences bouts of cyanide perfusion in the atmosphere. Due to winds and the fleeting nature of cyanide, each bout of perfusion may last only hours or even minutes. Other times, when industrial contamination is at a peak and winds are calm, the perfusion may linger for days. If winds are strong and blow from the direction opposite the source of contamination, then the atmosphere may be clean despite synchronous, industrial polluting.

Now then, imagine that an investigator is commissioned to prove that arson is occurring in the neighborhood that is experiencing numerous, brief fires. It is evident that several homes are charred, and there are even smoldering embers from place to place, but this particular investigator has been bribed by the arsonists. His intention, therefore, is to prove that no fire exists. In order to prove that no fire exists, the investigator takes pictures of the neighborhood with a special film that detects only flame. He takes these pictures either on days with heavy rains, or on days when the arsonists know that he will be taking pictures so that they can refrain from starting fires. Likewise, an environmental investigator may test the atmosphere for cyanide either on days when winds blow the opposite direction from the source of pollution, or on days when the industry doing the polluting has been advised that testing will be done. This is a simple means of seemingly proving that no cyanide pollution is present, although in actuality it is rampant.

Still further, imagine that an individual living in the neighborhood plagued by fires learns about the bribery between the investigator and the arsonists, so he hires a second investigator. To complicate matters, the first investigator learns that the second investigator has been hired, and he forewarns the arsonists whenever the second investigator approaches the neighborhood. In addition to this, the first investigator hires a third investigator, who he claims to be a nonpartisan expert, to examine the pictures he has taken and confer that there is no flame in the pictures and there must be no fire. The second investigator, meanwhile, sees that there is a significant proportion of charred wood in the neighborhood, and has no trouble finding several samples of smoldering embers. Where there is smoke, there is fire, so the second investigator tangibly proves that arson is evident in the neighborhood.

Comparable to the charred wood in the neighborhood, is the history given by patients suffering from chronic cyanide intoxication. The symptoms these patients have experienced are not erased by changing winds, and may even withstand subversive, political intimidation. Comparable to the smoldering embers, are levels of serum and urine thiocyanate found in patients tested for cyanide exposure. Blood cyanide has a short half-life, and is comparable to flame, but thiocyanate is a specific metabolite of cyanide that lasts considerably longer before excretion in the urine. Published literature definitely recommends testing for thiocyanate when investigating for chronic cyanide intoxication.

Two patients working at the Philadelphia Naval Shipyard were tested for serum thiocyanate. Chronic cyanide intoxication was suspected in both of these patients. The first patient was a very light smoker, smoking about three cigarettes daily. The second patient was a nonsmoker.

A comprehensive study found in 'Clinical Chemistry,' 20(10):1344-8, Oct. '74, furnishes established reference values for serum thiocyanate. One hundred sixty-seven nonsmokers were tested for serum thiocyanate on several occasions each. The average level in nonsmokers was 0.26 mg/dl, and the highest level in a nonsmoker was less than 0.6 mg/dl. The nonsmoker tested at the Philadelphia Naval Shipyard had a serum thiocyanate level of 2.1 mg/dl. This is not only definitely positive for cyanide exposure, it is high enough to represent exposure to a lethal quantity of cyanide. Furthermore, regarding chronic cyanide intoxication, it is the highest level that I know of on record.

The light smoker tested at the shipyard had a serum thiocyanate level of 1.0 mg/dl. Smokers normally have significantly higher serum thiocyanate levels than nonsmokers. In the previously cited reference article, several smokers were tested who smoked ten or less cigarettes daily. The average level among these light smokers was about 0.45 mg/dl, and the highest level was about 0.66 mg/dl. Thus, the serum thiocyanate level of 1.0 mg/dl in the light smoker at the shipyard definitely, along with his symptoms, signifies environmental cyanide exposure.

Besides myself, fourteen individuals at the shipyard were tested for urine thiocyanate levels. In the case of nonsmokers, true urine thiocyanate levels are normally less than 2 mcg/ml, and should definitely be considered positive for exposure to environmental cyanide at levels greater than 5 mcg/ml. Smokers normally have significantly elevated levels of urine thiocyanate, several times higher than the levels found in nonsmokers. In fact, nonsmokers suffering from clinical, chronic cyanide intoxication resulting from bouts of environmental cyanide exposure may be diagnosed with elevated urine thiocyanate levels which are well within the normal range for heavy smokers. Thus, symptoms may play an especially important role in diagnosing smokers with chronic cyanide intoxication.

Of the fourteen subjects tested for chronic cyanide intoxication at the shipyard, all of whom acknowledged symptoms of cyanide intoxication, five were smokers and nine were nonsmokers. The average urine thiocyanate level among the smokers was 8.6 mcg/ml, and the average urine thiocyanate level among the nonsmokers was 9.4 mcg/ml. [Note: there was one urine thiocyanate marked as "negative" among the smokers; and likewise, there was one urine thiocyanate marked as "negative" among the nonsmokers. Both of these results were entered as a "0" when calculating the averages. National Medical Services performed all of these tests, and that laboratory's stated detection limit for urine thiocyanate, at that time, was 5 mcg/ml. Pertaining to the fact that there were fourteen shipyard workers tested (not including me), and that only eleven shipyard workers are found listed at the beginning of chapter eleven, I would point out that missing from the list of eleven names at the beginning of chapter eleven are the names of two civilian workers, one with the first name of Anthony, and another with the first name of Jules (Jules is given the fictitious name of Chester Parkins in this book), and that also missing is the name of a military member with the first name of Donald. If I had included my own urine thiocyanate level when calculating the average among nonsmokers tested at the shipyard, then the average level of urine thiocyanate in nonsmokers would have been higher at 10.5 mcg/ml.] This is very significant; it indicates exposure to a sufficient quantity of environmental cyanide to nullify the normally dominant effect of smoking on urine thiocyanate levels. Even without reference levels, this concludes environmental exposure to cyanide.

After ten days as a patient in the Naval hospital, which is located about one mile from the shipyard, I experienced an acute episode of chronic cyanide intoxication which was verified by a serum thiocyanate level of 1.8 mg/dl. I am a strict nonsmoker. The cyanide contamination in South Philadelphia, then, is not restricted to the shipyard. Individual vulnerability to illness from cyanide exposure varies greatly from person to person, but I am certainly only one of many individuals suffering from this previously undisclosed, environmental contaminant.

Due to strong financial and political interests on the part of industrial and health organizations, ultimate solution to this problem may depend upon concentrated efforts by informed citizens and cooperative physicians.

*Sincerely,
Timothy Oesch, M.D.*

Besides helping to acquire the urine thiocyanate results, Lieutenant Norris was also instrumental in securing three affidavits from the shipyard dispensary. Two of the affidavits came from civilian nurses with whom I probably had more frequent contact than any other health professionals at the dispensary. The nurses' affidavits read as follows:

AFFIDAVIT OF JOYCE KELLY, RN
I, Joyce Kelly, a civilian, residing at 314 Greentree Drive, Philadelphia, am a registered nurse and have worked with the Philadelphia Naval Shipyard as an occupational health nurse from June, 1982 to present. During my employment with Philadelphia Naval Shipyard, I had contact with Dr. Timothy Oesch, MC, USNR, who worked at the civilian medical dispensary as a relief doctor during the months of July through November. Dr. Oesch would fill in when civilian doctors were out or when the case load was very busy.

I was very comfortable with Dr. Oesch's medical knowledge and clinical skills. Being a new employee, he did not see patients as quickly as a doctor more experienced with our practices but he improved with time and more experience. He picked up on the use of our numerous forms.

Patients never complained about Dr. Oesch's treatment, and I felt comfortable referring patients to him.

Dr. Oesch was quiet, cooperative, and sincere.

Dr. Oesch did express a personal interest in cyanide poisoning but it did not create a problem with his daily workload. He treated the problems which were presented to him in a capable manner.

Joyce Kelly
JOYCE KELLY

Maryjane R. Kelley
Witness: LTJG Maryjane R. Kelley, JAGC, USNR

AFFIDAVIT OF ELLEN BRULTE

I, Ellen Brulte, a civilian, residing at 1135 Alexander Avenue, Philadelphia, am a registered nurse and have worked with the Philadelphia Naval Shipyard as an occupational health nurse since July, 1982. During my employment with the Philadelphia Naval Shipyard, I had contact with Dr. Timothy Oesch, MC, USNR, who worked at the civilian medical dispensary as a relief doctor during the months of July through November, 1982. Dr. Oesch would fill in when civilian doctors were out or when the case load was very busy.

In my opinion, Dr. Oesch's medical knowledge and clinical skills were good. His notes on patients' charts were always clear; his treatment for injury was relevant and he was consistent in his care of patients. I never heard a patient complain about Dr. Oesch and he was always willing to explain procedures and answer questions patients had. He spent adequate time with each patient. Dr. Oesch would give straight answers and he appeared to be a man of integrity and honesty.

Dr. Oesch did not appear to be focused in on diagnosis and treatment of cyanide poisoning to the exclusion of all else.

Ellen Brulte

ELLEN BRULTE

Maryjane R. Kelley
Witness: LTJG Maryjane R. Kelley, JAGC, USNR

It was definitely comforting to read the favorable remarks of my medical comrades at the dispensary. Perhaps even more consequential, though, was the third affidavit. I do not remember ever meeting LTJG Maryjane R. Kelley, JAGC, USNR, but I presume she was an associate of Lieutenant Norris. Whoever she was, I certainly admire the proficiency and quality of the affidavit she provided:

I, LTJG Maryjane R. Kelley, JAGC, USNR, on 14-15 June 1983, checked the medical files of the Philadelphia Naval Shipyard Medical Dispensary, of the following persons to determine if the request and results of urine thiocyanate tests ordered by Dr. Timothy Oesch, MC, USN were noted in the files:

> *Luke Crane*
> *Windell Sweeny*
> *Bob Guviendo*
> *Randy Corraine*
> *Gilbert Furseille*
> *Ron Shapiro*
> *Todd Gates*
> *Earnest Rutherford*
> *Tom Gennings*
> *Peter Napazzi*
> *John Adams [The names of these eleven shipyard workers are fictionalized.]*

There was no indication in the files that such tests had been given. Ann Bettinger, R.N., Occupational Nurse Director at the dispensary could not explain why the files did not note the tests. All tests are to be recorded in the files. Verdi Douglas, Administrative Clerk of Record also indicated that test results should be in the file and nowhere else. She stated that the test results are never kept in CDR DeJesus's office.

I was referred to CDR DeJesus, MC, USN, Senior Medical Officer, who stated that she had the original tests requested and results in her desk because she did not want them to get lost. She admitted that no notation was in the file and she did not explain why copies of the tests requested and results were not placed in the file in place of the original.

I also questioned CDR DeJesus why Dr. Oesch's lecture in cyanide poisoning was abruptly cancelled. She stated that she did not remember the reason for its cancellation.

Attester: LTJG Maryjane R. Kelley, JAGC, USNR
Witness: LT Norris, JAGC, USNR

Needless to say, the above information indicated that rather extreme measures were taken to conceal facts—measures that amounted to much more than mere ignorance.

Chapter 16

```
AO 440 (Rev. 5/85) Summons in a Civil Action
```

United States District Court
─────── DISTRICT OF ───────

TIMOTHY R. OESCH, M.D.   ALIAS   SUMMONS IN A CIVIL ACTION

         V.   CASE NUMBER: 3-90-409
                                                          JARVIS
CITY OF HOUSTON

TO: (Name and Address of Defendant)

    CITY OF HOUSTON
    Kathryn J. Whitmire, Mayor

Accumulated Proof

Friday evening, February 26, 1983, I decided my wife and I had been apart long enough. I picked up the phone and dialed her parents' number:

"Hello, Mercer's residence, Melody Oesch speaking…"

"Hi honey!"

"Tim! What's going on?"

"I'm coming after you."

There was a pause. "What? You're coming after me? When?"

"Tomorrow. I'll fly over and drive your car back."

"But…what about the cyanide?"

"We'll move as soon as we get back."

"Have you found an apartment?"

"No, I thought you'd want to help me do that."

"Can we afford it?"

"I may have to borrow some money, but it's worth it."

The next morning I boarded a jet and flew to Iowa. The day after that, I began driving back to Pitman. We took our time coming back, not arriving in Pitman until March first. Then, with the help of Leighann

Deere, Melody located an apartment while I was at work at the naval hospital. The apartment was located about eighteen miles northeast of Pitman in a town not far from Cherry Hill, New Jersey. [*The apartment actually had a Marlton, NJ address. However, we later moved several miles east to another location with a Marlton address that was farther away from Cherry Hill. The distance between Cherry Hill and Marlton is 5.98 miles, or 7 miles by car.*]

On Saturday, March fifth, we moved to the apartment near Cherry Hill. There were beautiful woods to the west of our apartment, and as chance or providence would have it, there was an industrial park just on the other side of those woods. In addition to the industrial park, an electroplating plant sat about two miles west of our apartment. Still, we felt better at our new residence than before in Pitman. We did not perceive feeling ill when winds came from the west until several weeks later. Our discovery about the industrial park was not to occur until July 7th. We were probably not exposed to as much cyanide near Cherry Hill as previously in Pitman.

Even with reduced levels of cyanide exposure, an individual's sensitivity to cyanide can increase with time. Besides industrial literature recording increased sensitivity, my wife and I have personally experienced it. When we began our new residence near Cherry Hill, my wife had just spent several weeks recovering in Iowa, and I had just come from the relatively worse environment in Pitman. At first I seemed to improve living near Cherry Hill, though I never entirely regained my health, and at first my wife's health seemed stable.

As I experienced illness from time to time near Cherry Hill, I simply attributed the illness to cyanide exposures in Philadelphia. After assignment to *home subsistence*, however, I could no longer attribute my illness to Philadelphia. The settlement on our house in Pitman came on March 29, 1983. I was mentally relieved to find buyers despite our ominous reason for moving. I felt morally obligated to tell prospective buyers that we were moving because of an environmental contaminant, but the family that bought our house already lived in Pitman and did not seem to suffer ill effects like my wife and me—at least not that they admitted. At any rate, they were determined to remain in Pitman because of the good school system, so I felt okay about selling them our house. We decided to rent thereafter.

Lieutenant Norris encouraged me to obtain some news coverage that would put pressure on the naval officials at my upcoming hearing. So,

I contacted Stan Hewing of the *Philadelphia Inquirer*. Stan came to my apartment near Cherry Hill on April 26th; he was a special writer on environmental problems for the largest newspaper in Philadelphia. I held back almost nothing from Stan. He received copies of my naval rebuttals, my report from Houston, and numerous exposés on individual publications from medical libraries. Sometime later, Stan mailed all the material back to me; nothing was printed.

After witnessing beguiling manipulation of the public media in Houston, I was personally relieved when the Philadelphia Inquirer remained silent about the cyanide problem. At the same time, though, the silence was disquieting. Stan Hewing received copies of objective laboratory testing from at least five major laboratories that disclosed exposure to cyanide. In addition, he received article summaries from published medical literature affirming that the findings were pertinent and portentous. The fact that a public newspaper withheld such information from an uninformed society seemed cruelly complacent.

Besides the previously mentioned material that I turned over to Stan Hewing, I prepared a summary entitled *What American Citizens Should Know About Chronic Cyanide Intoxication*. The summary read basically as follows:

What American Citizens Should Know About Chronic Cyanide Intoxication

1. *Individuals living within a few miles of an electroplating plant which utilizes cyanide compounds are subject to possible chronic cyanide intoxication. Cyanide is also utilized in photographic processes, case-hardening of steel, and for extraction of gold and silver from their ores. If sewer drainage or prevailing winds come from the direction of a plant using cyanide, chances of intoxication are increased. Cyanide enters the atmosphere after being discharged into sewers or other water channels. [And of course, I now know that burning fossil fuels is a major contributor to airborne cyanide.]*
2. *Chronic cyanide intoxication is very selective among different individuals who are exposed to environmental cyanide. Some persons may be very ill, while other persons in the same, contaminated environment do not experience noticeable symptoms.*

3. Symptoms and findings of chronic cyanide intoxication include weakness, faintness, splitting headaches, nervousness, feelings of apprehension and suffocation, abdominal pain, disturbance of the intellect, vertigo, nausea, depression, psychological disturbances, low blood pressure, altered sugar metabolism, forgetfulness, lower back pain, fast heartbeats, numbness, weight loss, decreased appetite, restless sleep, lagging eyelids, muscle twitching and cramps, aching muscles and joints, chest pains, burning eyes, itching, rash, irritated mucous membranes, lack of motivation, anemia, hair loss, immune deficiency, secondary infections, decreased libido, easy bruising, bleeding tendencies, irregular menstrual periods, testicular pain, edema, irritability, changes in the taste of food or cigarettes, a lingering metallic taste, and unusually red venous blood. The number of these symptoms and findings an individual experiences depends upon his sensitivity to cyanide exposure. Some persons experience only tiredness and headaches. These symptoms may come and go, or may persist for extended periods of time. Individuals suffering from chronic cyanide intoxication tend to feel better after spending several days away from contaminated areas.

4. Persons chronically exposed to low doses of cyanide, who do not experience acute illness, may still suffer permanent neurological damage. Such damage may include decreased vision, nerve deafness, and other sensory losses.

5. Screening tests for cyanide exposure include blood cyanide, serum thiocyanate, and urine thiocyanate tests. Blood cyanide only has a half-life of about 30 minutes in the bloodstream, so testing must occur during or right after cyanide exposure. Thiocyanate tests are better in screening for chronic cyanide exposure, and may be positive up to several days after episodes of illness. Thiocyanate is a metabolite of cyanide. Smokers normally have increased levels of thiocyanate in their serum and urine, and the normal level of thiocyanate in smokers may be greater than the level of thiocyanate in nonsmokers who are seriously ill with chronic cyanide intoxication. It is important, therefore, to use specific, thiocyanate reference values for nonsmokers and entirely different reference values for smokers. It is best for individuals to stop smoking, and it is best to test nonsmokers rather than smokers in screening for chronic cyanide intoxication in an area of suspected contamination.

I.) Reference Values

A.) Blood Cyanide
   1.) Nonsmokers – less than 5 mcg/dl. Average is less than two micrograms per deciliter.
   2.) Smokers – if at least one hour has passed since smoking a cigarette, the blood cyanide level should be less than 10 mcg/dl.
B.) Serum Thiocyanate
   1.) Nonsmokers – less than 0.5 mg/dl. Average is about 0.26 mg/dl with a standard deviation of 0.096 milligrams per deciliter.
   2.) Smokers – average is about 0.84 mg/dl with a standard deviation of 0.28 mg/dl.
C.) Urine Thiocyanate
   1.) Nonsmokers – less than 5 mg/L. Average is less than two milligrams per liter. (5 mg/L are equivalent to 5 mcg/ml.)
   2.) Smokers –
   a.) 10 cigarettes per day – average about 3.7 mg/L.
   b.) 20 cigarettes per day (1ppd) – average about 7.9 mg/L.
   c.) 30 cigarettes per day – average about 12.1 mg/L.
   d.) 40 cigarettes per day (2ppd) – average about 17.5 mg/L.

Note: True thiocyanate levels are absolute, not relative, so laboratory reference values should be fairly consistent from one laboratory to another. At least one national laboratory is forwarding erroneously high reference values for thiocyanate. This may be due to political manipulation by those who consider the finding of widespread, chronic cyanide intoxication financially threatening. The reference values listed in this report are supported by substantially documented, published literature. Life and health must take precedence over fiscally-based subterfuge.

6. Treatment for chronic cyanide intoxication is cessation of exposure to cyanide, and prescribed doses of hydroxocobalamin, a particular type of vitamin B12. Also, sodium thiosulfate crystals dissolved in water may be taken orally for acute, minor episodes of cyanide intoxication.

7. Most physicians have not been educated regarding chronic cyanide intoxication; the following articles may be very helpful to one's private physician:

[Sixteen references are then listed in the report.]

Sincerely,
Timothy Oesch, M.D.

A Breath of Cyanide

Despite the rejection for publication by Stan Hewing and the Philadelphia Inquirer, the preceding summary still served well for informing individuals about cyanide intoxication. The individuals who seemed most pitifully deplete of such knowledge were physicians consulted by my prior patients in Houston. The following letter, written on March twenty-second and received by me on about May first, illustrates this sordid fact well. It was written by a woman who suffered from cyanide intoxication in the Heights:

Dear Dr. Oesch:

I got your address from Brenda Jenkins about three weeks ago. Maybe I can get this letter wrote today. I'm just hoping and asking that you can come back to Houston to help us. I'm still not feeling well and I have had a bad headache for 3 weeks straight. My eyes bother me a great deal. Plus other things. I've went to 2 Doctors here and they tell me they can't find anything wrong and maybe I should see a psychiatrist. They couldn't help me and besides I can't afford one. I still think I need an X-ray of my head and chest. I'm at a loss as what to do next. Can you tell me if I should still take the thiosulfate? Maybe I could still get that from Northwest Pharmacy. My nerves are so terrible I can't do anything. I have talked to Marie Black twice and that helps knowing she has the same problem. Do you remember me telling you about the man friend of ours who was sick like me? He had everything wrong with him that I did, yet he wouldn't have his self checked for cyanide. Well he has cancer of the right lung and I don't know if he will live the rest of this year.

Anyway Dr. Oesch I hope all is well with you and your wife.

I told Dr. P. Flouly of the Heights Clinic that 2 people who swallowed cyanide are still living and that the city and news media will someday have to apologize to you. I just get so angry at the Doctors here for not being concerned.

Dr. Hitt & Dr. Johnstone are the only ones I knew that are trying.

Again if there is anything you can do for me or tell me what to do, please let me know.

Thanks
Mrs. Pam Edwards

I was not so appalled by the understandable ignorance that many physicians had about cyanide intoxication, as by their flippant disregard for seriously suffering patients. Perhaps it was easier not to become involved with a politically activated illness, but perhaps the value of human life and health should have merited at least equal consideration. I read with interest what Mrs. Edwards penned about her friend contracting lung cancer. Little if any literary association is made between cancer and cyanide exposure, yet infamous cigarette smoke certainly contains a respectable quantity of cyanide. In addition to this, Gloucester County [*where Pitman is located*] has the highest cancer rate of any county in the nation, and Gloucester County is replete with industrial electroplating plants.

Another plague infecting Gloucester County is that of miscarriages and birth defects. I personally believe that cyanide intoxication plays a role in attributing to these maladies. A published article lending support to this belief is found in *Teratology*, 24:289-291 (1981). One specific birth defect mentioned in the preceding report is microcephaly. I was informed that an alarming number of women in Gloucester County delivered babies with microcephaly.

Mrs. Edwards also referred to patients that survived cyanide poisoning in Chicago, poisoning attributed to sabotaged Tylenol tablets. I found it curiously interesting that cyanide was not discovered in Tylenol tablets in every instance in Chicago—or so I heard—and that the agent blamed for the poisonings [*namely Tylenol*] was perhaps the most common treatment accompanying individuals who suffer from headaches. Patients suffering from environmental cyanide intoxication are likely to use frequent doses of pain medication, such as Tylenol, and are likely to have the medication nearby during an acute attack of cyanide intoxication. Knowing the extremes of moral turpitude exhibited by industry and government in Houston, why not consider the possibility that a *Tylenol scare* was being used to evade the truth of industrial, environmental contamination with cyanide? Having never lived anywhere near Chicago, I decided to suggest the possibility to an official involved with the investigation.

I mailed a copy of *What American Citizens Should Know About Chronic Cyanide Intoxication* along with the following message:

I was investigating environmental cyanide poisoning months before the 'Tylenol scare.' You may wish to check into the industry in the area of Chicago where the cyanide victims were (individuals with cyanide intoxication tend to have headaches and therefore would likely take Tylenol) and make sure you were not used for a scapegoat.

In response, I received a reply from a medical director thanking me for my letter and claiming that industrial poisoning had already been considered in Chicago. He insinuated that industrial poisoning was dismissed from consideration because all the poisonings were *clearly consistent with acute cyanide intoxication*, and because their investigation for potential industrial pollution in the area was negative. Interestingly he also stated that differences in blood cyanide and serum thiocyanate levels between smokers and nonsmokers were an important consideration in their investigation. He closed the letter by again thanking me for my correspondence. [*I later learned that Tylenol capsules were found that had been emptied, or partially emptied, and then filled with potassium cyanide. Some capsules reportedly contained 65 mg (milligrams) of "poison." One may speculate, however, that with increased testing for cyanide in the community, there may have been some positive findings for cyanide poisoning that resulted from environmental exposures rather than from the unfortunate and nefarious poisoning that resulted from sabotaged Tylenol tablets.*]

In reading the medical director's reply, several points became evident. First of all, he inferred that clinically acute cyanide intoxication rules out an industrial source, which it certainly does not. Secondly, the types of environmental testing performed were not specified. Urine and serum thiocyanate screening of nonsmoking residents would probably serve much better than attempting to find elusive cyanide in the air or drinking water. Finally, if the clinical findings were clearly consistent with acute cyanide intoxication, then what were the laboratory findings? This question becomes weightily significant in light of the medical director's claim that the blood cyanide and serum thiocyanate differences between nonsmokers and smokers were an important consideration in the investigations. Perhaps some of the objective laboratory results in these lethal cases were similar to laboratory results from living patients in Houston and Philadelphia.

Subsequent to writing the preceding paragraph, I called the medical director's office and asked his secretary if I could acquire the laboratory results from those victims tested in Chicago. The date was August 23, 1983. At first the response was promising. The medical director was in a meeting, but his secretary said that she would mail me the results if the medical director gave her his permission. The next day, however, the secretary called me back and said that the legal authorities in Chicago would not give the medical director permission to release the results.

From April 14th to April 17th my wife and I were both ill at the same time and with the same symptoms. Although our illness was painfully reminiscent of cyanide intoxication, I did not want to believe that we were again inhaling air polluted with hydrogen cyanide gas. One new factor appeared in association with our sickness that I had not positively linked with cyanide intoxication previously. Our urine turned distinctly green in color rather than yellow. The illness returned time after time, and we learned that it was associated with westerly winds. Our urine continued to turn green on occasion during these illnesses. [*My wife and I suspected that some sort of exposure caused the green urine, but it was several weeks before we realized that we again experienced cyanide intoxication in our new location near Cherry Hill. Meanwhile, I felt some better and began exercising, and I may not have taken any antidote to cyanide exposure during this time. After finally deducing that we again suffered symptoms of cyanide intoxication, I developed some speculation in regard to cyanide and green urine. The next paragraph jumps ahead in time to after we realized that we were again experiencing cyanide intoxication, and note that this realization was subsequent to my First Hearing.*]

With the rueful revelation that cyanide again vexed our bodies, I contemplated the green tint to our urine more demurely. This brought a past patient from Houston to my mind, Cheril Moody. Cheril had to leave Gulf Coast Bible College after the fall semester of 1981 due to failing health. Although she saw another physician besides myself, I know that she complained of green urine and green stool.

Putting several facts together: liver damage from cyanide exposure in fish autopsies, liver tenderness in some of my patients suffering cyanide intoxication, the baby that developed toxic hepatitis at the naval hospital, and abnormal liver tests in some of my patients at the naval base; I decided that the green urine probably resulted from toxic effects of cyanide on the liver. One of the more sensitive processes in the liver is transferring conjugated bilirubin into the bile. With slight to moderate liver damage, this bilirubin may spill back into the blood, become oxidized to biliverdin—which is green—and then be excreted into the urine. Lactic acidosis, which sometimes occurs with cyanide intoxication, may boost the oxidation of conjugated bilirubin to the green-colored biliverdin. Green-colored stool may also occur when the total amount of conjugated biliverdin is increased by hemolysis, the breakdown of red blood cells. Increased copper in the blood may cause increased hemolysis, and copper may be increased by cyanide intoxication which releases it from storage sites in the liver.

Despite the accuracy or inaccuracy of my medical speculations regarding green urine in cyanide intoxication, my wife and I faced another round of illness while living near Cherry Hill. This became especially minacious in light of political technicalities explained to me by my new attorney, Lieutenant O'Hanlan. Lieutenant O'Hanlan was stationed in Philadelphia where he served to represent defendants such as myself in *fair hearings*. Such hearings took place before a special panel of judges known as the *Physical Evaluation Board*. My Physical Evaluation Board would consist of a naval captain, a naval commander, and a marine colonel.

I never actually met Lieutenant O'Hanlan until the day before my hearing in Philadelphia. [*Note: I met with Lieutenant O'Hanlan, on the day before my hearing, in Philadelphia. The actual hearing, the next day, was in Bethesda, Maryland.*] Lieutenant Norris informed me that I was fortunate to have Lieutenant O'Hanlan's services, and future events led me to agree wholeheartedly. Lieutenant O'Hanlan called me several times from Philadelphia and gave me advice toward preparing for my upcoming hearing. I also gave Lieutenant O'Hanlan some suggestions, and he followed up on them superbly. One political technicality explained to me by Lieutenant O'Hanlan, which sounded rather inauspicious, was that the Physical Evaluation Board would simply decide whether or not I was *fit for duty*; they would not question my psychiatric diagnosis in the event that I was not found *fit for duty*. In other words, I would either be declared *fit for duty* or *severely paranoid*; there would be no allowances for a physical disease that was caused by cyanide intoxication. Furthermore, I was not aware that my wife and I again suffered from cyanide exposure living near Cherry Hill until after the hearing on May nineteenth.

My health was, at first, considerably better near Cherry Hill than prior to that in Pitman. I thought that the minor symptoms of cyanide intoxication that I experienced were probably setbacks from my prior illness. Perhaps this was wishful thinking. At any rate, there was obviously no choice in the matter; I would have to declare myself *fit for duty*. This seemed to risk reassignment in Philadelphia where I might again suffer from severe cyanide intoxication, but I preferred such a risk to allowing the enactment of a farcical frame-up. Besides, there were thousands of lives to consider besides my own. [*I now know that stating* **millions or billions of lives to consider besides my own** *would be more accurate.*]

Together, Lieutenant O'Hanlan and I compiled several exhibits to present as proof that I was not crazy and that I had suffered from cyanide intoxication. These exhibits would later be designated by the letters *B* through *N*. Exhibit *B* was a psychiatric evaluation from a civilian psychiatrist dated 05/03/83. It read as follows:

PSYCHIATRIC EVALUATION

Reason for Referral:
Dr. Oesch is a 28 year old white married male who presented to the clinic for psychiatric and psychological evaluation. The evaluation was requested by his attorney who is representing him in a hearing concerning his dismissal from his duties as a Navy physician at the Philadelphia Naval Hospital. He relates that the dismissal resulted from his presenting his concerns about a potential environmental problem.
Mental Status Examination:
Dr. Oesch was neatly and appropriately dressed in a three piece suit. Initially tense, he relaxed maintaining good eye contact through the interview. He was friendly, warm, and cooperative. Normal in its rate rhythm and tone, his speech was spontaneous, coherent and goal directed. His mood and affect overall was full, expressive and appropriate. There was no evidence of perceptual disturbances, no symptoms of depression, no ideas of reference or influence, no magical thinking or thought insertion or broadcasting. There was no evidence of derealization or depersonalization. He denied suicidal ideation. His sensorium was intact, revealing an above average intelligence and an ability to use abstract thinking and reasoning. There was no impairment in his judgment.
Summary:

Dr. Oesch is a 28 year old white married male. He presents himself in a warm friendly manner. There were no abnormalities in his speech, mood or affect. There was no evidence of a thought disorder nor of an underlying organic process. He manifested above average intelligence and an ability to think and reason abstractly. His judgment ability was intact.
<u>Assessment</u>:
No significant underlying psychopathology detected.

Cheryl L. Sanfacon, M.D.
Psychiatrist

Exhibit C was a psychological evaluation by two civilian psychologists, one a Ph.D. and the other a psychometric technician. It read as follows:

<u>Reason for Referral</u>:
Mr. Oesch is a medical doctor, presently in the Navy and assigned to the Philadelphia Naval Hospital. Due to his concern and questioning of a potential environmental problem, Dr. Oesch was dismissed from his duties pending a hearing. The Navy is questioning his sanity, and, therefore, psychiatric and psychological evaluations are requested of Dr. Oesch's attorney. Dr. Oesch is married and is originally from Oklahoma. He has been in the Navy since 1978 and is presently a lieutenant. Dr. Oesch attended the University of Texas Medical School in Galveston.
<u>Behavioral Observations</u>:
Dr. Oesch is a pleasant and cooperative 28 year-11 month old male with red hair, wearing glasses for myopia. Dr. Oesch initially is physically tense but quickly and progressively becomes more relaxed and more verbally spontaneous. On most tasks, Dr. Oesch works precisely and systematically, yet demonstrates a variety of approaches to the various presented tasks. No nervous nor overly anxious proclivities are observed. During informal interviewing, Dr. Oesch is relaxed, open and spontaneous. His Christian beliefs and principles transcend his personality, views, and behavior and are essential aspects of his vocation and avocation.
<u>Test Results</u>:
  Tests Administered:
Wechsler Adult Intelligence Scale-Revised (WAIS-R)-selected subtests

Clinical Interview
The Rorschach Test
Draw-a-Person Test
Curtis Incomplete Sentence Test
Minnesota Multiphasic Personality Inventory (MMPI)-computer scored by NCS Interpretive Scoring Systems

Selected subtests of the WAIS-R are administered to screen Dr. Oesch's intellectual skills and to observe his personality styles and approaches on a variety of tasks. The majority of his skills are above average. His most efficient ability areas are his auditory attention and concentration (immediate recall), his social judgment in practical situations, and his analytic/synthetic reasoning (non-verbal problem-solving). Slightly above average are his abstract (verbal) reasoning and his visual sequential perception of a total social situation. Dr. Oesch's resultant score on a task measuring visual perception/attention to his environment is within the average range. His scores and styles of performance reflect above average intellectual ability and a keen analytic approach to problem solving in both practical and social settings.

The personality assessment reflects a young man with a normal personality with satisfactorily developed and integrated affectional needs, adequate impulse control, and no significant indicators of any psychopathology. Dr. Oesch is a thoughtful and pensive person who is overly sensitive to emotional stimulation but with adequate "outer" controls. This emotional sensitivity may actually be an asset in interpersonal relationships, but Dr. Oesch tends to suppress and/or deny negative feelings. Aggressive and hostile tendencies are indicated (normal levels) but are viewed by Dr. Oesch as unacceptable action tendencies. Therefore, these proclivities are suppressed and controlled. His projective test responses indicate good creative potential, excellent problem-solving ability, and a highly religious approach to life. His Christian ethics are evident throughout his test results, partially explains his suppression of negative feelings, and are especially influential on the incomplete sentence test. The test patterns also reflect a high energy level, an achievement orientation, and significant level for work performance.

(As of the writing of this report, the MMPI results had not been received from the computer service. When received, an addendum report will be submitted.)
<u>Diagnosis</u>:
No significant psychopathology is psychometrically revealed.
<u>Summary and Conclusion</u>:
Dr. Oesch is a bright 28 year old male who demonstrates good creative and intellectual ability, excellent problem-solving and reasoning skills, and exceptional judgment in both social and practical situations. Some denial and/or suppression of negative feelings is evident, but this along with his control of impulses and external expression of affect may be a reflection of the influence of his Christian ethics upon his life. No significant psychopathology is evident, nor any salient personality features which would impede his social, emotional, or intellectual functioning.

Dr. Edward G. Daniels   *Aaron Botbyl, Ph.D.*
Psychometric Technician   *Licensed Clinical Psychologist*

I appreciated the report issued by the psychologists, and it was useful in supporting my claims. It seemed surprisingly accurate, though there are instances when someone would be mistaken to give the insinuation that Christian ethics call for the suppression of aggression. The Bible teaches that Christian should cooperate in punishing evildoers (I Peter 2:13-14), and should not forgive those who do not repent (Luke 13:3 & Luke 17:3). Jesus said: Think not that I am come to send peace on earth: I came not to send peace, but a sword. (Matthew 10:34). [*Note: this verse is not in conflict with Luke 2:14. A direct translation of Luke 2:14 would be,* **Glory within to most high God and upon earth peace within to men of good will**. *Thus, Luke 2:14 speaks of peace to men of good will, not peace to an evil world where a sword is needed in order to deliver human beings from evil bondage and grant them the freedom to know and worship Jesus Christ. It follows, then, that the term peacemakers in Matthew 5:9 should be interpreted as those who establish freedom to know and worship Jesus Christ and who foster a society where men are encouraged to be of godly disposition. This subject is addressed in my book:* **New Testament Supernatural & Inerrant: Proof per Hebrew Idiom** *by* **Timothy Swiss**.] The love and peace of God reign in righteousness, they do not withdraw before evil or surrender to wicked tyranny.

Exhibit *D* was an Interpersonal Behavior Survey (IBS) Profile Form filled out by Chaplain Baggott while I was in the naval hospital on December 9, 1982. It was a graph indicating the prominence of particular behavioral traits. Under the heading of *Relationship*, three traits were listed: conflict avoidance, dependency, and shyness. Chaplain Baggott told me that persons with paranoia should rank high in these areas, but I ranked very low—averaging below the fifteenth percentile. Two other qualities also fell below the fifteenth percentile in other sections of the evaluation, they were *expression of anger* and *passive aggressiveness*.

Exhibit *E* was the Discharge Summary written by Commander Gilmore when I was released from the naval hospital on 12/17/82. It stated that *several serum thiocyanate levels were obtained*, yet only one such level appeared in my hospital record. It also stated that I was *admitted for evaluation of proported environmental cyanide detoxification*. I cannot find any such word as *proported* in the dictionary [*this is, of course, is a real word—it simply must not have been in the dictionary that I consulted*], but I never made any claims of being *detoxified* by my presence at the naval hospital. Just the opposite occurred during both my first and second admittances to the naval hospital: I was toxified by environmental cyanide.

The first sentence of the last paragraph in Commander Gilmore's summary reads as follows: *Psychiatric evaluation was obtained, and at the time of discharge was felt to have a fixed paranoid delusion*. I could not help laughing after reading that my *psychiatric evaluation* had a *paranoid delusion*. I suspect, however, that the misdiagnosis stemmed from more than just delusion. The remainder of that same paragraph read as follows:

However, it was felt that there was a personality disorder involving the conviction that cyanide poisoning was occurring, in the absence of significant evidence of this and, in spite of, reassurance of essentially normal screening for cyanide, both in himself, the environment that he was working in, and in a number of individuals who he obtained screening tests on. The patient was discharged on 17 December 1982 with 30 days convalescent leave pending a medical board.

The preceding two sentences are quite fascinating when one considers how much false information they contain. Commander Gilmore had in her possession a copy of my blood cyanide test from

Houston showing a level of 104 mcg/dl. She wrote herself, in the first paragraph of the summary, that my thiocyanate levels were pending at the time of discharge—how can one be reassured that the results of tests are essentially normal when those results are not yet known? Furthermore, the screening tests on individuals at the shipyard were not negative for cyanide exposure, they were conclusively positive.

Exhibit *F* was copies of nursing notes from my hospitalization at the naval hospital. Exhibit *G* was a handwritten statement from the corpsman who drew my venous blood on December eleventh, verifying that the blood was bright red in color. Exhibit *H* was a telephone deposition taken from a licensed practical nurse, Mrs. Marion L. Bryant. She stated that my lips and fingernails became noticeably blue during my hospitalization, and that she noticed my blue coloration even before I mentioned it to her. I was thankful to receive this deposition since my hospital records failed to include any episodes of cyanosis.

Exhibit *I* consisted of two data summaries: one for symptoms of cyanide intoxication, and one for reference values for urine thiocyanate in nonsmokers. Lieutenant O'Hanlan suggested that I construct these summaries and list specific references to support each item. The symptomatic summary read as follows: [*I listed twelve different scientific references for symptoms of cyanide, and listed the symptoms stated by each reference. To list all of these would be rather redundant in consideration of what has already been penned in this book, but suffice it to say that they definitely supported the fact that my symptoms in the hospital were consistent with cyanide intoxication.*]

The urine thiocyanate summary read as follows: [*Again, I will avoid redundancy in listing the seven sources that followed in regard to urine thiocyanate levels in nonsmokers. However, I do want to include the concluding paragraph for Exhibit I. It read as follows:*]

One point to especially note in the above summary is that industrial workers with known, documented exposure to hydrogen cyanide gas had urine thiocyanate averaging 6 to 13 mcg/ml. These were derived from a completely separate study from the one NIOSH cited for reference values of urine thiocyanate in nonsmokers, values which may have been so notably low because the subjects tested were on special diets avoiding foods such as cabbage and broccoli. [The average urine thiocyanate in nonsmokers in this NIOSH study was only 0.17 mcg/ml plus or minus 0.136 mcg/ml.] The industrial workers who were tested included both smokers and nonsmokers. This makes the findings among workers at the naval shipyard very significant, definitely indicating exposure to cyanide. [*The average urine thiocyanate among ten nonsmokers tested at the shipyard, including my own urine thiocyanate level, was 10.5 mcg/ml.*]

Exhibit *J* provided copies of lab reports confirming hypogammaglobulinemia in myself and elevated urine thiocyanate levels in my wife. Melody's urine was collected in Pitman, and my gammaglobulin test was performed on blood drawn during my hospitalization in the naval hospital. Exhibit *K* was a phone deposition from Chester Parkins' personal physician in Philadelphia, Doctor Lester J. Groverman, M.D. In it, Doctor Groverman verified that Chester had a serum thiocyanate level of 21 mcg/ml [*2.1 mg/dl*] and that this is a high level. He also confirmed that Chester was a nonsmoker, having stopped smoking about two years before that time. [*Note that Chester's serum thiocyanate level was even higher than the upper range of normal in a smoker.*] Furthermore, Chester was discharged from a civilian hospital [*Harrison Hospital*] on February 14, 1983, with the diagnosis of *chronic lung disease, chronic cyanide intoxication*.

Exhibit *L* was a telephone deposition from Doctor Hitt in Houston. All of these depositions were taken by Lieutenant O'Hanlan. In his deposition, Doctor Hitt definitely confirmed his belief that a problem with cyanide contamination existed in Houston. He discussed his own positive testing for cyanide exposure among patients, and strongly supported the testing which I ordered while in Houston. In addition, he mentioned that many of his patients with cyanide intoxication had low immunoglobulin levels, especially low IgG (hypogammaglobulinemia). This same finding appeared in testing done on myself in the naval hospital.

Exhibit *M* was actual copies of the test orders and test results of patients tested for thiocyanate at the naval shipyard. I put the reference *Code 2* on many of the test orders, meaning that these patients were carefully questioned and had not smoked at all during the preceding two weeks. Most of them, of course, were simply nonsmokers. Exhibit *N* was a telephone summary between Lieutenant O'Hanlan and my attorney in Houston, Brenda Jenkins. The summary read as follows:

SUMMARY OF TELEPHONE CONVERSATION DATED 18 MAY 1983 BETWEEN LT O'HANLAN, JAGC, USNR, AND BRENDA JENKINS, ESQUIRE

Ms. Jenkins with the law firm of Werner and Rusk, 3636 San Jacinto, Houston, Texas, is the attorney for Timothy Oesch et al., in a law suit pending against the City of Houston for cyanide poisoning in the environment.

Ms. Jenkins assured me that in addition to test results from both Dr. Oesch and Dr. William Hitt, that she has additional evidence including water testing, soil testing and foliage tests showing unusually high levels of cyanide in the Houston area.

The suit has not yet been filed.

An initial lawsuit, actually against General Electric Company, was filed on June 29, 1983. Thirty-five plaintiffs were named in the suite, including my wife and me.

Our opposition in the upcoming hearing in Philadelphia, namely the officers who signed my original Medical Board, would submit two documents on their behalf. One was the initial Medical Board itself, presented previously in chapter twelve. The other was a report by Dr. Jason Mills, Laboratory Director for National Medical Services. This, of course, would not be my first conflict with National Medical Services. Dr. Mills' report read as follows:

Dr. Dr. Gilmore:
In accordance with your request, I have reviewed the Medical Board Report Rebuttal of January 13, 1983 and attachments of laboratory reports.

You asked for my expert opinion as a pharmacologist and forensic toxicologist as to whether or not the conditions and circumstances in the above constitute evidence of acute cyanide poisoning episodes or chronic cyanide poisoning due to alleged wind-borne general environmental ambient air contamination with cyanide arising from electroplating (or other) operations at some distance from the site of occurrence of alleged cyanide-caused illness.

It is my scientifically reasonably certain opinion that the described circumstances do not support any reasonable contention of acute or chronic excessive exposure to cyanide in the ambient general environmental air as a competent cause of acute or chronic cyanide poisoning for the following reasons.

At ambient temperatures, Hydrocyanic acid (HCN, Hydrogen Cyanide) is a gas which is slightly lighter than air and thus is rapidly dispersively diluted relative to its originating source. For an acutely toxic concentration to prevail at any significant distance down-wind from a cyanide source, obviously and classically grossly acute to fatal cases would abound in the area between the source and the complainant.

There is no corroborated or accepted experimental, epidemiologic or clinical evidence that idiosyncratic hypersensitivity – acute or chronic – exists to trace concentrations of cyanide in general environmental ambient air such as are postulated in the present case. Therefore, the absence of mass illness in personnel in the same location as the complainant also mitigates against cyanide in the ambient air as the cause of the complaints.

There a numerous <u>dietary</u> sources of cyanide (as cyano gluconides) and thiocyanate, in addition to their normal metabolic formation by man and in addition to such other common sources as tobacco smoke, power engine emissions, combinations of nitrogen containing organic materials and microbial formation. The possibility that chronic occupational exposure to an average of 6 to 10 ppm cyanide in the breathing zone for long periods (up to 15 years) may produce thyroid anomalies is controversial. Similarly, it has been suggested that chronic heavy smoking (tobacco smoke contains cyanide concentrations which may reach over 100 ppm!) and ineffectively detoxified cyanogenic staples (cassava) may cause certain neurologic disease.

The present case, therefore presumes unlikely – not just unorthodox – assumptions in order to implicate a hypothetical toxic environment, without objective environmental measurement evidence, in the cause of claimed illness.

Sincerely,
Jason Mills, Ph.D.
Laboratory Director

It interested me that Dr. Mills used some of the same arguments as the Houston Health Department, such as claiming that many people would have to be dead in order for large amounts of cyanide to disseminate from a given source. The simple explanation that cyanide compounds are dispersed in the environment before generating cyanide gas, so that the gas does not come from a point source, should not be too complicated for a Ph.D. to comprehend [*such as with the discharge of cyanide wastes into drainage waters from a plating operation*]. [*Also, consider how the smoke and fumes from an incinerator are dispersed into the air from the top of a stack, and how exhaust fumes from automobiles are dispersed.*] Of course, in some instances, the dispersed compounds may still be concentrated enough to cause death. Besides this, Dr. Mills was wrong to insinuate that hydrogen cyanide gas is lighter than air and will float upwards: the weight of hydrogen cyanide gas is 27 grams per mole, and the weight of nitrogen gas, which composes 80% of our atmosphere, is 28 grams per mole. The weight of oxygen gas is 32 grams per mole, so according to weight—hydrogen cyanide gas may blend more stably with our atmosphere than oxygen.

There is quite an inconsistency in denying idiosyncratic hypersensitivity to cyanide in the air among particular individuals and then turning around and stating that certain neurologic diseases may result from *ineffectively detoxified cyanogenic dietary staples*. If someone is ineffective in detoxifying cyanide from a dietary source, then he will also be ineffective in detoxifying cyanide from the air: cyanide is cyanide. Dr. Mills sent two references with his report which themselves revealed his report to be erroneous. These references included *Patty's Industrial Hygiene and Toxicology*, pp. 4845-53; and *Drill's Pharmacology in Medicine*, pp. 1180-1203.

Utilizing the two articles forwarded by Dr. Mills, I wrote the following essay:

Literature From National Medical Services Regarding Environmental Cyanide

My serum thiocyanate level from blood drawn on 11DEC82 was 1.8 mg/dl. I pointed out to my naval physician that the average serum thiocyanate level in three dogs sacrificed by cyanide poisoning was 1.9 mg/dl. A fourth dog in the study, that became unable to stand or walk without difficulty—but did not die—had a serum thiocyanate level of 1.3 mg/dl. This data is found in an article from the **Journal of the American Medical Association***, March 6, 1978, Volume 239, p. 946. My naval* *physician responded by saying that dogs are more sensitive to cyanide than humans. I was unaware of any data regarding such a statement, so I made no objection to the remark.* [*Of note, a study published in 2007, namely Cyanide-metabolizing enzyme rhodanese in human tissues: comparison with domestic animals,* **Comparative Clinical Pathology***, March 2007, Volume 16, Issue 1, pp 47-51, Mahmoud Aminlari, Ali Malekhusseini, Fatemeh Akrami, Hadi Ebrahimnejad; reports that the rhodanese activity in the liver of dogs is comparable to that in humans: and another article, found at the following internet site:* https://www.researchgate.net/publication/290656066_Cyanide_Detoxifying_Enzyme_Rhodanese; *reports that the liver is believed to be the major site of cyanide detoxification. I will concede that dogs reportedly have lower rhodanese activity in the kidneys than humans.*]

On pages 4851 and 4852 of **Patty's Industrial Hygiene and Toxicology***, which is literature forwarded by a toxicologist from National Medical Services, one finds a comparison between the sensitivities of human beings and dogs to cyanide exposure. Air levels reported as rapidly fatal are 315 ppm in dogs, and 270 ppm in humans. Dogs may tolerate 30 ppm cyanide, and humans may develop slight, acute symptoms at 18 to 36 ppm cyanide.* [*Note that these air levels likely refer to normal, average human beings rather than to human beings with exceptional sensitivity or vulnerability to cyanide exposure.*] *In short, it appears that dogs and human beings have very similar sensitivities to given quantities of acute cyanide exposure. This reemphasizes the pertinence of data from the dog study found in the* **Journal of the American Medical Association***. It also adds additional evidence toward the severity of cyanide exposure I experienced at NRMC Philadelphia.*

In other literature forwarded by the toxicologist from National Medical Services, taken from **Drill's Pharmacology in Medicine***, several pertinent factors are disclosed. The article mentions that industrial effluents and other waste waters at times contain high cyanide concentrations. It reveals that industrial and other sources make cyanide a fairly widespread potential hazard of industry as well as of the non-occupational environment (p. 1190). The same page also states that hydrogen cyanide constitutes a highly volatile inhalation hazard, that it has vapor density about the same as air, and that it will readily permeate a room. In addition, page 1191 affirms that most* *intoxications by HCN are a result of inhalation, and that the most rapidly developing form of poisoning occurs from inhalation. This is explained by pointing out that the more rapidly HCN is absorbed, the less it takes to cause a given effect. Deaths by inhalation may result from as little as 0.7 mg of cyanide per kilogram of body weight; this is about 50 mg in an average, adult male.*

Drill's Pharmacology in Medicine *further explains why venous blood is almost as bright red as arterial blood in acute cyanide poisoning, and why rapid breathing occurs (p. 1190). Sodium thiosulfate and hydroxocobalamin are both noted as treatments for cyanide intoxication (pp. 1191, 1193, & 1194). ST electrocardiographic changes are associated with acute poisoning, which is pertinent since a nonsmoking patient from the Philadelphia Naval Shipyard presented with ST depression, was sent to Locality Hospital [there may have been a hospital referred to as Harrison Hospital, based upon one affidavit I found—Locality Hospital is a fictitious name], and was tested positively for cyanide exposure. His urine thiocyanate level was 9 mcg/ml, and his serum thiocyanate level was 2.1 mg/dl. This signifies exposure to a sufficient quantity of cyanide to cause death.*

Patty's Industrial Hygiene and Toxicology *also offers pertinent information. It lists symptoms which may appear with lower dosages of cyanide, namely weakness, headache, confusion, and occasionally nausea and vomiting. Rapid pulse is also noted (p. 4846). Regarding acute cyanide poisoning, it states:* **The most specific pathologic finding in acute cases is the bright red color of venous blood**. *Urine thiocyanate concentrations are given for both smokers and nonsmokers not exposed to cyanide, the level for smokers being 4.4 mg/L, and the level for nonsmokers being 0.17 mg/L (p. 4848). Bear in mind that the units mg/L are equivalent to the units mcg/ml which are used by National Medical Services.*

Soon after becoming aware of a problem of cyanide intoxication at the Philadelphia Naval Shipyard, I was scheduled to lecture the physicians and physicians' assistants at the shipyard dispensary regarding cyanide poisoning. On page 4845 of **Patty's Industrial Hygiene and Toxicology***, the following is stated: 'It is essential that all personnel working with processes involving cyanides or nitriles be specially trained so that they are fully aware of the hazards and follow faithfully all rules laid down for safe handling. It is also essential that* *special training be given in the specific first aid measures, and that adequate specific antidotes be available for first aid and for use by physicians.' Additionally, a sentence from page 4849 states: 'In order to use effectively such first aid and medical therapy, it is necessary that all personnel and all physicians and nurses be thoroughly familiar with the toxic effects of cyanide and with the specific first aid therapy.' Thus, the lecture I planned to give at the dispensary was medically indicated, if not mandated. This was not only true because cyanide was utilized on the base, but also because patients were presenting to the dispensary with symptoms of cyanide intoxication. A captain in the environmental department at NRMC Philadelphia forbid my lecturing on the subject of cyanide. The lecture was never given.*

Sincerely,
Timothy Oesch, M.D.

Another article I wrote which pertained to both the Houston Health Department and National Medical Services was one entitled *Misuse of Information by the Houston Health Department and National Medical Services*. The article followed my investigation of the references alluded to by both of these agencies in supporting their claims. I made some notably pertinent discoveries. The essay follows:

National Medical Services, and the Houston Health Department, each forwarded misused information from single, published references pertaining to cyanide intoxication. The article chosen by National Medical Services is found in **Archives of Biochemistry and BioPhysics**, *Vol. 39, pp. 292-299, 1952. That selected by an ad hoc committee in Houston, entitled* **Cyanide Exposure In Fires**, *is found in* **Lancet**, *08JUL78, 2(8080):91-2. All the literature on chronic cyanide intoxication as a whole, definitely supports the presence of poisoning in Houston and in Philadelphia. By looking closely at the two articles mentioned above, one may ascertain how misuse of information and misrepresentation of facts falsely belittled the seriousness and extent of cyanide contamination in the Houston and Philadelphia environments.*

*First, National Medical Services used the article they selected to forward a reference value of **up to 20 mcg/ml** for urine thiocyanate levels in nonsmokers. To my knowledge, no other major laboratory in the United States uses a reference value above 5 mcg/ml, and both Bio-*

A Breath of Cyanide

Science Laboratories and Metpath Laboratories designate 2 mcg/ml [2 mg/L] as the upper limit in nonsmokers. Furthermore, by examining the selected article, it is easy to see that the article gives absolutely no grounds or basis for establishing a normal reference value for urine thiocyanate in nonsmokers. A total of seven urine thiocyanate levels are disclosed in the entire report, only three of which are stated to come from normal subjects. There is no mention whatsoever as to whether any of these subjects are smokers or nonsmokers. In addition, the summary to this report reveals that the thiocyanate was measured indirectly, after rapid oxidation of thiocyanate to cyanide, rather than by direct measurement of thiocyanate itself. All in all, the defectiveness of this report for obtaining reference values for urine thiocyanate in nonsmokers is blatantly apparent.

Secondly, the article selected by the ad hoc committee in Houston forwards the highest reference values for blood cyanide of any legitimate-appearing article I have read; it does not forward values in keeping with the majority of literature on the subject. Nonetheless, the article still strongly supports the presence of cyanide exposure to patients tested in Houston. How the article supports cyanide contamination will be pointed out, as well as how the Houston Health Department misused the article.

First of all, the control group used to derive blood cyanide levels consisted of individuals attending an outpatient clinic at a hospital. It is very conceivable that many of these individuals were ill or had some type of chronic medical problem. Despite this fact, the Houston Health Department claimed these reference values were from normal, healthy individuals. Besides this, the average level of blood cyanide among control nonsmokers in this study, namely 7.5 mcg/dl, is still 44% lower than the average level among thirty-seven nonsmokers tested in Houston, namely 13.5 mcg/dl. Furthermore, the average level among nonfatal-casualty nonsmokers given in the article, referring to individuals exposed to fumes presumably containing cyanide gas, was 27.1 mcg/dl. Notably, twenty-five of the thirty-seven nonsmokers tested in Houston, who had positive results for cyanide exposure with levels above 4 mcg/dl, yielded an average level of 27.5 mcg/dl, a level greater than the nonfatal-casualty reference above.

The ad hoc committee in Houston emphasized that thiocyanate levels are better for evaluating exposure to cyanide than are blood cyanide levels. I agree with this statement. The article they selected for reference gives levels of blood thiocyanate as well as blood cyanide. The average blood thiocyanate in control nonsmokers was 0.18 mg/dl, corresponding to a serum thiocyanate of about 0.3 mg/dl. The nonfatal-casualty level in nonsmokers was 0.39 mg/dl, corresponding to a serum thiocyanate level of about 0.65 mg/dl. The average serum thiocyanate among fourteen nonsmokers tested in Houston was 0.49 mg/dl, 63% greater than the above reference [meaning the reference for the average in control nonsmokers]. Furthermore, the average among nine of the fourteen tests, which were designated as positive for exposure to cyanide, was 0.61 mg/dl, an average near that for nonfatal-casualties in nonsmokers listed in the above reference. Thus, the thiocyanate levels given in this article definitely support the conclusion that patients in Houston experienced cyanide exposure.

One or two additional points about the article selected by the ad hoc committee in Houston merit consideration. The average blood cyanide for smokers in this article was more than twice that of nonsmokers. Among my patients in Houston, the average blood cyanide was higher in nonsmokers than smokers. This indicates that environmental exposure to cyanide was sufficiently high to override the normally higher blood cyanide in smokers. Also, the article gives an average blood cyanide level of 65.8 mcg/dl for cases of fatality following exposure to fumes. The article does not attribute these deaths solely to cyanide, but this level still serves to accentuate the seriousness of cyanide exposure in Houston.

Thus, when the Houston Health Department circulated information which suggested that blood cyanide levels up to 31 mcg/dl should be considered normal in nonsmokers, they were being deceptively misleading. The very article they used to obtain this figure discloses that lower levels than this can indicate exposure to cyanide-containing fumes. The failure to reveal the truth about information which they obviously had in hand, may have cost lives, and almost certainly contributed to extensive human suffering. Likewise, the apparent, fallacious reference value forwarded by National Medical Services may have already permitted otherwise remediable, human suffering.

Sincerely,
Timothy Oesch, M.D.

Although I suggested using the above article as evidence at my May nineteenth hearing, Lieutenant O'Hanlan advised against it. He seemed to want the case kept as simple and straight forward as possible; but he received quite a surprise from our opposition.

Chapter 17

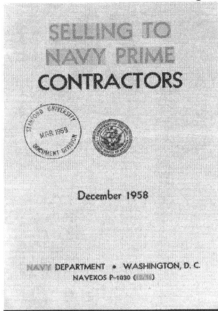

(Note: the following address to the plating plant that was located in the Timbergrove region of Houston, next to the Heights, is found on page 121 of the book of Navy Contractors that is featured to the left. The author was unaware of this connection between the plating facility and the U.S. Navy during the time of his military service in Philadelphia; and in fact, did not find out about this connection until the year 2020.

First Hearing

My wife's blood was drawn on May 3, 1983, and tested for Histoplasma yeast antibodies; the test was positive. [*I have definitely associated chronic cyanide intoxication with reduced function of the immune system.*] I think her doctor was concerned that the multiple lymph swellings all over her body might be cancer, but my mother-in-law diagnosed my wife correctly by telephone before any tests were run. I am not sure when more specific cyanide symptoms such an anxious depression first reappeared, but my wife's fungal disease probably postponed recognition of cyanide intoxication. Furthermore, I was not looking for cyanide intoxication—I wanted it behind us so badly that I refused to see it until it became undeniably obvious. With the navy accusing me of paranoia, the last thing I wanted to do was discover that the area near Cherry Hill was also affected by cyanide contamination.

My wife began taking Nizoral every morning to treat her fungal infection. The swelling gradually decreased and she began improving consistently, except that now and then she experienced puzzling episodes of illness which seemed to come and go for no apparent reason. With time, these episodes worsened into the typical syndrome of cyanide intoxication—despite the improvement in her histoplasmosis. I started keeping track of wind direction, and it was easy to ascertain that westerly winds brought illness. My own health was somewhat better than my wife's, but I could definitely tell the difference between a day with easterly winds and a day with westerly winds.

The new discovery of cyanide contamination did not take place until after my hearing on May nineteenth. I drove to Philadelphia on the eighteenth and met for a while with Lieutenant O'Hanlan. His appearance did not surprise me; he looked like a young, Irish boxer in spring training. We went over the strategy for the next day's hearing, which would be the very first hearing the following morning. With all the evidence we had in hand, Lieutenant O'Hanlan was quite optimistic about a successful outcome.

I met with Lieutenant O'Hanlan again at about 6:30 a.m. the next day: "Just talk with them person to person, they're usually fairly reasonable," he advised. [*This hearing was with the Regional Physical Evaluation Board, Naval Medical Command Bethesda Hospital, Bethesda, Maryland.*]

Copies of our exhibits were completed just in time to supply one copy to each member of the Physical Evaluation Board. Lieutenant O'Hanlan and I entered the board room and I was seated at the end of a long table. Another table was centered perpendicularly at the other end of this table, forming a *T* configuration. The three board members sat along the adjoining table facing me.

In the center of the adjoining table sat Colonel Clark, USMC, President of the Board. He was stalky and solid with weathered skin and thin, grayish-white hair. To his left sat Commander Wyvill, USNR, a considerably younger reserve officer who sat in on the hearing because I was a reserve officer: it was a matter of policy. To the right of Colonel Clark sat Captain Wilson, MC, USN. He was a replacement for the usual medical officer who sat in on cases for reserve officers. Apparently the usual medical officer was unable to attend.

To my left, at the side of the first table, was Lieutenant O'Hanlan's position. To my right, along the other side of the table, sat Lieutenant

Reynolds, JAGC, USNR, and Mr. Preen [*I'm quite certain that* **Preen** *is a fictitious name*], the recorder. Lieutenant Reynolds was a female attorney assigned to represent my opposition. When Lieutenant O'Hanlan and I entered, everyone else was already seated in their positions. Introductions were made, then Lieutenant O'Hanlan had to leave the room to retrieve something he had forgotten.

During Lieutenant O'Hanlan's absence, an awkward silence beset the room. I tried making eye contact with the Board members, but when this failed, I decided not to even attempt initiating conversation. Everyone seemed intent on studying their fingernails, toes, or gazing blankly in the direction of inanimate objects. Finally Lieutenant O'Hanlan returned and took his position. Opening formalities were taken care of; I *affirmed* to tell the truth, and the hearing was underway.

Lieutenant Reynolds presented the opposing evidence: "In addition to Exhibit A, I offer into evidence the report by Jason Mills, Ph.D., Laboratory Director for the National Naval Medical Laboratory, as Exhibit B."

This was the first time I ever heard National Medical Services called National Naval Medical Laboratory. Considering the location of the laboratory in the same town as a Naval Air Base, however, it was not too surprising.

Colonel Clark responded: "Exhibits A and B are, subject to any objection, received in evidence."

"Would you further identify Exhibit B," directed Captain Wilson.

"It was sent to Lieutenant Gilmore. Could Lieutenant Oesch further identify this exhibit?" inquired Lieutenant Reynolds.

I was startled to be asked to identify the opposition's evidence. Having been informed about the letter by Lieutenant O'Hanlan, though, I did know more about the letter than Lieutenant Reynolds seemed to know.

"Lieutenant Gilmore is actually Commander Gilmore," I pointed out. "She is an internist at NRMC, Philadelphia."

"It is my understanding that his material was forwarded to us from the Naval Hospital, Philadelphia, as further information," inserted Captain Wilson.

It was quizzical that Captain Wilson basically answered his own, previous question. Furthermore, he eyed me questioningly as he did so.

"As far as I know," I responded to Captain Wilson's interrogating stare.

"He has no idea," spoke up Lieutenant O'Hanlan. His voice was chastising.

"Exhibit B then pertains to documents from the hospital at Philadelphia," surmised Colonel Clark, as if to settle the issue.

"Yes," attested Lieutenant Reynolds.

Lieutenant O'Hanlan was not satisfied with such a settlement. "I'd like to object to Exhibit B," he asserted.

"On what grounds?" questioned Colonel Clark.

"It's not clear from that letter exactly what was reviewed by Doctor Mills and exactly what was presented to him or how it was presented to him."

Colonel Clark seemed rather embroiled. "This Board will recess to consider your objection."

What Colonel Clark's *recess* actually meant was that Lieutenant O'Hanlan, Lieutenant Reynolds, and I had to go out in the hall and wait while the Board members decided what to do. It also meant that the Board members would carry on a discussion that would not be recorded.

"Do you think they'll throw it out?" I asked Lieutenant O'Hanlan as we stood in the hallway.

Lieutenant O'Hanlan's attitude about the case already seemed altered. "They'll probably just note the objection and go on."

We were summoned back to our position. The hearing resumed:

"This Board will come to order," announced Colonel Clark. "Exhibit B is accepted in evidence, your objection is noted. Counsel for the Board, you are instructed to further examine the genesis of Exhibit B and where it came from and what we are doing with it."

"Okay," obliged Lieutenant Reynolds. "May I please be excused to my office?"

"Request granted," pronounced Colonel Clark, and Lieutenant Reynolds quickly left the room. "Counsel for the member, proceed."

Lieutenant O'Hanlan addressed the Board undauntedly. "Right at the outset, sir, I would like to make another objection and that is to both Exhibits A and B as not following the standards set for diagnosis of mental disorders as set out in the VA Code under which this Board is charged to work, specifically Section 4.126. It states that: *It must be established first that a true mental disorder exists*. Then it goes on to state that normal reactions, discouragement, anxiety, depression, et cetera, must not be accepted by the rating a Board is indicative of.

"More importantly, right here," expounded Lieutenant O'Hanlan, addressing literature he held opened in one hand, "*mere failure of social and industrial adjustment or the presence of numerous complaints should not, in the absence of definite symptomatology typical of a psychoneurotic or psychophysiologic disorder, become the acceptable basis of the diagnosis in this field.*" He looked up from the literature toward the Board members. "There is evidence in Exhibit A that Lieutenant Oesch exhibited specific symptoms, mainly elevated thiocyanate levels in his bloodstream, to indicate that there is something wrong with him and these are not symptoms that can rise about through psychoneurotic or psychophysiologic disorders, and he has not been properly diagnosed. From the start, I would like to object to the whole Board."

"Okay," said Colonel Clark, "I understand your objections to Exhibits A and B, and the Board will take those objections into consideration during deliberations."

"Thank you," returned Lieutenant O'Hanlan. "Right now I would like to introduce into evidence exhibits for the member..."

At this point in the hearing, Lieutenant O'Hanlan presented the exhibits *B* through *N* which were discussed in the preceding chapter. Afterwards, Colonel Clark accepted them as evidence. Following this came the portion of the hearing denoted *Examination By Counsel For The Member*. Lieutenant O'Hanlan asked me a large number of questions in order to elicit new, pertinent evidence...

"Lieutenant Oesch comes before the Board today asking that he be found fit for full duty," stated Lieutenant O'Hanlan. Then he turned to me: "Lieutenant Oesch, how do you feel today?"

"All right," I replied.

"Specifically, the symptoms that you complained of in your Medical Board, in the hospital, have they cleared up?"

"Yes, they have."

"Could you describe for the Board exactly what those symptoms were?"

"Weakness, lethargy, foggy-mindedness, inability to remember things well or concentrate, bad headaches, shortness of breath, and some chest pain."

"Where are you living now?"
"Marlton, New Jersey."
"Have you recently moved?"
"Yes."
"Why did you move?"
"I moved because my wife had a severe illness which was threatening death. I had to send her to Iowa for six weeks of recovery and then bring her back to the apartment in Marlton rather than Pitman."
"What was the problem in Pitman?"
"Cyanide intoxication."
"Do you know that there was industry there that was putting cyanide in the air?"
"Yes. We found out that we were within a mile and a half of a plant which utilized cyanide and, nearby, to the north, were five more electroplating plants that used cyanide in a neighboring town. And there was still another electroplating plant in another town to the northwest."
"Is your wife doing better now in Marlton?"
"As far as cyanide goes she is much better and is doing fine. However, she now has a relapse of histoplasmosis, which is a fungal disease, which, when someone's immunity system is decreased or compromised—it can regrow again, and we feel that probably the cyanide intoxication harmed her immune system so that the fungus was allowed to grow again."
"*We*, meaning you and who?"
"She and I. Her doctor, Doctor DeEugenio, said that he would put histoplasmosis on the top of the list as the most likely cause—she now has lumps growing on her neck, axillae, inguinal region, and along the inner aspect of her arms. He was also the doctor that wrote down the diagnosis of cyanide toxicity for what she had last fall."
"When you sent her home to Iowa, did she start improving?"
"She immediately started improving when she left. After six weeks, she was not completely back to normal, but she was improved enough that I brought her back to New Jersey—only this time to Marlton, where we moved."
"Did she exhibit the same symptoms you discussed earlier?"
"When I first brought her back from Iowa we still lived in Pitman. Within three days of returning to Pitman, she began demonstrating symptoms of cyanide intoxication again. And when we moved to Marlton, the symptoms cleared quickly and have not returned."

"And these are the very same symptoms of cyanide intoxication which you described earlier for yourself?"

"Yes."

"But as far as your health, are you working out now?"

"About two weeks ago I started working out again for the first time since I grew too ill to do so in November, or actually at the end of October."

"What do your workouts involve?"

"At this point I'm just walking, jogging, doing some pushups, leg lifts, jumping jacks, and things like that. When I get in better shape I'll start more strenuous activity again."

"What did you do before you became ill? What sort of activity, athletics?"

"Well, I've been in sports all my life, high school, college, and AAU. Once I got out of college I continued sprinting and started body building. I do pretty strenuous workouts when I'm not ill."

"When you were released from the hospital on December 17th, what did you do then?"

"I was put on 30 days of convalescent leave, and I went out of state for two weeks. After two weeks I came back for a medical appointment with Commander Gilmore. And then, I planned to go out of state again, but Commander Gilmore said I had to stay in order to sign my Medical Board."

"When did you go back to work?"

"I went back to work approximately January seventeenth."

"What did you do?"

"I was put on the eighth deck in Command Education. There I taught courses to EMT's, corpsmen, nurses and physicians. I taught subjects such as fluid and electrolytes, head and neck injuries, eye injuries, and cardiovascular risks. I also revised, well, I actually redid the indoctrination course for new physicians at NRMC, Philadelphia. It was a 210 page production giving a 10 day orientation program. The reading, activities and all were included."

Since decreased production ability is one feature of paranoia, Lieutenant O'Hanlan and I purposely pointed out my productivity while working in Command Education.

"When you were working on the eighth deck, did you start exhibiting these symptoms again?" posed Lieutenant O'Hanlan.

"To an extent, but I took daily treatments of antidote, you know—for cyanide. During the first six weeks, or perhaps the first two months of my illness, I did not know what I had, and was not treating myself—and I was unable to continue working. Once I found out that I had cyanide intoxication, I started taking the antidote. As long as I was taking the antidote, I never missed a day of work—but I was still sick, yes."

"Are you still working there?"

"No, I am not."

"Why not?"

"On approximately April first I was put on home subsistence."

"Why?"

"I don't know. I introduced an Article 138 Complaint and almost immediately afterward was put on home subsistence."

"What was the article 138? Did that involve any of what we are talking about today?"

"Yes, it did."

"Can you give us briefly what you encountered? What happened?"

"Before issuing the Article 138 Complaint, I requested that the Commanding Officer at NRMC Philadelphia drop my psychiatric diagnosis and change the diagnosis to chronic cyanide intoxication. This was not granted, so I submitted the Article 138 Complaint."

"What sort of antidote were you taking?"

"I was taking mostly sodium thiosulfate, which is a salt containing sulfur. It's nonprescription, so basically anyone can purchase it who wants to, and it doesn't have any harmful side effects unless you take gobs and gobs of it, except perhaps for some diarrhea. The other thing that I took was hydroxocobalamin, which is a particular type of vitamin B12. The doses I took were not really sufficient to treat cyanide intoxication by themselves, but they were still helpful when used in addition to sodium thiosulfate, and they were also helpful since cyanide can interfere with the body's normal use of vitamin B12."

"Were you giving yourself shots or anything?"

"I was taking shots of hydroxocobalamin for a while, but then I decided to start drinking it since there is no reason that a normal person—by normal I mean someone without intrinsic factor deficiency—cannot absorb vitamin B12 from the stomach. Hydroxocobalamin is only available in injectable form, but I just started drinking it anyway because, the shots—I don't like taking shots."

"When did you first get to Philadelphia?"

"July twenty-second, nineteen eighty-two."

"When were you called to active duty?"

"Approximately, I think it was approximately May of nineteen eighty-two that I was called to active duty beginning on July fifth." [*Note: I'm quite certain that my memory was mistaken in regard to the month of May. I think I received the orders, which were actually dated February 4th, by at least sometime in April.*]

"Where were you between July fifth and July twenty-second when you reported to Philadelphia?"

"I first reported to Corpus Christi where I was sent for indoctrination. I stayed there about ten or eleven days and then traveled to Philadelphia."

"Did you have any problem in Corpus Christi?"

"No. In fact, I improved there quite rapidly and was able to start working out."

"After having left Houston?"

"Right. I started working out every day."

"When you reported to Philadelphia, what was your first assignment?"

"I was placed at the dispensary in the shipyard, working primarily with civilian employees."

"Is this when you ran across the employees whose tests you ordered, that are exhibit *M*?"

"No, because there were no such tests ordered for about two months. I did run across patients with the same symptoms of chronic cyanide poisoning, but at the time I did not know about the electroplating plant on the base."

"So the dispensary is where you ran into people with these symptoms?"

"I ran across the symptoms, yes, but I did not suspect cyanide because I did not know there was any around."

"But at the same time you were starting to exhibit a few of the same symptoms yourself?"

"Yes. I grew gradually worse."

"And you were being seen by whom?"

"I was seen by a number of different physicians at first. I went to sick call either at the hospital or at the dispensary, and there were three, four, or five different physicians who saw me. When my illness grew bad enough that I was sent to internal medicine, then I was seen by Doctor Wendle. Then, when I went into the hospital, I was transferred to Doctor Gilmore."

"So the onset of these symptoms is gradual, they don't all come on as soon as you are exposed?"

"No, they came on gradually and worsened with time."

"When did you decide to order those tests?"

"At the end of my first hospitalization, Doctor Gilmore questioned me about the cyanide intoxication in Houston. She also asked me for copies of the blood cyanide and thiocyanate tests that were done in Houston on my wife and me. In addition, she informed me that all the tests for other things besides cyanide intoxication had come up negative. My wife brought me a copy of my report from Houston, *Metropolitan Effects of Environmental Cyanide*, to give to Doctor Gilmore. I reread the report myself before giving it to Doctor Gilmore, and noted that the symptoms I experienced in the naval hospital were exactly the same as those I experienced in Houston. I also noted that all of my general laboratory tests were consistent with cyanide intoxication up to that point, basically all being negative. I gave Doctor Gilmore the report, and decided at that time that with all the evidence given by my six to eight weeks of illness, I had better check into the possibility that I was again experiencing cyanide intoxication."

"How do you interpret the results of those tests?"

"Which tests?"

"The ones that you ordered on the civilian employees at the Philadelphia Naval Shipyard?"

"Definitely positive."

"On several of the people tested?"

"Yes."

"Do you know Doctor Groverman?"

"No, I don't."

"Have you ever spoken with him?"

"Yes, once or twice over the phone for a short period of time."

"Why?"

"I was asking him if he had records of some tests that had been done on one of his patients—which were ordered by a Doctor Schmidt at the Locality Hospital Emergency Room." [*I think this was Harrison*

Hospital Emergency Room. I used a fictional name for this hospital when I first penned this book.]

"You didn't order the tests on Chester Parkins?"

"I suggested that they be ordered. I didn't actually write the order, no."

"And Doctor Groverman, what did he tell you? What did you all discuss? Did he confirm what you thought?"

"Yes, he did."

"Is that what is reflected in the deposition with him, Exhibit *K*?"

"Yes."

"Did he confirm your diagnosis of chronic cyanide intoxication in this patient?"

"To be honest, I'm not really...I don't really remember what is written on those pages. But he did with me on the telephone."

"Do you agree with your Medical Board?"

"No, I don't."

"Why?"

"Because I do not believe that I have any primary psychiatric problems, and I do believe that I have a physical problem resulting from an environmental contaminant—and I have evidence to support those claims."

"Were the doctors ever able to account for your thiocyanate levels being high?"

"No. They made the suggestion that the sodium thiosulfate caused elevated thiocyanate, but they were not able to back this with any factual evidence. Furthermore, I had a serum thiocyanate level of 0.3 when I went into the hospital, and I did not take any antidote for ten days before my blood was drawn on December eleventh after having acute symptoms of cyanide intoxication—and the level of serum thiocyanate then was 1.8. So, considering that I took no antidote during my hospitalization, it would have been impossible for it to have contributed to my elevated serum thiocyanate level."

During this long episode of questions and answers, Lieutenant O'Hanlan and I faced one another and the Board members looked on. Finally, at the mention of my objective serum thiocyanate test from December eleventh, a reaction was elicited from Captain Wilson: "What are the units of measure with this level of 1.8?" he posed.

"One-point-eight milligrams of thiocyanate per deciliter," I answered.

"Milligrams per deciliter?" reiterated Captain Wilson.

"Correct," I affirmed.

Captain Wilson looked down toward the table and made no further remarks.

Lieutenant O'Hanlan resumed his questioning: "Was it ever explained to you why your globulin levels in your bloodstream were so low?"

"No, it wasn't."

Lieutenant O'Hanlan turned briefly toward the Board: "I might add that hypogammaglobulinemia is confirmed and noted in the Medical Board, as well as medical notes from Doctor Oesch's hospital record." He then turned back facing me. "Were you ever removed from that environment to check for possible environmental causes of you illness?"

"No, I wasn't."

"Were you suffering from these symptoms you described earlier—the light-headedness, the foggy memory loss you mentioned earlier—at the time the naval psychiatric evaluation was written?"

"Definitely. My antidote was withheld during my second hospitalization and my symptoms grew very severe."

"Since you were ordered home, have you consulted a psychiatrist?"

"Yes, I have."

"Is that what is in Exhibits *B* and *C*, Doctors Sanfacon and Botbyl?"

"Correct. There was also one other psychologist who conducted psychometric tests."

"What sort of psychometric testing did they do?"

"They did testing to try to analyze my ability to make social judgments about things going on between people. They also tested to try and analyze my ability to make judgments on analytic data, and also tested to see how much attention I pay to my environment, and things such as that."

"What was their conclusion?"

"They said that my highest capabilities were in making social judgments and analytical judgments, and that I was not below average in anything. My lowest rating was in paying attention to my environment."

"Did they find any evidence of psychoneurotic problem?"

"No, they did not."

"Do you agree with the Medical Board's appraisal of the cyanide question in Houston?"

"No, I don't."

"Is there still a question in Houston or a controversy over whether or not cyanide intoxication did exist or still exists?"

"Some people feel there is still a question. I feel that the question has been answered. There is definitely cyanide intoxication in Houston."

"In what way are you still involved in that controversy?"

"I'm a plaintiff along with a lot of other people in a lawsuit down there."

"Do you know Doctor Hitt?"

"Yes, I do."

"How do you know him?"

"I met him through a patient in Houston who had cyanide intoxication—actually, it was through an ex-paramedic who was associated with that patient."

"Have you read the deposition, Exhibit L, that I took from Doctor Hitt over the telephone?"

"Yes, I skimmed it."

"Do you agree with his appraisal of the situation?"

"Yes."

"And the symptoms that he recited as exhibited by you and your wife?"

"Yes."

"Is it true that when you and your wife would leave Houston to visit either her family or your own family that these symptoms would go away?"

The only members of my own family we had visited while living in Houston were my grandmother in Tulsa and my cousin in San Antonio. Still, Lieutenant O'Hanlan's statement was a true one: "Yes, they did. In fact, they went away back then much more rapidly than after we had suffered cyanide intoxication for a longer period of time."

"When you returned again to Houston, would these symptoms come back again?"

"Yes."

"What area of Houston did you live in?"

"Primarily the Heights and Spring Branch, the Heights being east of a particular electroplating plant and Spring Branch being west of the plant—these areas are where we experienced notable illness. We finally moved to Katy in order to escape illness."

"Is that outside of Houston?"

"Yes, it is."

"How far?"

"Not too far, about ten miles."

"Is the areas you mentioned the same area where many of the patients Doctor Hitt examined also lived?"

"Yes, it is—the Heights and Spring Branch."

"Did Doctor Hitt do control studies and everything to test and see whether patients not living in these areas would test differently?"

"Yes, he did."

"What did he find out?"

"The last I spoke to him, and he has progressed since that time, he had tested about 200 controls and got only one positive. That one positive control turned out to be a patient who worked or lived near a plant that used cyanide in another town. Of those persons who were found positive for cyanide poisoning through blood cyanide or serum thiocyanate tests, he found about 50 percent of them had developed—in addition to whatever symptoms you can get from cyanide without being allergic to it—they had also developed sensitivity to cyanide, like allergy to cyanide. So out of his control group only one out of 200 showed allergy to cyanide, and of the patients who were ill in the contaminated areas of Houston, over 50 percent tested positive for allergy to cyanide."

"And was he able to isolate the area involved?"

"To some extent he was, yes."

"And that was the Heights area?"

"Heights and Spring Branch."

"Would you agree also with Doctor Hitt that a lot of the symptoms that these patients exhibited had to do more specifically with the effects of cyanide on the mental processes and memory and thought?"

"Well, yes they did—because cyanide affects almost every tissue in the body, including brain tissue."

"Who prepared the exhibits on the cyanide reference levels?"

"I did."

"Have you done extensive research in this field?"

"Yes, I have."

"Why?"

"Because a large number of my patients in Houston were affected by it, so I felt behooved to find out about it on their account. Also, my wife and I both experienced cyanide intoxication and that gave me a personal interest in the subject."

"Have you also done research into dietary causes of cyanide intoxication?"

"Yes, I have."

"What have you concluded?"

"I have done research in literature on the subject, and have also tested people after having them eat unreasonably large amounts of types of plants that are supposed to contain cyanide. The results of these tests, along with the literature, showed that these were not a factor in the cyanide intoxication occurring in Houston."

"Such as?"

"Such as broccoli and cabbage. Both the literature and testing I performed revealed that normal cyanide levels in people who eat these foods are far below the levels found in Houston or over here."

"Over here meaning where?"

"At the naval shipyard and naval hospital in Philadelphia—in myself and other patients. Also, in the literature, the normal reference values for cyanide and thiocyanate include those amounts resulting from eating foods such as cabbage and broccoli. There is one study where such foods were removed from the diets of those subjects tested, but in that study the normal levels for thiocyanate were considerably lower than the levels which I listed as norms."

The *one study* I was referring to above is found in *Br J Ind Med* 32(3):215-9 Aug. '75. The average urine thiocyanate output in this study is about 0.074 mg/L. This is over twenty times less than the upper limit of 2 mg/L given by Metpath Laboratories, Inc. and Bio-Science Laboratories. What was evaluated in the study was the change in urine thiocyanate levels among industrial workers exposed to measured levels of cyanide in the air. If the level of HCN in the air was 10 ppm cyanide, then the urine thiocyanate level increased by approximately 4.34 mg/L. HCN concentrations over 0.3 ppm are considered too high in Russia. What do the Russians know that we do not?

"Have you read Doctor Mills' letter?" continued Lieutenant O'Hanlan.

"Yes, I have," I acknowledged.

"Would you agree with it?"

"No, I don't."

"Any particular reason?"

By this time, I was making considerably more eye contact with the Board members, and speaking to them as well as to Lieutenant O'Hanlan as I answered questions. When I stated that I disagreed with Doctor Mills' letter, Captain Wilson noticeably perked up.

"There are two major reasons," I expounded. "For one thing, Doctor Mills ascertained that if cyanide was being generated from a given location, then people should be dropping dead between the point of origin and where I was experiencing illness. The problem with this is that Doctor Mills is assuming that the poison is coming from a particular point of source, when in fact, what I am saying is that cyanide compounds are first dispersed in the environment, as in the sewer system or other waterways, and that hydrogen cyanide gas is produced from these compounds after they are already spread out. Thus, the actual hydrogen cyanide gas comes from chemicals which are first discharged and spread out. It is not coming from a point source."

"What about his statement that cyanide gas would not affect people very far from its source because it is lighter than air? He implies that it would quickly rise up."

"Yes, he seems to give the implication that hydrogen cyanide would act like helium or hydrogen and float quickly upward. The fact is, hydrogen cyanide has a weight of 27, almost the same weight as nitrogen gas, which is 28—and nitrogen composes about 80 percent of the atmosphere. Oxygen gas has a weight of 32, so there is four times greater difference between the weight of oxygen gas and nitrogen gas than between the weight of nitrogen gas and hydrogen cyanide gas. In other words, hydrogen cyanide is practically the perfect weight to blend stably with the atmosphere, almost as stably as nitrogen."

Colonel Clark and Commander Wyvill looked on with seeming interest and occasional astonishment. It was easily detectable, though, that Captain Wilson held the upper hand in determining my verdict. This was probably because Captain Wilson was a physician, and was presumed to have more knowledge and insight about my case. When I explained why hydrogen cyanide gas blends well into the atmosphere,

Captain Wilson frankly blushed. He looked downward and faintly laughed—it was as if my comments had affronted him directly. [*Remember that 98% of airborne cyanide remains in the earth's lower atmosphere, as documented in the introduction to this book.*]

Lieutenant O'Hanlan seemed to pick up on Captain Wilson's obvious, nonverbal communication.

"What he is referring to," Lieutenant O'Hanlan addressed the Board, "is that Doctor Mills said in here…ah…*hydrogen cyanide is a gas which is slightly lighter than air and thus is rapidly dispersively diluted relative to its originating source*. That is the statement about the weight of it. He said: *the absence of mass illness in personnel in the same location as the complainant also mitigates against cyanide in the ambient air as the cause of the complaints*."

"There is another point with which I disagree," I spoke up. "There was not an absence of illness besides my own illness. I talked to one employee at the electroplating shop, building forty-one, and he was taking large doses of Tylenol for severe headaches. He had decreased vision over the preceding six months, he got short of breath just walking up stairs, and he had some chest pains—he said the chest pain got so bad once that it nearly made him cry."

"Did you attempt to bring any of this to the attention of the authorities at the Philadelphia Shipyard?" Lieutenant O'Hanlan resumed questioning me.

"Yes, I did."

"What was the immediate result of your mentioning this?"

"The immediate result was—I was basically told not to mention it."

"What would happen if you did mention it?"

"I was told three different things that would happen. One was that I would be put into a psychiatric hospital, another was that other people would probably think that anyone who would treat himself for cyanide intoxication should not be practicing medicine, and the third thing was that it could be very dangerous to be involved with that kind of thing."

"Very dangerous to whom?"

"He just told me it could be very dangerous."

"Who told you this?"

"Should I give his name?"

"Yes, you should give the name."

"Captain Galasyn."

I noticed a troubled look mount Captain Wilson's face as I revealed Captain Galasyn's name. Whether he was troubled on my behalf, or not, I was uncertain. Now I am quite sure that his discomfiture stemmed from concerns other than my well-being. [*Note: in regard to Captain Galasyn, it is certainly true that he made several threats against me and that he had my lecture on cyanide intoxication cancelled. What I have not mentioned, up to this point, is that I remember having the impression that he actually admired my courage and dedication. I did not learn until this year, the year 2020, that there was a direct tie between the U.S. Navy and the GE plating plant on 12th street in Houston, Texas. To the best of my knowledge, I was supposed to serve as the chief medical witness in the lawsuit against GE; and given the connection between GE and the U.S. Navy, Captain Galasyn may have been under pressure from his superiors to deal with me in a manner that would hinder my contributions to the lawsuit against GE, or at least keep me from gaining further information that would benefit the plaintiffs in the lawsuit against GE. I am not trying to excuse what Captain Galasyn did, and I certainly believe that what he did was unethical and even criminal; but nonetheless, he may have been under a great deal of pressure to behave in the manner that he behaved.*]

"Who is he?" continued Lieutenant O'Hanlan.

"He is head of the Department of Environmental Health."

"At the Philadelphia Naval Shipyard?"

"Correct."

"When did you join the Navy?"

"February of 1978."

"Why didn't you go on active duty when you graduated from medical school?"

"I applied for active duty, but the Navy postponed it for two years."

"And you were called in May?"

"I was called to go on active duty in July, I believe I received my orders in May, I think."

"Do you like the Navy?"

"Yes, I like it when I'm not being poisoned with cyanide."

"Why do you want to stay on active duty?"

"I would like to finish the commitment that I have made to the government in an honorable and respectable manner."

Lieutenant O'Hanlan settled back in his chair. "That is all of the questions that I have of Lieutenant Oesch. I would like to state something for the record. I spoke on the phone to several laboratories on the east coast, especially regarding reference levels for the tests done on the employees at the Naval shipyard. They all agree that the level stated by National Medical Services is too high. Even the toxicologist at National Medical Services said that the ceiling level, the level above which toxicity is indicated, is only half what is stated on the laboratory reports. So, the reference value listed on the tests is not in keeping with the values stated by other toxicologists at other laboratories, and it does not signify the severity of the problem at the shipyard. Doctor Dan Lockett of National Medical Services, the laboratory which actually performed those tests, said that actually 10 mcg/ml rather than 20 mcg/ml was the upper limit for urine thiocyanate. He also said that the trend nowadays in toxicology is for lower and lower levels to be accepted as toxic. I think the reference value listed by National Medical Services is misleading, and I wanted to clarify that, so I checked with other laboratories, SmithKline Laboratory, Bio-Science Laboratories, and Metpath Laboratories, Inc., and they all confirm that the lower levels are actually the ones that are more accepted by the field today. That is all the questions that I have."

With Lieutenant O'Hanlan finished, there was some minor commotion and Lieutenant Reynolds was summoned back to the room. Once she was seated, Colonel Clark instructed her to identify Exhibit B, the letter from Doctor Mills.

"I spoke to the Staff Judge Advocate for the Philadelphia Naval Hospital, who is the one who sent us Exhibit B," stated Lieutenant Reynolds, "and he said that Doctor Gilmore, who was Lieutenant Oesch's treating physician, consulted with Doctor Mills throughout her treatment of Lieutenant Oesch, and that basically what is written on there is what he had already told her orally throughout the consultation. Additionally, from the Staff Judge Advocate for the Philadelphia Naval Hospital, he is putting a packet in the mail of information he has received from Houston and of additional information regarding Lieutenant Oesch's work while he was at Philadelphia, that is probably pertinent to the case and may require there being a continuance."

"Thank you," said Colonel Clark, then immediately called upon the medical officer to his right: "Doctor Wilson?"

"What is the nature of the material that is being forwarded from Houston or Philadelphia?" inquired Doctor Wilson?

"Basically, the nature of the information being forwarded from Houston includes news articles, results of tests by the Houston Health Department, et cetera, that they did in exploring the possibility of whether or not Lieutenant Oesch's claim of cyanide poisoning had any grounds," replied Lieutenant Reynolds.

"And from Philadelphia?" coaxed Captain Wilson.

"They are basically reports and I believe they are reports that Lieutenant Oesch has written out that would seem to indicate somewhat of a bizarre thought process."

"Are there any other official investigation results available?"

"I'm not positive whether they are official or not, what is coming in, they may be. May I be excused?"

"Request granted," Colonel Clark again allowed.

Next, after Lieutenant Reynolds again left the room, Captain Wilson turned his attention to me. This began the section of the hearing noted as *Examination By The Medical Member*. As with Lieutenant O'Hanlan before, Captain Wilson asked me a large number of questions which I answered in sequence.

"How did you spend the two years between your graduating from medical school and entering the Navy?" began Captain Wilson.

"In medical school, I finished all the requirements for graduation in three years, and then I did a year of externships. After graduating in 1980, I applied to go directly into active duty with the Navy—and from the way my recruiter talked, I thought that I would be accepted. The Navy postponed my active duty, though, and I then applied to go overseas to Africa as a missionary. I was accepted by the mission board and commissioned to go to Nalerigu, Ghana, West Africa—but even after working on my visa for five months, the mission board was unable to obtain the visa. The next thing I did as far as medicine goes, which was about a year later, was to start my own private practice in Houston."

"What did you do...a year later...what happened during that year?"

"Well, they took five months trying to get me to Africa..."

"In this period of time you weren't practicing?"

"No, I wasn't. I wasn't practicing medicine. I did take some additional college courses. I took mainly communication courses because I preach as well as practice medicine."

"And the second year?"

"Then I had a private practice in Houston. For about the first four or five months I had only my own private practice. After that, I still had my private practice and I also worked for an industrial clinic. I served as the company physician for oil companies, the police, firemen, construction companies, and such as that."

"How did you get into that line of work?"

"I applied for it through…actually it was through a special employment agency for physicians. That is how I got it."

"Was it after this that you became interested in cyanide?"

"No, I was already interested in cyanide. The first practice I was in, my private practice, was where I first found patients with cyanide intoxication. The first patient I found, in fact, worked at a plant which used cyanide—and that was how I first got onto it. I had seen patients with symptoms of cyanide intoxication for some time, but I had never suspected cyanide. I had the patient who worked at the plant bring me a list of things he was exposed to, and then I read about each one of them. Then, I tested him for the ones that sounded suspicious, and the only one that came out positive was cyanide."

"You haven't been concerned about cyanide then before you started your own practice?"

"No."

"The symptoms that appear constantly in your record and the ones that you mentioned are, of course, quite vague, and could represent a whole host of disease processes other than cyanide. I'm sure you are well aware of that?"

"Most of them, yes, that is true."

"How is it then that you are so certain that it's cyanide rather than some other problem?"

"Well, one reason is because of my experience. I've seen a lot of cyanide intoxication and have dealt with it in the past. Also, there are certain symptoms and findings which are quite specific for cyanide. Bright red venous blood, for example, would only be found in carbon monoxide poisoning or cyanide intoxication. (Note: in carbon monoxide poisoning, the blood is actually *cherry red* or *pink* in color.) Elevated thiocyanate levels are specific for cyanide. I've done quite a bit of thiocyanate testing, and the levels found in Philadelphia were definitely high. In fact, my serum thiocyanate level of 1.8 mg/dl was higher than any level in the literature associated with chronic cyanide poisoning, and higher than any patient tested in Houston."

"In nonsmokers?"

"Or smokers. I have never tested a smoker with a level that high."

"It seems to me that the levels that seem to have been documented, either on yourself or your wife or some other patients, are below that which is established as…"

"As the upper limit for smokers?"

"Yes."

"The levels of thiocyanate given in the literature which indicate chronic cyanide poisoning in nonsmokers are well within the normal levels listed for smokers. However, the ceiling level given for smokers is much higher than what you will generally find. The average level is usually less than a third of what the ceiling level is. You may have some smokers that smoke three packs of cigarettes a day, and their levels might be quite high. I have never seen a smoker tested in the literature that had a serum thiocyanate over 2 mg/dl, nor have ever tested any that high. In fact, I have never tested any smoker with a level over 1 mg/dl."

"The material that you submitted to the Naval shipyard also doesn't specify whether…I think there is one in there that says he was a nonsmoker."

"There were seven nonsmokers and five smokers. [*This First Hearing was apparently prior to my receiving all of the results from urine thiocyanate testing at the shipyard. There were nine nonsmokers, or ten including myself, and the average urine thiocyanate among nonsmokers still remained higher than the average urine thiocyanate among smokers.*] The average urine thiocyanate level among the smokers was about 8.9 mcg/ml, and the average among the nonsmokers was about 9.1 mcg/ml—it was a little higher among the nonsmokers than smokers, which indicates that the environmental exposure to cyanide was high enough to override the normally higher level in smokers."

"Is there any documentation of that other than your own testimony?"

"Well, besides their medical records, which you could check to see if they were smokers or not, I asked each of them before they were tested how much they had smoked during the last two weeks—and if they had not smoked at all, I wrote down *Code 2*. I didn't want to write down that they were nonsmokers because I was afraid the laboratory would see that and think that they should find a low level. I just wanted the laboratory to run the tests and find what was actually there. So, I wrote down *Code 2* if they had not smoked at all during the preceding two weeks."

"Why were you assigned to industrial medicine, Department of the Shipyard, when you first came to Philadelphia?"

"They asked me what I had done in the past, and when I mentioned that I had worked in industrial medicine in Houston, they very quickly decided to send me to the dispensary."

"Would you have rather been working in the hospital?"

"No. I prefer satellite or clinical work to work in a hospital. I like firsthand, primary care. Assignment at the dispensary was exactly what I wanted. I was very happy with that."

"You say your wife was sickened close to death, was that because of cyanide poisoning or because of histoplasmosis?"

"At that time she was ill from cyanide poisoning. The symptoms of cyanide poisoning and histoplasmosis are very different."

"And it is your contention that her immune system was affected?"

"That it was compromised by the cyanide, yes. Dr. Hitt, who is a specialist in that field, maintains that in fact chronic cyanide exposure can compromise the immune system."

"These are things, this business about cyanide and the immune system, are not well documented as far as I am aware."

"Well, besides Doctor Hitt and my tests on patients at the shipyard, I don't know that anyone else has tried to document it."

"Both you and Doctor Hitt have spoken and discussed this matter in terms of allergies. Are we talking in terms of a tightly defined allergy where you are dealing with cyanide as an allergen, and where the cyanide affects people because they are allergic to it, or some other concept?"

"He does and I don't. My feeling is that the allergy testing in Houston primarily served to prove that people were being exposed to cyanide. You develop an allergy to something from being exposed to it. You do not have to be allergic to cyanide to suffer more symptoms than someone else sitting beside you. You may be a slower converter of cyanide to thiocyanate, so that you do not change cyanide which enters your body into something else less harmful as quickly as most other people do."

"Of course that was my next question, why do your wife and you, for instance, get sick and everybody else doesn't?"

"Well, we are not the only ones that get sick, it's just that most people are not diagnosed with cyanide intoxication. In the literature, it says that there is great variability between individuals in their resistance or sensitivity to cyanide, but it does not really explain why. My opinion is that it has to do with the individual's turnover rate in changing cyanide to something else. Also, I believe that persons exposed to low doses of cyanide may suffer damage to their systems so that their capabilities of metabolizing cyanide at a certain rate can become reduced."

"But you could say that is conjecture on your part at this time…"

"Well, yes, you could say that. It is based on evidence, but I suppose you could call it conjecture."

Later, I regretted making the statement above. The fact was, I really did not know or did not remember the dictionary meaning of the word *conjecture*, and I should have said so. Conjecture is based on little or poor evidence, and the difference in rates of metabolizing cyanide between different individuals is based on very strong evidence. Besides other sources, NIOSH plainly states a variance of rate between individuals on their study on cyanide. Furthermore, there may not be a single, biological function that different individuals do not perform at different rates. Captain Wilson finagled me into practically testifying against my own case, as well as against the truth.

"There was some indication that you and your wife had been taking antihistamines," continued Captain Wilson.

"I had not taken any because the only time I take them is during ragweed season, August and September. I did not take any in November or December or thereafter," I plainly stated.

"Since antihistamines are notorious for making people drowsy, I was just wondering if perhaps that is one reason why you and your wife were drowsy, not due to cyanide but to antihistamines."

After telling Captain Wilson that I was not taking any antihistamines during November or December, the months that I was hospitalized, his persistence in attempting to blame my illness on antihistamines probably evidenced an obstinate adherence to premeditated tactics. Doctor Gilmore had tested my urine for antihistamines, methadone, quinone, morphine, barbiturates, meperidine, glutethimide, D-amphetamine, propoxyphene, codeine, cocaine, and chlorpromazine. All of these tests were negative. I do not even drink coffee.

"That may be one reason why I was slow to suspect the presence of cyanide back in August and September," I replied, hoping to eventually gain a favorable report from Captain Wilson despite his obvious prejudice. "If I felt a little ill in September, I probably just blamed it on my allergies. By the time October and November arrived, I no longer had the runny nose and itchy eyes that I get with my hay fever, so I quit taking antihistamines. My illness, though, continued to get worse."

"Are there other allergies you suffer from?"

"I'm allergic to celery."

"What else?"

"That is all I know of that I react to, ragweed and celery."

Captain Wilson seemed very quick to change the subject when the answers to his questions lent support to my claims. "Your Board is signed by three physicians. Doctor Jacobs, who is Doctor Jacobs?"

"He is the Captain in the psychiatric department at NRMC, Philadelphia."

"Doctor Gilmore?"

"She is a Commander at NRMC, Philadelphia, in the Department of Internal Medicine. She was my attending physician when I was hospitalized, both times."

"So that both Doctor Jacobs and Doctor Gilmore are thoroughly familiar with your case?"

"Doctor Jacobs interviewed me once. Doctor Gilmore saw me quite often."

"Were you seen by other psychiatrists in Philadelphia?"

"I was seen by Doctor Mangrum and also by…he was not a psychiatrist…I'm not even sure he was a psychologist…but they have someone else there by the name of…" Try as I might, I could not remember the name of the other officer who saw me. His evaluation, however, did not appear in my hospital records. I have no idea what he wrote about me. "I don't remember his name. They didn't mention it did they?" No one replied. "In the department they have psychiatrists and psychologists. I think he was a psychologist."

"Doctor Mangrum spoke with you very extensively then I would imagine?"

"He only spoke with me once, but I think he did spend around an hour or an hour and a half talking to me."

At this point, the transcribed record of the hearing neatly omits a claim by Captain Wilson that Captain Galasyn was my Commanding Officer, which he was not. I am uncertain exactly how the subject was introduced. To the best of my memory, Lieutenant O'Hanlan brought up the subject.

"Why is Doctor Galasyn's name on your Board?" inserted Lieutenant O'Hanlan. He was aware of Captain Galasyn's criminal, political behavior and his primary role in instigating my Medical Board.

"I don't know," I replied.

"Did you ever talk to him?"

"He is the one who threatened me about the environmental situation."

Captain Wilson was notably annoyed by the information Lieutenant O'Hanlan elicited. "Captain Galasyn's name is on the Medical Board because he is Lieutenant Oesch's Commanding Officer," he derided authoritatively. He spoke so matter-of-factly that I thought he might be correct, but he was not. The record resumes with his next statement: "If I'm not mistaken, on my reading of your record, Doctor Galasyn gave you the environmental counseling after considerable time and controversy had gone by with this whole issue…"

"Two and one-half days after I started testing for cyanide intoxication he told me not to order one more test. I did not order any more tests after he told me not to. All of the results that we have were tests ordered before he spoke to me, except for the one man who was sent to the emergency room. His tests were ordered by Doctor Schmidt at Locality Hospital."

My reply did not seem to please Captain Wilson at all, though I noticed that Lieutenant O'Hanlan smiled.

Captain Wilson elected to change the subject. "Did you research environmental cyanide before you moved to Marlton?"

"I asked around. I asked if there were any electroplating plants near where we wanted to move. It seemed to be one of the safest directions to go, and that's why we moved there."

"What have you available to submit as official documentation as far as health authorities go? Obviously we are talking about a potentially serious public health problem. What is available through public health officials in Houston, or from Philadelphia or surrounding areas, or from Philadelphia Naval Shipyard in support of your allegations?"

"You can speak to authorities on the subject, for example, the Atlanta Poison Control Center. All they can give you is…"

"I'm not talking about generalization," interrupted Captain Wilson. "I'm talking about official documentation specifically addressing the problem that you have."

"Correct," I persisted. There were at least seven major laboratories having yielded official documentation of unusually high cyanide exposures, so I presumed that Captain Wilson was asking for an authoritative source to vouch that the test results were indeed high. In actuality, this may not have been the case. Captain Wilson may have simply wanted to divert attention away from positive laboratory findings, and focus upon the negative claims of the Houston Health Department and the Naval Environment Department at Philadelphia. "The Atlanta Poison Control Center can give you specifics as far as my findings go, because they have information that I sent them. I guess I'm one of the foremost investigators in the field right now. They can also give blood cyanide levels in patients who are taking a drug called nitroprusside which generates abnormally high levels of blood cyanide. The average level of blood cyanide in patients I tested in Houston was even higher than the average in these patients taking nitroprusside."

"What about the Houston Health Department?" posed Captain Wilson. It was becoming apparent that the only opinions he cared to consider were those supporting my Medical Board. Lieutenant O'Hanlan became more and more aggravated as the hearing went on.

"The Houston Health Department may be sued before long," I stated frankly, "and they would probably be glad to see me tagged with a psychiatric diagnosis."

"There is no documentation available to support your position from them?" asked Captain Wilson.

"From the Houston Health Department?"

"Yes, from the Houston Health Department."

"Goodness no, they are liable to get sued," I reiterated. "There is evidence that they were in cahoots with the industry that was doing the contamination. In fact, they even licensed the industry to dump cyanide into the sewer system." [*At the time of this hearing, I had no clue that testing by the Houston Health Department revealed cyanogen chloride, a cyanide war gas, in effluent water from the electroplating plant that they licensed to discharge industrial effluent into the sewer water. This plating plant was located in the Timbergrove area between the Heights and Spring Branch. Such testing was conducted at least as early as May of 1982. Judging from records that I have examined, it may be that the Director of the Houston Health Department never came to the realization that inhalation of cyanogen chloride results in positive laboratory testing for cyanide and thiocyanate. I say this because one of the many enclosures sent to the Navy from the Houston Health Department was an interoffice correspondence dated 24 FEB 1982, and that is the date of a correspondence that denies any excessive levels of cyanide in effluent discharged into the sanitary sewer, but that also reveals the finding of cyanogen chloride in that same effluent.*]

"And in Philadelphia?"

"In Philadelphia—I haven't reported it to the health department there."

"How about the Philadelphia Naval Shipyard?"

"I doubt that they have reported it."

"Did they investigate these complaints?"

"One day they took a couple of specimens that were collected by members of the Naval Environmental Health Department, and sent these to National Medical Services. I think one of the specimens may have been drinking water, I don't know, it was taken from a building other than building forty-one, and they reported negative findings. The other tests they did were from air samples taken one morning that yielded very low results, not high enough to account for my illness—at least the specimen they turned over to the laboratory had low cyanide levels."

It was not until weeks later when I learned that the water tested by National Medical Services came from rinse tanks in building 25 [*not building 41*], rather than from the actual electroplating tanks where cyanide was added and allowed to overflow into the sewage system [*in building 41*]. This disclosure resulted from a conversation with an OSHA employee.

"No other questions," stated Captain Wilson.

Colonel Clark carried on. "Commander Wyvill?" he queried, informing the only reserve officer on the Physical Evaluation Board that his turn for asking questions had arrived.

"I have none," defaulted Commander Wyvill.

Then Colonel Clark addressed me himself. The next, brief portion of the proceedings were noted: *Examination By The President Of The Board.*

"Lieutenant Oesch, if this problem is so widespread in Houston and in Philadelphia, as you have indicated that you feel that it is, why aren't there more incidences of illness?" asked Colonel Clark.

"There are many instances of illness, there are just not many known instances of illness," I replied. "Chronic cyanide intoxication causes basically no consistent changes in usual laboratory testing, and the most common symptoms it causes are just depression and headaches, which are often passed for viral illnesses or emotional problems. For instance, I saw many patients in Houston who had chronic cyanide intoxication before I found out about the cyanide contamination through the patient who worked at the electroplating plant, and I did not diagnose them with cyanide intoxication because I did not know to look for it. Unless specific tests for cyanide exposure are done, such as serum thiocyanate or urine thiocyanate, then there is no reason that a physician would find the problem because it does not show up on other tests. It's a very elusive problem, in other words."

That was the only question Colonel Clark asked me. He then addressed Lieutenant O'Hanlan: "Counsel, do you have anything else to add?"

"Argument, sir," responded Lieutenant O'Hanlan with suppressed furor: noble and admirable furor.

"Proceed."

"I think that Lieutenant Oesch has been unjustly punished by the Medical Board, it's more than an inaccurate diagnosis, I think he has really been wronged by it. I think the situation in Houston and Philadelphia are interesting, they are very interesting, and they are important in understanding the problem of cyanide intoxication—but they beg the question here. The question here is: is this diagnosis correct or is this man fit for duty? First of all, he has come before you with psychiatric evidence, tests done by a licensed psychiatrist and psychologist finding no underlying psychopathology detected. This immediately confronts the findings of the Medical Board. That, alone, casts enough doubt on it that I think this Board should find him fit for duty. He came up with findings that are directly contrary to the Medical Board.

"But even further than that, I think if you look at the Medical Board—it was dictated on 10 January 1983 on a psychiatric evaluation that was begun on 02 December 1982, just a little over a month before, while he was hospitalized, while his thiocyanate levels were up, and at a time when he was observed to have blue fingernails and lips. The corpsman that drew his blood noted the bright red color of the venous blood, which is not the color it should have been except if something was wrong. The Medical Board states that the thiocyanate levels were up itself. It also states that the globulin levels in his blood were low, which is a physical rather than a psychological finding, and it doesn't account for either of these. There was something wrong with him, it wasn't psychosomatic, you can't change the thiocyanate levels in your bloodstream because of a mental illness.

"There was no check of the validity of Lieutenant Oesch's claim that the symptoms he had were symptoms of cyanide intoxication. Lieutenant Reynolds made the statement that Doctor Gilmore consulted Doctor Mills throughout Lieutenant Oesch's examination. She did not say how many times the toxicologist was consulted, nor is there any check of the validity of the symptoms Lieutenant Oesch complained about against those of cyanide intoxication. There is no check of the wind effects that he complained of. His illness was taken as prima facie evidence of a mental problem, but he was complaining of objective findings and objective environmental factors, and there was no check to see if he was right or wrong.

"He explained that he got better when removed from the area of cyanide contamination, and got worse again when he returned to it, and yet he was not removed from the environment to see if it was indeed a factor. You are not supposed to diagnose someone as having a mental illness until you are positive that the symptoms are not from a physical cause. He does have these things, elevated thiocyanate, decreased globulin, cyanosis, and bright red venous blood in his Medical Board—and they are unexplained. Furthermore, it has been shown by the exhibits today that many symptoms of cyanide intoxication arise from cyanide affecting mental processes. It would inhibit normal performance on a psychiatric analysis. The confusion, disorientation, memory loss, and all of these facts should make psychiatrists wary about giving a psychiatric diagnosis. These mental effects of cyanide intoxication are, of course, going to affect what comes out on a psychiatric examination. This casts even more doubt onto the evaluation of the Medical Board.

"Then, Lieutenant Oesch comes up with a new psychiatric evaluation at a time when he was in an environment away from the hospital, when he was feeling better and not exhibiting these symptoms. This evaluation says he is psychologically normal. In a question of reliability, I think these factors come out in support of the civilian diagnosis, or at least they cast enough doubt into the Medical Board to make it unsound to find him unfit for duty and have him discharged with a psychiatric diagnosis.

"Then you have the next four exhibits after the psychiatric and psychological evaluations. The discharge summary by Doctor Gilmore, the nursing notes, the handwritten statement from the corpsman who drew the bright red venous blood, and the deposition from the nurse about the blue lips and fingernails—these give positive evidence that Lieutenant Oesch exhibited symptoms which were not addressed in the Medical Board. Next come the data summaries on symptoms of cyanide intoxication and reference values of urine thiocyanate. These summaries give the present state-of-the-art as far as the scientific world goes concerning these symptoms and reference values. Then come copies of actual tests done on Lieutenant Oesch and his wife. The tests performed on his wife were obtained by another physician, and served to corroborate what he suspected.

"Then you have two telephone depositions from Doctor Groverman, a physician, and Doctor Hitt, an immunologist. Doctor Groverman confirmed cyanide intoxication in a patient that Doctor Oesch diagnosed in Philadelphia, and Doctor Hitt confirmed cyanide intoxication in patients in Houston. Doctor Hitt states that he has done controlled tests before, and has previously been able to isolate areas of a community where there are problems. He was able to identify an area in Houston which was contaminated with cyanide. This area was where Doctor Oesch and his wife lived.

"Obviously, the Houston Health Department is not going to be helpful in this because of the implications of a lawsuit. With their ties to the problem, such as licensing the dumping of cyanide compounds into the sewer system, they are cornered into denying the problem. They are not a reliable party to consult regarding claims made by Lieutenant Oesch, and yet they are the only source of information about the problem in Houston which the Naval people in Philadelphia acknowledge.

"Then you have the tests of the shipyard workers themselves. Several of them, not all, but several of them show positive results for cyanide exposure. This gives objective reason to believe that the symptoms Lieutenant Oesch suspected as cyanide intoxication, even though he did not suspect cyanide at first, were indeed caused by cyanide. So, there you have it. The objective test results uphold Lieutenant Oesch's claims.

"Lieutenant Oesch asked to be found fit for duty and claims that he is fit for duty. I think, at the very least, this Board should not accept this psychiatric diagnosis and that he should be evaluated further if there is any question. This is a man with extensive knowledge and experience who could be of use to the Navy. I think the Board should recognize the problems with the Medical Board, should not accept the diagnosis of paranoia, and should find Lieutenant Oesch fit for duty."

This last presentation of dialogue from Lieutenant O'Hanlan began baring the underlying contention between him and the Physical Evaluation Board—a Board which for all practical purposes consisted of Captain Wilson and Colonel Clark. Up to that point, Lieutenant O'Hanlan respectfully pleaded fair consideration of the facts. In response, Captain Wilson disclosed with unabashed deliberateness that the entire session was a masqueraded kangaroo court. Colonel Clark sat stolidly impermeable to any reason or logic which stood contrary to input from the medical adviser to his right. Finally, Lieutenant O'Hanlan decided to state the issue plainly, and allow the inevitable decision of the Board to appear as ludicrous as it apparently would be, regardless of the alienation such an undertaking would create between himself and the Board members. I sat in admiration.

When Lieutenant O'Hanlan finished speaking, Colonel Clark turned his gaze toward me. "Do you have anything else you would like to add?" he asked.

"No sir," I answered. Lieutenant O'Hanlan had advised me not to make any additional remarks.

"This Board will close for deliberations," stated Colonel Clark.

Lieutenant O'Hanlan and I again left the room so the Board members could talk privately. Before long, we were summoned back to our places, and so was Lieutenant Reynolds.

"This Board is reopened," pronounced Colonel Clark. "Let the record show that all persons who were present when the Board went into deliberations are now present and that Lieutenant Reynolds, Counsel for the Board, has rejoined this deliberation.

"In its deliberations, the Board determined that in order to arrive at a full and fair decision, that we would have to look at the additional material that is being forwarded from Philadelphia that Counsel for the Board indicated was forthcoming.

"Counsel, did they give you an indication when that material might arrive?"

"The Staff Judge Advocate said he would place it in the mail today. He said that he was under the impression that this hearing was not going to be conducted until next week," stated Lieutenant Reynolds.

"The Staff Judge Advocate for the Philadelphia Naval Hospital was told that this hearing was going to be this morning, by me, on Friday a week ago," interjected Lieutenant O'Hanlan.

"According to him, the last he heard was from Lieutenant Maronai, and she said it would not be until this week…ah, I mean until next week," maintained Lieutenant Reynolds.

Colonel Clark interceded. "We won't argue the point of what week it was or when it was, but the Board would like to look at the material to see what it may add in determining this case. We can't rule on the material unless we see it."

"Did the Staff Judge Advocate say what that material was?" asked Lieutenant O'Hanlan.

"He said it was reports from the Houston Health Department and said it was reports which Lieutenant Oesch has written while he was on duty at the hospital that indicated bizarre thought patterns."

As it turned out, there were never any notes forwarded that I had written while on duty. There was, however, a great deal of propaganda from the Houston Health Department which eventually managed to reach the Physical Evaluation Board.

"I would like to object to continuing this Board in order to wait for this material," stated Lieutenant O'Hanlan.

"Your objection is noted," proclaimed Colonel Clark.

By this time I surmised that the Board could note all manner and number of objections without it making much difference.

"I have a brief argument on that," persisted Lieutenant O'Hanlan. "The NRMC in Philadelphia has had good notice that his hearing was going to take place. They were required to submit their evidence before the case went into the Disability System and they failed to do that. But, more importantly, the question in Houston or the question in Philadelphia of cyanide intoxication is only begging the question that is before this Board. This Board is to determine this man's fitness or unfitness for duty and not whether or not there is cyanide intoxication in Houston. Whether or not there is cyanide intoxication in Houston is relevant, but not necessary to the determination before this Board today. Furthermore, it is beyond the competency of this Board to determine whether or not there is cyanide intoxication in Houston. Do you gentlemen feel that you can determine whether or not there is cyanide intoxication in these communities?"

"That is not the question," objected Colonel Clark.

"It appears that is the question if you are waiting to see material from Houston," resumed Lieutenant O'Hanlan. "The question is: is this man being properly evaluated by this Board? There have been several discrepancies pointed out in the Medical Board that are enough to have it thrown out without any further evidence. They will not be affected in any way by what the Houston Health Department has to say about the situation down there. What is important about what happened in Houston has already been flushed out by testimony and submitted exhibits. I object to further study about the situation. The question is whether or not this hearing supports the diagnosis of paranoia. Sufficient testimony and evidence has been presented to discount the diagnosis of paranoia and show this man is fit for duty. Anything else is merely tangential and will unduly delay a decision. That is the basis of my objection."

"Your objection is noted," stated Colonel Clark. "The Board's position remains the same. We want to look at all the material available in order to determine a fair rating under this particular case."

"Does this Board feel that it has the competency to determine whether or not there is a question of cyanide intoxication in Houston or Philadelphia?" Lieutenant O'Hanlan questioned directly.

"That is not the point," maintained Colonel Clark. "The point is, we want to look at the material in relation to Lieutenant Oesch."

The fact was, the material presented in the hearing was so heavily against the Medical Board that the Physical Evaluation Board would have appeared sadly inane to have simply supported the Medical Board at that point. Statements written by Captain Wilson, and later discovered by Lieutenant O'Hanlan, revealed that Captain Wilson decided to support the Naval diagnosis of paranoia before a second meeting was ever held. This directly contrasted with Colonel Clark's claim that they wanted to look at all the material available in order to determine a fair rating. It causes one to question the real reason why the meeting was extended. Whatever the reason, it probably worked out for my good. There was considerably more evidence in my support by the time a second hearing was arranged.

"Does Counsel for Member feel competent to overthrow a psychiatric diagnosis?" interjected Captain Wilson, coming to the aid of Colonel Clark. Since Lieutenant O'Hanlan had a law degree, rather than a medical degree, Captain Wilson's question was obviously designed to degrade Lieutenant O'Hanlan's remarks as compared to his own.

"Counsel for the Member comes to this hearing with a psychiatric diagnosis which does just that," returned Lieutenant O'Hanlan, "and this Board fails to recognize that fact. Furthermore, this Board is looking at circumstances that happened in the last year and a half without any competency to evaluate them or determine the validity of them. On the other hand, this Board does have sworn testimony from this man, and a diagnosis by a licensed psychiatrist directly in conflict with the diagnosis given by the Medical Board. That alone casts enough doubt on the Medical Board that he should be found fit for duty and returned to either full duty or for additional evaluation. It is clear that he is not properly diagnosed by the Medical Board."

"I also add that the Board members may also wish to seek additional information other than that which is being forwarded from Philadelphia as a result of examining that material," remarked Captain Wilson.

"I'm fully aware of what you are saying, but continuance just on the basis that you want to see reports from Houston is not warranted," argued Lieutenant O'Hanlan. "Also, if you continue the Board in order to see reports of bizarre behavior by Lieutenant Oesch while he was stationed at Philadelphia, that action is likewise unwarranted. Lieutenant Oesch has already stated that cyanide intoxication causes mental disorders, so any evidence that he did suffer mental disorders will simply be cumulative. The fact is, Lieutenant Oesch has suffered from cyanide intoxication which manifested itself not only with mental disorders but with proven, verifiable, physiological evidence. It is not proper for this physiological evidence to be overlooked and unexplained by a Medical Board which forwards the diagnosis of paranoia. The Board is just wrong."

"We understand your objection, and we will take it into consideration," stated Colonel Clark. "Do you have anything further to add?"

"Nothing except to urge that the Board decide this issue in favor of Lieutenant Oesch's fitness for duty once and for all. This man has been living under a cloud with this situation for the last six months, and it's not giving him a full and fair hearing to continue it further. It can be resolved today and it should be if this Board will just carry out its assigned responsibility."

"I understand your position," declared Colonel Clark. "This Board is continued."

Chapter 18
Medical Times
80 Shore Road, Port Washington, N.Y. 11050 • 516-883-6350 • A Romaine Pierson Publication

Editor-in-Chief: Internal Medicine
Alfred Jay Bollet, M.D.
Clinical Professor of Medicine
Yale University;
Chairman, Department of Medicine
Danbury Hospital
Danbury, Connecticut

Editor-in-Chief: Family Practice
Allan H. Bruckheim, M.D.
Assoc. Prof., Clinical Family Medicine
State U. of NY at Stony Brook;
Director of Family Medicine
St. Mary Hospital
Hoboken, New Jersey

April 16, 1984

Timothy R. Oesch, M.D.
4348 Barton Run Blvd.
Marlton, NJ 08053

Dear Dr. Oesch:

I'm happy to inform you that your article, "Cyanide Intoxication: A Possible Etiology of Reye's Syndrome," has been accepted for publication in Medical Times. I am, therefore, enclosing our honorarium check for $200. As soon as the article is set in type, we will send you galleys to approve.

Revelation

Soon after returning home to the apartment near Cherry Hill, I ascertained that westerly winds brought enough hydrogen cyanide gas to our new apartment that my wife and I would again have to move. This was still several weeks before I learned that there was one electroplating plant a mile to the west of us, and another electroplating plant two miles to the west of us. The new discovery of cyanide intoxication was disconcerting, to say the least. In addition to the crushing effects of the illness itself, I was counting on the improvement of our health in the apartment near Cherry Hill to help demonstrate an environmental etiology to our disease.

I thought that treatment with larger doses of hydroxocobalamin might enable my wife and me to remain in our apartment near Cherry Hill, so I contacted the drug agency that manufactures alphaREDISOL. I found out that the company produces hydroxocobalamin powder which may be taken orally, and which would give much more detoxifying capacity than the diluted alphaREDISOL, but the company would not allow me to have any. [*Sublingual 5,000 mcg hydroxocobalamin tablets are now available without a prescription per Amazon, as are the less expensive 5,000 mcg sublingual methylcobalamin tablets.*] Apparently it has not been approved by the Food and Drug Administration. Not even as a licensed physician was I able to obtain the comparatively harmless powder which may have provided vital relief. Each additional day brought the threat of westward winds and renewed suffering.

In time, my wife and I would move about seven miles to the southeast and find that our health improved a great deal. Meanwhile, between the time of my first hearing on May 19th and a second hearing scheduled for June 28th, we traveled west to visit relatives in other states. Our bodies were stressed, run down, and particularly sensitive to cyanide exposure. There were two places in our travels where we suffered symptoms of cyanide intoxication. First, in Lexington, Kentucky, where we learned there were at least five electroplating plants. Then secondly, in Greeneville, Tennessee, where we learned that we were not too far from a governmental electroplating plant for plating pennies.

My wife began crying in her sleep in Lexington. My head was swimming and my breathing was labored. It was about 4:00 a.m. After waking my wife, who felt ill but did not realize that she was crying, I arose and walked into my brother's den. The television was connected to a cable weather station; the wind was coming from the direction of downtown Lexington. [*Remember that, although my focus at that time was upon electroplating, cyanide is also released from smokestacks and other sources.*]

[*At this point, before continuing the manuscript that was typed out in the 1980s, I would like to insert some information in regard to airborne cyanide intoxication and crying. After moving to Tennessee, and sometime during the 1990s, I came across an interesting plea on the internet. A lady from Australia was reaching out for help, trying to find the cause of crying spells that she claimed would last eight hours a day. This lady's name was Maureen Hurley, and she subsequently sent me a rather extravagant copy of her family tree, revealing that her maiden name was Maureen Hynes, and that her ancestors had immigrated to Australia from Ireland. Her home was in Ashburton, a suburb of Melbourne, Victoria, Australia. When I read about her symptoms, I believed that she could definitely be suffering from cyanide intoxication, and I responded to her by email. She greatly benefitted from treatment with sodium thiosulfate and hydroxocobalamin, and we became longtime, long distance friends. Following is some correspondence from her physician in Australia, Dr. Geoffrey Kemp, which was postmarked 7 JUN 1999:*

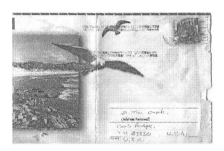

BURKE ROAD MEDICAL CENTRE
Dr. G. C. M. Kemp *M.B., B.S. (Melb)*
Provider Number: 212141K
Dr. M. G. Soccio *M.B., B.S. (Melb)*
Provider Number: 238254Y

681 BURKE ROAD
CAMBERWELL 3124
P.O. BOX 498
CAMBERWELL
Tel: 882 1366

15th March 1999.

Dr. Tim Oesch,

Oak Ridge,
TN 37830,
U S A

Dear Tim,

    I have been wanting to write to you to thank you for your kindess to Kevin and Maureen Hurley, and also myself in sharing your knowledge and through me, all the patients whom I have been able to assist with the methods you indicated could be used.

    Maureen Hurley has been stable for some months now.

    Another patient of mine who had been the victim of a catastrophic inclinator (a diagonal lift) accident, suffering a ruptured aorta, fractured femora, cerebral and spinal anoxia, believes that the throsulph and B12 have given him another few hours a day in which he can function without severe, debilitating fatigue.

    80% of Melbourne people tested are above the limit including myself. I am without symptoms.

    Burke Road is a major North South artery in a city of 3,000,000 people with an area similar to that of Los Angeles. Most families live on quarter acre blocks - there is not much residential high rise accommodation, thus a lot of people drive a long way every day - hence a lot of pollution.

Yours sincerely,

[signature]

When doctor Kemp wrote that **80% of Melbourne people tested are above the limit**, *I am quite sure that he was referring to urine thiocyanate testing. This does not surprise me. Note that he claimed that he did not experience symptoms of cyanide intoxication himself, and this is consistent with the fact that some persons feel ill from given levels of airborne cyanide, and other persons do not feel ill while breathing the same air. So then, back to the story penned in the 1980s...*]

Fortunately, the winds in Lexington did not come from the direction of downtown for too large a segment of our visit there. Checking the Lexington phone book, I found five electroplating plants listed in the yellow pages under *plating*. Inquiring into their locations, I learned that they were all located in basically the same direction—the direction of downtown. Our relatives had experienced some of the same symptoms from time to time, and were quite interested in learning more about chronic cyanide intoxication. By this time, I was thoroughly convinced that cyanide contamination and cyanide intoxication are nationwide problems. Though it seemed unlikely to accomplish much good, I notified the health department in Lexington.

Our illness in Greeneville, Tennessee was vaguer than in Lexington. Occasional symptoms of cyanide intoxication may have been associated with winds from the east or northeast, but I did not pinpoint a specific direction during our visit. There had been an electroplating plant about a thousand feet northeast of where we were visiting, but it was no longer in operation. An industrial park was situated just beyond the closed electroplating plant, but I did not learn whether or not any electroplating took place there. Another potential source of cyanide contamination was the government penny plant, several miles to the northeast.

An employee at the penny plant, where copper coatings were electroplated onto zinc plugs, told me that discharge water was dumped into a pool behind the plant. The pool drained into a stream. This was highly interesting when coupled with information given to my wife by Betty Stiel. Betty was suffering with headaches, gastrointestinal problems, fatigue, sleepiness, muscle aches, joint aches, irritability, restless sleep, sharp pain in the right side of her abdomen, and pain under her shoulder blades. She lived near the penny plant, and her problems started with a bad headache which she developed while participating in a tour of the plant. The symptoms she described are classic for chronic cyanide intoxication.

I supplied Betty Stiel with a copy of my report, *What American Citizens Should Know About Chronic Cyanide Intoxication*, and my wife and I departed for the apartment near Cherry Hill. Before ever leaving the apartment on vacation, we had submitted blood and urine to be tested at a nearby hospital. The blood was sent to National Medical Services, and the urine was sent to Metpath Laboratories, Inc. Upon returning to our apartment, we found the test results in our mailbox. My blood was tested for cyanide and found negative. Melody's blood was tested for thiocyanate and found to contain 2 mcg/ml [*I assume this was a serum thiocyanate level, though I have not been able to find the original test report or a copy thereof*], which is equivalent to 0.2 mg/dl. Her urine was tested for thiocyanate and found to contain 3 mg/L.

The only test which was abnormally high was Melody's urine thiocyanate test, and it was only slightly elevated at 3 mg/L since the upper limit for nonsmokers was 2 mg/L. This seemed to indicate that our bodies had become so vulnerable to cyanide exposure that very small quantities of cyanide induced illness. I wondered if perhaps our bodies were depleted in sulfur, which is necessary for converting cyanide to thiocyanate, so after returning to our apartment I took large doses of sodium thiosulfate for several days. Then I submitted another urine for thiocyanate testing. This time the hospital sent the urine to National Medical Services, and they found my urine to be negative for thiocyanate.

Even though National Medical Services did not measure urine thiocyanate levels below 5 mcg/ml [*now, in 2020, they give a Reporting Limit of 0.10 mcg/ml for urine thiocyanate*], it was still obvious that the *negative* level was nowhere near the 21 mcg/ml which was detected in my urine submitted at the Philadelphia Naval Shipyard. It was also evident that lower thiocyanate levels were not just resulting from depleted levels of sulfur in our bodies; my wife and I were apparently becoming ill from relatively smaller doses of environmental cyanide. My wife's previous urine thiocyanate level in Pitman was 6 mg/L, twice as high as that found near Cherry Hill. Yet her illness near Cherry Hill, and mine too by this time, was growing progressively worse. If just National Medical Services alone had reported such relatively low findings, I may have doubted the results due to the entanglement of politics. With a relatively low level reported from Metpath Laboratories, Inc. too, however, I concluded that the results were authentic.

The apparent increase in our vulnerability to cyanide exposure troubled my wife and me. Not knowing that electroplating plants were situated one and two miles to the west of us, we wondered where we could move in order to escape harrowing illness. Meanwhile, Lieutenant O'Hanlan and I were collecting additional evidence to present at a second hearing scheduled for June 28th. In addition, Lieutenant Norris came brilliantly to our aid by obtaining the affidavits presented at the end of chapter fifteen. These were the affidavits disclosing that civilian test results were withheld from civilian medical charts at the Philadelphia Naval Shipyard, and presenting support from civilian nurses on my behalf.

Perhaps the first new exhibit I prepared following my first hearing on May 19th was a paper entitled *Variability in Metabolism of Cyanide*. The paper read as follows:

In a book entitled **Laboratory Diagnosis of Diseases Caused by Toxic Agents**, *edited by F. W. Sunderman and F. S. Sunderman, Jr., p. 290, one finds the following statement:* **There is a great variation in resistance of different individuals to cyanide intoxication**. *I personally believe that rates of cyanide metabolism may vary manyfold among different individuals. A threefold difference is indicated by data in Recommendations For Cyanide Standards by NIOSH, which gives the half-life of cyanide in blood as from 20 minutes to one hour. [Also note that after cyanide flees the bloodstream in favor of body tissues, what happens to cyanide in those tissues may also vary greatly from one individual to another.] The article also gives an approximate detoxification rate for hydrogen cyanide injected intravenously, namely about 0.017 mg/Kg/min. In an average-sized man, this would amount to the detoxification of about 1.2 mg of cyanide per minute.*

Considering a threefold variance in cyanide metabolism, two different men may detoxify inhaled cyanide at rates of 0.6 mg/min and 1.8 mg/min. If both men inhaled cyanide at the rate of 1.4 mg/min for one hour, then by simple mathematics, one man would have basically no cyanide in his body while the other man would be left with 48 mg of un-detoxified cyanide in his body. After several hours of such exposure, one man may experience little or no illness while the other man becomes fatally ill. Furthermore, on page 228 of **Industrial Toxicology**, *Hamilton and Hardy, Third Edition, Publishing Sciences Group, Inc., 1974, the following is stated:* ***After development of chronic symptoms, the worker should be made to change his work****. This supports my own observation that previously unaffected individuals who are repeatedly exposed to low doses of cyanide may develop vulnerability to cyanide exposure. Perhaps it would be more accurate to say that such individuals suffer injury to their innate abilities to detoxify cyanide.*

Although the preceding paper is profound in demonstrating differences in cyanide metabolism between individuals, the actual figures given were attributed to differences between healthy individuals. Persons who suffer from chronic cyanide poisoning may detoxify cyanide far less proficiently than any of the above figures indicate. Without any doubt, the data from NIOSH confirmed my belief that different persons detoxify cyanide at different rates, along with several other published articles. Such a belief was not just *conjecture*, as Captain Wilson had implied. Furthermore, the three references sited in the paper definitely disproved Dr. Jason Mills' insinuation that no references existed which evidenced one person having more sensitivity to cyanide than another. In fact, many references substantiate this observation.

Another exhibit added to my collection was the Minnesota Multiphasic Personality Inventory (MMPI). The report read as follows:

This report is an addendum to the original 5/2/83 psychological report, summarizing the results of the Minnesota Multiphasic Personality Inventory (MMPI) which was computerized by NCS Interpretive Scoring Systems.
According to the MMPI, Dr. Oesch is an outgoing, sociable individual with a strong need to be around others. Behavioral stability is good, and no definite diagnosis of any significant psychopathology is evident. Although Dr. Oesch is gregarious and effective at gaining recognition from others, his personal relationships may be somewhat superficial. Although demonstrating outward emotional control, Dr. Oesch actually has difficulty dealing with some affect, especially anger. Therefore, rigidity and inflexibility are evident and may be passive expressions of his anger. Dr. Oesch dislikes confrontation and

will tend to be more passive or compliant in emotionally arousing situations. A little rebelliousness is suggested and, combined with his passive-aggressive proclivities, may cause him problems with authority figures. He tends to blame others and demonstrates less efficient introspection.
The MMPI results reveal no significant psychopathology. The proclivities delineated are merely salient personality features within a normal personality. These results are similar and comparable to the other personality assessment results.

Dr. Edward G. Daniels	*Aaron Botbyl, Ph.D.*
Psychometric Technician	*Licensed Clinical Psychologist*

My wife could hardly believe that the above report claimed I had a *strong need to be around others*. The fact is, I like to work alone, exercise alone, and even enjoy spending evenings alone. I certainly enjoy being with people at times, but I also enjoy time with myself and God. The Interpersonal Behavior Survey (IBS), another psychological test which I took the preceding December, was more in keeping with my wife's opinions. It concluded that I was highly independent: it ranked dependency as the least evident quality in my entire survey.

Another point where the two psychological tests reached vastly different conclusions was the subject of passive aggressiveness. The MMPI deduced that I had *passive aggressive proclivities*; whereas, the IBS scored me far below average in passive aggressiveness. The IBS also deduced that I was low in general aggressiveness, but it scored me high in general assertiveness and frankness. All in all, I think the IBS reached far more accurate conclusions than the MMPI. At any rate, the large difference in results probably reflects the element of human opinion in modern psychology.

I consider myself to be a deeply introspective individual, and perhaps the most affronting comment on the MMPI result was that I *tend to blame others and demonstrate less efficient introspection*. Furthermore, even though the MMPI interpretation designated this as merely a salient personality feature within a normal personality, I figured that the Physical Evaluation Board would capitalize upon those particular words from the MMPI report. The reason I figured such is because *blaming others* and *lack of introspection* are associated with paranoia. Doctor Sanfacon, my civilian psychiatrist, adroitly discounted paranoia: *there was no evidence of perceptual disturbances, no symptoms of depression, no ideas of reference or influence, no magical thinking or thought insertion or broadcasting.* Nonetheless, I mentally predicted that the Board would ignore Doctor Sanfacon's clear remonstration, and focus upon the affronting comment in the MMPI report. This prediction proved true. [*It never struck my mind until now, in the year 2020, that the summary of the MMPI report may have been influenced through the persuasion of naval officials. As alluded to in chapter 13 of this book, the health official who interviewed me at the New Jersey State Health Department in Trenton, New Jersey, disclosed how naval officials had contacted him prior to my visit there, and had given a very derogatory report about me. I don't even know how the naval officials were aware that I was going to the health department in Trenton, New Jersey. But in regard to my MMPI report, which unfortunately is not dated apart from stating the original date of my psychological examination, it is obvious that naval officials had the identity of the mental health professionals who provided the report in Exhibit C of my Physical Evaluation Board hearing on May nineteenth. These mental health professionals practiced in Marlton, New Jersey, which is notably closer to Philadelphia than Trenton, New Jersey. The summary report from the MMPI concluded a normal personality, but the salient personality features mentioned in the report were in direct contrast to the conclusion in the first report from these same mental health professionals:* **No significant psychopathology is evident, nor any salient personality features which would impede his social, emotional, or intellectual functioning**. *Not only was this MMPI report in stark contrast to all other psychiatric or psychological tests that had ever been administered to me (note that the naval diagnosis of paranoia was not backed up by any actual psychological testing); but also, the report seemed obviously inaccurate to both my wife and to me.*]

With the unexpected emphasis on the cyanide problem in Houston by the Physical Evaluation Board, Lieutenant O'Hanlan advised me that we should acquire some additional support from Houston. He felt this was necessary in order to counterbalance the propaganda solicited from the Houston Health Department by the Philadelphia Naval Hospital. By this time I possessed copies of the material forwarded by the Houston Health Department, or at least most of it. There were many newspaper or magazine articles, with titles such as: *Cyanide nonexistent in the Heights; Probers Find no cyanide poisoning; City officials say cyanide not sure cause of symptoms; Cyanide levels are negligible, Houston Health Department health officials say; Health director skeptical about poisonings; Results negative in the Heights cyanide testing, city health officer reiterates; Panel of medical experts finds no cyanide*; and, *The doctor who took on City Hall*. More interesting than the newspaper articles, though, was information published by the Houston Health Department that the newspapers never printed.

Included in the forwarded material was an abstract written by Dr. Judith Craven, Director of the Houston Health Department, and coauthored by Dr. Belinda Friggs [*Belinda Friggs may be a fictitious name*], Assistant-Director of the Houston Health Department. The abstract was entitled, *An Account of the Handling of a Potential Environmental/Medical Crisis by a Local Health Department*. As might be expected, there were some notably unsubstantiated and misleading statements in the report. I will note some of these statements as they occur. The report follows:

The Houston Health Department has recently responded to a community environmental crisis precipitated by the findings of a local physician that low levels of cyanide were detected in the blood samples of a small number of his patients, all living in close proximity to one another. Note: this report begins by suggesting that the *environmental crisis* was the result of my *findings*, rather than the cyanide contamination itself. Furthermore, the blood cyanide levels were not *low levels*, and the patients identified with poisoning were found to live as far as ten miles apart. *The physician suggested that environmental factors were responsible for the presence of the substance in these patients' bloods. Subsequent fear and outcry from the community necessitated the Public Health and medical community's performance of a full-scale investigation of the matter. The complexity of the crisis was compounded by the involvement of the press; a parochial educational institution; and a church-based community action organization, each receiving separate and contradictory reports from the Houston Health Department and the local physician, who was a part-time employee of the educational institution*. Note: notice how the emphasis of the report is quickly shifted to politics, rather than to the scientific and medical implications of the laboratory findings.

In chronological sequence, the events and response of the major players are presented below.

On Tuesday, November 24, 1981, a telephone call was placed to the Environmental Control Division of the Houston Health Department by the physician. In this conversation, the physician indicated that he had sampled ten patients' bloods for cyanide and had received laboratory reports indicating small to toxic levels of the substance in those samples. Note: I only reported three patients found with cyanide poisoning before leaving for Tulsa on Thanksgiving vacation. Although I did call John after departing, I did not speak to anyone else in Houston after my departure until I returned following the Thanksgiving holidays. *Upon further questioning, the physician indicated that the testing for cyanide resulted from his encounter with a patient who worked for a metal-plating industry. The patient had presented with symptoms of depression, fatigue, headaches, dizziness, and nausea, and had suspected that his illness was due to chronic exposure to cyanide used at his plant.* Note: this is a starkly false statement. John first presented with the major complaint of pain in his hands and fingers, and he had no idea what was causing it. Cyanide was not suspected until I began reading about different agents John was exposed to at work. *Having received the laboratory report indicating some cyanide in the patient's blood, the physician proceeded to test nine other persons who complained of similar symptoms.* Note: again this is false. The second person I tested was John's wife, who I tested at his attorney's request. Not until her test came back positive did I realize the environment might be contaminated with cyanide. *Lab tests ranged from 2 to 28 micrograms per deciliter. In addition, the physician determined that all ten patients were, in some way, associated with the parochial educational institution, either as student, staff, or family member.* Note: the preceding sentence failed to mention that the eleventh patient found with cyanide poisoning had nothing to do with the ***parochial educational institution***, nor did most of the cyanide victims identified thereafter in Spring Branch.

Between November 26th and 29th, over the Thanksgiving holiday, the Houston Health Department collected samples of sewage, water, and air and proceeded to analyze them. Note: there is no disclosure of where these samples were taken, or of how sensitive the testing procedures were for detecting cyanide.

On November 30, the parochial educational institution appointed a committee which would meet on the next day to discuss the potential problem.

On December 1, the physician's announcement of his findings to the press precipitated numerous inquiries by the media to the Public Information Office of the Houston Health Department. Note: I was not the one who broke the story to the press, though perhaps I should have been.

Also on December 1, the Environmental Control Division of the Houston Health Department, seeking a comprehensive evaluation of the emerging problem, requested the involvement of the Department's Epidemiology Section.

Both the Public Information Officer and the Assistant Director of the Environmental Control Division of the Houston Health Department were requested to be at a meeting held by the physician on December 2, at the educational institution. Upon arrival at the meeting, Houston Health Department representatives discovered that members of the media were present and that a press conference was to be held. Note: I was asked by a Gulf Coast Bible College official to prepare a report to present to the student body on December 2nd during chapel service. Not until shortly before that service was I informed there would be a news conference instead. I was certainly not the one who invited the Houston Health Department officials, and I do not know who did. *The physician answered questions from reporters concerning his previously announced findings. A statement was also requested of the Assistant Director of Environmental Control from the Houston Health Department. This statement indicated that samples of various environmental agents had been taken and were currently in the process of being analyzed.*

The Houston Health Department's Epidemiology Section, in response to the request for its services, initiated a study in the community. At this point, the need to replicate the blood sampling was seen as appropriate to ascertain that cyanide levels found in the first tests had not been subject to an error in laboratory procedures. Note: such an ascertainment, of course, would be blatantly erroneous. The half-life of cyanide is only about 30 minutes in the bloodstream. Basically, at best, blood cyanide tests only reveal exposures to cyanide that occur on the same day that the tests are performed. *It was also decided that tests should be made on asymptomatic members of the population for the purpose of comparison. [Of note, high blood cyanide levels in a person who does not demonstrate notable illness would not prove that high blood cyanide levels are normal; and in fact, would indicate that there is a significant source of cyanide from somewhere.]*

Samples were drawn from the original ten patients of the physician. In addition, a control group of eighteen asymptomatic volunteers from the educational institution were sampled.

Under carefully controlled conditions, each of the blood samples were divided into three parts and were tagged to permit blind study analysis. Three laboratories were commissioned to evaluate results. These were the official State Health laboratory housed in the Houston Health Department, the laboratory of the County Coroner, and the private laboratory which had submitted the original results. A brief questionnaire was also administered to the twenty-eight participants. Included were questions concerning symptomatology, demographic characteristics (age, race, sex), duration of illness, location of home and job places, incidence of illness in immediate family, and other questions relating to sources of exposure.

On December 3, the epidemiologists checked Carbon Monoxide levels in the community as a possible alternate cause determinant of the illness reported. Note: the testing for carbon monoxide on December 3rd is interesting in light of the fact that one of the Houston Health Department officials witnessed the bright red color of venous blood drawn from my arm on December 2nd. Carbon monoxide is the only agent besides cyanide, to my knowledge, that can cause the venous blood to turn red. In actuality, though, carbon monoxide causes more of a *pinkish* color, whereas cyanide causes a redness the color of arterial blood.

The physician also confirmed that two more of his cases showed cyanide in the blood samples. [Notice that there is no mention of the fact that the two additional cases revealed blood cyanide levels of 55 mcg/dl and 104 mcg/dl, with the 104 mcg/dl being found in the blood that was bright red in color and that was shown to a Doctor from the Houston Health Department who pointed out that the bright red color was from cyanide blocking oxygen uptake by the tissues.]

A Breath of Cyanide

On December 4, the Director of the Houston Health Department, a physician formally-schooled in Public Health, having been made aware of the medical aspects of the cases only through information in the press, requested an audience with the local physician who had reported the cases. Including her Assistant-Director, also a physician, her Assistant Director of Environmental Control, the Chief of her Epidemiology Section, the Chief of the Department Laboratory and her Public Information Officer, the Director of the Houston Health Department sought to clarify the facts surrounding the patients reported to have cyanide present in their blood samples. She also requested of the local physician that new information be channeled through the Houston Health Department prior to its release to the press in order to avoid unwarranted anxiety within the community. In addition, a routine check was made of the local physician's credentials which indicated that he had graduated as a student in good standing, but had never served an internship or residency of any kind. Note: my year of externships prior to graduation was simply not mentioned.

During this time and due to increased publicity, the Houston Health Department was being bombarded by concerned inquiries from persons living in the community surrounding the educational institution. Over four hundred calls per day were received from pregnant women, lactating mothers, persons working in the area, and other physicians. [The health department never informed me that they were getting calls from physicians, and certainly never gave me the names and phone numbers of those physicians.]

Later that same December 4th afternoon, the Director of the Houston Health Department held a press conference suggesting that a full epidemiologic investigation of the problem was necessary and appropriate due to the heightened level of public anxiety concerning the problem. She also stated, that based on a preliminary investigation of the data, she was unable to confirm the alleged outbreak of cyanide poisoning. In addition, on that same day, after the press conference, representatives of the church-based community action group demanded a private conference with the Director of the Houston Health Department and also pressed for her appearance at a community meeting. Such meetings were granted. The community action group and the community-at-large were apprised of relevant information and future plans. Note: December 4th was the day that the

Director of the Houston Health Department, Dr. Craven, appeared on public television and stated that I had acted prematurely in contacting the news media. She made this statement despite my clear remonstration earlier that same day in my office that I was not the one who initially contacted the news media. In addition, she basically led the public to believe that there was no cyanide problem at all.

On December 6, the local physician indicated that he now was aware of the source of cyanide. He released information to the press that the cyanide was in the pecans found in the community. Note: this has got to be the nuttiest remark in Dr. Craven's report (excuse the pun). I maintained that the cyanide was airborne from the first day I reported the problem to health officials. The fact that it may have been absorbed into plant life, as well as animal life, did not change my stance on the cyanide being airborne. I never claimed that pecans were the source of the cyanide. Such a statement is absurd. I became ill on several occasions myself without eating a single pecan. *This information was based on a statement from an out-of-state individual who had received a gift of pecans from a friend in the community under investigation for cyanide poisoning. The individual reportedly ate the pecans, became ill, and was alleged to have a high cyanide level.* Note: I was informed by John Minowsky that his relative was tested for blood cyanide about a week after her illness and found to have a blood cyanide level of one microgram per deciliter. This is not a high cyanide level. *The name of the physician, hospital, patient, and laboratory involved in this incident were never furnished to the Houston Health Department or the press, although this information was requested by each.* Note: I never knew the name of the physician, hospital, patient, or laboratory, and I do not remember the Houston Health Department ever asking me to turn over any of them. *The local physician intimated that the Houston Health Department was responding to his findings in a **combative**, defensive manner. He suggested that the Federal Government should search for the source of illness.* Note: it appears that the idea of arraigning me with a mental disorder may have originated before I ever arrived in Philadelphia. Not only am I accused of naming pecans as the source of a cyanide epidemic, it is suggested that I defended this claim with hostile belligerence. I doubt that the Houston Health Department intended for this information to ever reach my hand. [*In retrospect, they may not have cared.*]

On December 7, the Director of the Houston Health Department contacted the Dean of the School of Public Health and requested his assistance in evaluating the problem. She stated that the Houston Health Department would gladly meet with any persons the Dean recommended to apprise them of the chronology of events that had transpired. She also stated her feelings that it was necessary for any persons assisting to form separate and objective conclusions to those formed by the Houston Health Department. Note: as long as the data supplied came from the Houston Health Department, what difference did it make that other agencies were called upon to interpret it? *The Dean immediately called back with the names of five individuals who would form a 'blue ribbon panel' and who would meet with the Director of the Houston Health Department that day. Each appointee represented a discipline which would be necessary for a comprehensive evaluation. Included on the Ad Hoc Environmental – Occupational – Toxicology Committee, as it was called, were professors of Occupational Medicine, Environmental Science, Toxicology, Industrial Hygiene, and Epidemiology.*

The Director of the Houston Health Department also contacted the County Medical Society and the two local medical schools to request technical/clinical assistance, if such were deemed necessary. The Medical Society and schools expressed their willingness to cooperate in any way possible. The State Health Department, as well as the State Water Quality Control Board, were alerted to the problem. Both agencies felt that the expertise of local health department officials was sufficient or better than their own for scientifically evaluating the problem. The Environmental Protection Agency and the Center for Disease Control (CDC) were also called. After having heard preliminary data, the spokesperson for CDC indicated that she saw no problem. Note: there is no mention of autonomous environmental testing by any agency other than the Houston Health Department in the preceding paragraph.

Later that day, a procedure for investigating the alleged cyanide problem was outlined by the appointed Ad Hoc Committee. Note: to my knowledge, this outlined procedure proposed scheduled medical examinations and laboratory tests on individuals volunteered by Gulf Coast Bible College. *The Committee also requested and received available scientific documentation from the Houston Health Department environmentalists, lab personnel, and epidemiologists.*

Because the cyanide issue was before the public and open to close scrutiny, the media began receiving anonymous information which was passed on to the Houston Health Department. Note: the Houston Health Department was apparently desperate enough to admittedly publish gossip. *For example, it was said that the parochial educational institution wished to expand its campus. A devaluation of property by persons moving from the area and selling cheaply would be to the advantage of the school.* Note: in actuality, the college had considered relocating in Oklahoma not long before that time, and had attempted selling its properties. A devaluation of property was probably the last thing they wanted. *Other information had to do with the local physician wanting to quickly build his practice, with his participation in other politically sensitive issues, and with the questionable intentions of the church-based community group. None of the allegations made were substantiated.*

By the 10th of December, the Ad Hoc Committee was ready to make a preliminary report, based on their own findings and the blind study blood sampling data. At a press conference, the panel indicated that results of all testing were essentially negative for cyanide.

The local physician who initially detected the 'problem' indicated he had now sent his samples to Mayo Clinic Laboratories and was awaiting the results.

On December 16, after reviewing all blood samples and environmental test results, the Ad Hoc Committee issued a more current report, indicating there was no evidence to support a diagnosis of cyanide poisoning in area residents, nor was it possible to support an impression of an acute outbreak of a specific illness.

The local physician charged, several days later on December 24, that vegetation was being covered with cyanide as a result of rain mixing with emissions from industrial plants. Note: I did not say that vegetation was being 'covered with cyanide.' There is evidence, however, that plants may absorb cyanide from the environment and contain it for short periods of time. *He stated that his own blood sample indicated 104 micrograms per deciliter of blood. The physician indicated that he and his wife would leave the area if the cyanide controversy were not resolved. An attorney, who was not being retained by the physician and who had personally paid for the vegetation studies, noted that the junior senator for the State had been contacted in hopes of involving the Federal government in the investigation. It was disclosed that the local branch of the State Air Control Board intended to sample the community. It also was admitted that four of the five blood cyanide levels from Mayo Clinic Laboratories were negative.* Note: four of the five blood cyanide levels returned from Mayo Clinic Laboratories by that time were less than 10 mcg/dl. The other one was highly positive at 30 mcg/dl, and occurred in a nonsmoker. Furthermore, one of the individuals with a blood cyanide level less than 10 mcg/dl was still found to have a serum thiocyanate level of 0.48 mg/dl. This is about twice the average level and was higher than that occurring in the individual with a blood cyanide level of 30 mcg/dl. [*Note that the Houston Health Department neglected to mention that the fifth blood cyanide tested by Mayo Clinic Laboratories was significantly high at 30 mcg/dl.*]

Nearly two months later, in mid-February, a local television station reported that an illegal drug operation was located in a private home in the community, in close proximity to the parochial educational institution. Note: to the best of my memory, the designated home was located several blocks east of Gulf Coast Bible College. *It was suspected that methamphetamines, as well as certain silver compounds, were being manufactured at the home. The television story put forth the hypothesis that a cyanide by-product of such manufacturing could be a possible source of the still-perceived problem of cyanide poisoning in the area.* Note: the story about the private home producing methamphetamine and silver compounds was publicized after soil samples were found to contain elevated silver levels. The story may have been fabricated to create an alibi for the plating plant in the Timbergrove region, which was suspected of dumping silver cyanide (AgCN) and other compounds. By far the highest silver level, though, was found in the east end of the ditch directly in front of the plating plant in the Timbergrove region. The second highest silver level came from an outlet on the west side of White Oak Bayou, which indicates the plating plant in the Timbergrove area rather than the 'private home' as the source of disseminated silver. *The Houston Health Department investigated the operation, concluding that, for individuals within the home, itself, there was certainly the potential danger of a reaction to cyanide, a by-*

product of the procedure being used. Nevertheless, it was felt, by Houston Health Department officials, that individuals outside the confines of the home-based operation were not likely to feel the effects of these procedures. Testing contraindicated hazardous community environmental correlates to the isolated incident.

On February 14, the educational institution contacted the Director of the Houston Health Department, requesting an audience with her and the coordinator of the Ad Hoc Committee from the School of Public Health.

On February 16, when the meeting was held, the officials of the educational institution indicated that they felt there was a cyanide problem—an epidemic of sorts. Note: notice the obvious focus on Gulf Coast Bible College. The entire report never mentions that persons unassociated with Gulf Coast Bible College were also found with elevated cyanide and thiocyanate levels. *This conclusion was based on having received complaints from a total of twelve to fifteen students or faculty members in a total population of approximately 375 persons. It was stated that one faculty person left school due to allergic reactions.* Note: this faculty member was found to be very allergic to cyanide by Dr. Hitt. She had a blood cyanide level of 55 mcg/dl when tested on December 2, 1981. [*It is my understanding that, like beryllium, cyanide alone is not something an individual can be 'allergic' to. The allergy, or sensitivity, is something that develops in some persons in response to their own bodily proteins being bound with cyanide, causing an antigenic protein that is the combination of cyanide bound to the native bodily protein. The type of testing that Dr. Hitt performed is comparable to the testing for beryllium sensitivity.*] *Other faculty and students complained of weakness, forgetfulness, drowsiness, and inability to concentrate. Some undetermined number of persons saw a non-physician allergist* [*who happened to be a Ph.D.*], *while at least one person saw an osteopath. The Houston Health Department epidemiologist, having identified types of medical resources available and key medical manpower in the community, was able to clarify the background of the diverse professionals who saw the students and faculty as the educational institutional officials related their information.* Note: I received word from an individual in Houston that Dr. Darrell Crasky [*I do not recall this individual's real name*], a member of the Gulf Coast Bible College Board of Trustees, instructed students to withhold insurance money that they received from their insurance companies for payment to Dr. Hitt. The students were advised to call Dr. Hitt and tell him that he and Dr. Oesch made up the whole story about cyanide poisoning, so they were not going to pay him. Apparently Dr. Hitt was deeply hurt [*I remember Dr. Hitt as being a compassionate and sensitive individual, who happened to be married to one of the teachers I previously had when I attended Frank M. Black Jr. High, now known as Frank Black Middle School, in Houston*], but he did not abandon the problem. May God have mercy.

Being made aware of the need for uniform and reliable methodology of approach, it was requested by the educational institutional representatives that a more formalized process be initiated to conduct the work-up of medical histories on the latest students and faculty members that had become ill. The Director of the Houston Health Department agreed that such an approach would be appropriate, especially since no clearly-defined medical problem had, as yet, been identified. The Director of the Houston Health Department promised that medical school involvement would be sought. In addition, she requested of the Ad Hoc Committee that an interview and medical protocol instrument be devised which would encompass all known possible factors which might contribute to the symptomology described.

The Director of the Houston Health Department, reestablished contact with one of the medical schools. Since the Ad Hoc Committee was comprised of faculty belonging to the same superstructure as one of the two medical schools in town, it was decided that requesting assistance from the school not yet involved would be the best means of preserving objectivity. That school and members of the Ad Hoc committee from the first school met to decide what information should be elicited from the group which would be referred by the parochial educational institution.

When the final interview instruments and the medical epidemiological protocol were developed and the services of staff physicians secured, the president of the educational institution was contacted for the list of persons he referred to at the February 16th meeting. His response to the Director of the Houston Health Department came via an informal list forwarded to the Houston Health Department epidemiologist by his executive president's aid, with no cover letter and on plain (not school) stationary. The list was *comprised of twenty-seven names which were largely those names originally submitted by the local physician claiming to have found cyanide poisoning. The list also included the names of the physician and his wife.*

The Director of the Houston Health Department became concerned as to the validity of this list since it had been agreed that those to be referred should come from persons still at or associated with the parochial educational institution and still reporting symptoms. Note: cyanide victims, according to the preceding sentence, were not considered 'valid' by the Director of the Houston Health Department unless they were associated with Gulf Coast Bible College. My wife and I, both having positive tests for cyanide exposure in Spring Branch, were not considered acceptable candidates. *As has been stated, the February meeting with the president of that school revealed that the physician no longer was employed by the school or living in the area.* Note: I lived a few miles west of Gulf Coast Bible College, on the other side of the plating plant in the Timbergrove area.

The Director of the Houston Health Department then sent a certified letter requiring return acknowledgement of signature to the president of the educational institution, requesting an official list, on institutional stationary, and signed by the president.

An identical list, exclusive of the names of the physician, his wife, and one other individual was sent. Note: I do not know the identity of that 'one other individual' who was excluded. *Appropriate endorsement was included.*

The listed persons were sent a letter from the Director of the Houston Health Department, indicating that a free and comprehensive medical/epidemiological test battery would be available to them. These patients were asked to make an appointment for a given day at the medical school clinic. Note: this is a poor way to test for an agent that is only present and detectable at given times. Unless, of course, one is purposely trying not to find that agent. *They were also instructed to call the Houston Health Department or the clinic if they wished more detailed information.*

After review of all pertinent data by the medical school and the Ad Hoc Committee, it was concluded that no commonality among diagnoses and no evidence of an epidemic existed at the parochial educational institution. Blood cyanide and thiocyanate evaluations were found to be within normal limits. Note: why are the exact levels that were found not given? What is the Houston Health Department calling normal limits? [*Also, I see no indication that any urine thiocyanate testing was performed, which is more sensitive for detecting fairly recent cyanide exposure than either blood cyanide or serum thiocyanate.*] *The medical school, as a result of these examinations, was able to identify several instances of correctable or treatable conditions.* Note: the chairman of the Department of Medicine from one of the local medical schools was quoted as saying that the ailments in the 14 people evaluated from Gulf Coast Bible College could be attributed to such common problems as stress, diabetes, pneumonia and urinary tract infections. Interestingly, diabetes had already been associated with chronic cyanide poisoning by another investigator besides myself, and I had definitely seen an increase in stress, pneumonia, and urinary tract infections among individuals suffering from cyanide intoxication.

The local physician, it was found, had joined a branch of military service, after which he sent a manuscript to various members of the media alleging that a cyanide problem still exists. Note: I joined the Navy on February 3, 1978, years before that time.

One off-the-road opinion of a member of one of the investigative teams was that the persons in the community had not received adequate medical workups. Others expressed the need for an evaluation of the area in terms of accessible physician manpower and quality of care.

This chronology expresses events as they have occurred to the present time. It is uncertain as to whether this issue will surface again as a result of further need or controversy. [*Note that, in this report, there is no mention, whatsoever, of the finding of a cyanide war gas, namely cyanogen chloride, in the effluent being released into the sewer by the plating plant in the Timbergrove region. I did not find out about the cyanogen chloride until a notably later date, and I believe it is safe to assume that neither the Houston Health Department nor the United States Navy ever intended for me to know about the finding. Further, I have no reason to think that Lieutenant O'Hanlan was ever made aware of the finding. Cyanogen chloride is so volatile, meaning that it is easily evaporated into the air at normal temperatures, that each time it was found in laboratory testing, it could not be found a second time due to its being released into the air before a second test could be completed. So then, one may ask what organization actually conducted the tests that found cyanogen chloride? The answer—it was the Houston Health Department, with positive testing for cyanogen chloride at least as early as May of 1982—prior to my even leaving Houston for active duty in the Navy. Also of note, one of the enclosures sent to the Navy by the Houston Health Department was an interoffice correspondence dated 22 FEB 1982, and this may have been the report that denied the presence of cyanide in the discharge water from the General Electric plant, but that also acknowledged the finding of cyanogen chloride. I never received this report while in Houston, and I never received this report while in Philadelphia. I only received this report later, living in Tennessee, through the efforts of Walter Davis. Walter acquired data that had been collected by the Werner and Rusk law firm prior to the suit in Houston being unfortunately abandoned and then prohibited, and Walter mailed the data to me.]*

[*Of note, the Director of the Houston Health Department apparently considered the accomplishment of squelching concerns about environmental cyanide to be a feather in her cap. She even went so far as to attempt having the matter published in a medical journal:*

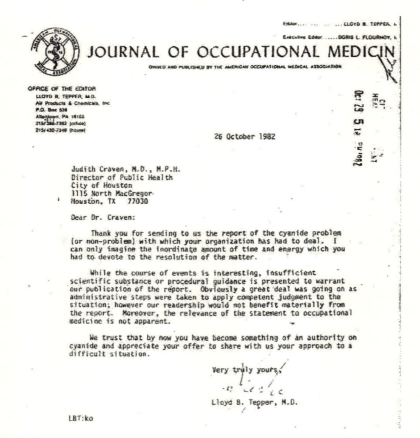

The article was rejected.]

Of the fourteen individuals associated with Gulf Coast Bible College who were examined at the medical school clinic, copies of the final reports mailed to eleven of them were forwarded to the naval hospital by the Houston Health Department. I do not know why the remaining three were omitted. In each of the reports, the last sentence of the first paragraph concluded by stating: *your cyanide levels as well as the remainder of your laboratory studies were essentially normal*. There were no specific values stated for either cyanide or thiocyanate. Furthermore, there was no indication of the ranges that the term 'essentially normal' was used to incorporate.

Among the eleven individual reports, eight of them stated detected abnormalities. These abnormalities included: [*Note that each of the following numbers, one through eight, indicates an individual patient.*

What each patient was found to have follows the number that is listed for that individual patient.] 1.) Anemia. 2.) Pus in urine and low blood potassium. 3.) Abnormal heart valve (mitral valve prolapse) and possible liver damage (elevated SGPT). 4.) High vitamin B12 level and possible liver damage (elevated SGPT). 5.) High vitamin B12 level. 6.) Possible hypertension (actual blood pressure not given). 7.) Abnormal urine (abnormality not specified) and elevated blood glucose level of 158. 8.) High vitamin B12 level and anemia.

The elevated B12 levels seen in three of the eleven patients probably indicated that these patients were taking hydroxocobalamin as an antidote to cyanide intoxication. In the presence of cyanide within the body, hydroxocobalamin is converted to cyanocobalamin, which is the form of vitamin B12 normally found in vitamin pills. [*Thankfully, vitamin tablets are now available that contain other forms of vitamin B12 such as methylcobalamin and hydroxocobalamin.*] Other abnormalities occurring more than once among the eleven patients included abnormal urine findings, anemia, and apparent liver damage. Elevated SGPT, which is a specific liver enzyme [*not really, it may also be elevated from vigorous muscle strain*], was also present in several patients at the Philadelphia Naval Shipyard who likely suffered from cyanide intoxication: (At first, I thought the patients in Philadelphia might have had some type of hepatitis. In a way, liver damage from cyanide is a type of hepatitis—it is toxic hepatitis rather than infectious hepatitis.) All in all, the findings of the medical clinic seem quite supportive to the presence of cyanide intoxication among the evaluated individuals. Apparently, the assigned investigators lacked either the knowledge or the willingness to point out how well these findings correlated with chronic cyanide intoxication.

I suppled Lieutenant O'Hanlan with the names of several additional persons who consented to supply information from Houston regarding the cyanide problem. Lieutenant O'Hanlan contacted a few of those persons by telephone. Copies of three resulting telephone depositions are in my possession. The depositions consist of a series of questions and answers. Following are depositions from Mrs. Marie Black, Mrs. Eileen Bland, R.N., and David Thompson. [*Note: I now possess more than three affidavits and/or depositions.*]

A Breath of Cyanide

Counsel For The Member: Good morning, Mrs. Black. My name is Lieutenant O'Hanlan, and this is a deposition by telephone taken on 14 June 1983. Could you state your name, please?
Witness: Marie Black.
Question: And your address.
Answer: 836 Hidden Gorge Lane. [Note, this woman lived near the Timbergrove region. The given address is fictitious. Her house was located about 1.45 miles, as the crow flies, northwest of the GE plating plant on 12th street. Given that the most predominant wind direction in Houston is from the southeast, it makes sense that she was found to have the highest urine thiocyanate level of anyone tested, even though she was a nonsmoker. In fact, since her house was situated more north than west of the plant, the emission of cyanide gasses from the sewer line flowing east from the GE facility put her in likely atmospheric pathways to receive cyanide-laden winds. Northwest winds are reported as occurring in Houston during fall and winter months as they tend to be associated with cold fronts, and this may explain why Marie tended to feel better during the winter. Gulf Coast Bible College, in comparison to where Marie lived, was located about 2.0 miles, as the crow flies, due east of the GE plating plant. The college administration building was situated between 11th street and 12th street. It was not common for winds to be blowing from due west, as they were on the day that the Houston Health Department conducted blood testing in the college administration building. Whether these winds that were blowing from due west constituted a momentous coincidence or an act of God, I do not know. I certainly believe, of course, that God is more than capable of causing winds to blow from whatever direction he so chooses, and it is remarkable that the very highest blood cyanide levels ever obtained were obtained on the day that the Houston Health Department conducted blood testing in the college administration building.]

Q. And what is your occupation, Mrs. Black?
A. I am a Shackley distributor.
Q. Shackley is?
A. Vitamins, nutrition.
Q. Mrs. Black, do you swear that everything that you state in this conversation today is the truth?
A. Yes, I do.
Q. Thank you very much. Do you know Dr. Timothy Oesch?

A. Yes, I do.

Q. How well do you know him?

A. Well, I...he was recommended to me by a Barbara Preskin [Barbara Preskin is a fictional name—her real name is disclosed toward the end of this book], and the reason I have gone to Barbara Preskin is as I've said before, I have been in nutrition for some time and I was on a very good nutritional program and still feeling bad— having headaches, being very, very tired and drained—and she was the one that suspected that I was allergic to the cyanide and she had sent me to him.

Q. What is 'she'? She is a nutritionist?

A. She is a nutritionist, yes...

Q. Okay, let me get this in the right time frame; when was this?

A. This was last year. I guess it was in March.

Q. Of 1982?

A. Of '82, yes.

Q. And can you tell us a little bit more about the symptoms you were feeling then?

A. Well, I was extremely tired and this is a weird tired, it's not a tired like when you work hard and you're tired—that's a good tired to me. This is a tired where your body just feels like there's lead in it and you also ache inside. It feels like the bones are aching, or close to the bones, or something like that; and you have extreme headaches, and of course when you have these extreme headaches you can't see straight; and, you know, this was just...I couldn't understand why I was so tired when I was on such a good nutrition program.

Q. Do you take vitamins regularly?

A. Yes. Three times a day plus at night; and she was the one that asked me...first of all she asked me where I lived, and I told her in the northwest part of town, and she had me draw a map exactly where I lived compared to where she was, and she suspected that I had the cyanide and she called Dr. Oesch right then and there and told me to go over to his office, which I did.

Q. Do you live near the Heights?

A. I live about a mile from the Heights, but I live about a mile from a company that supposedly was dumping cyanide.

Q. And she sent you to Dr. Oesch then?

A. Well, he listened to all my symptoms and everything and checked me over, and he also felt like this was what I was affected by, but he would not say...but he wanted to get my urine sample because I was leaving for Hawaii and he said after I came back from there I would probably be free of it and they wouldn't be able to tell the level that I had in my body, so they took it right then and there and then I left the next day for Hawaii.

Q. When you left did you feel better when you were in Hawaii?

A. Oh, yeah, I felt great over there.

Q. No more headaches?

A. No more headaches. I even stayed up late and we got up early which down here I get up and I drag; and I slept good up there. I just...I didn't really eat that well up there...I did take my vitamins, you know. I was very faithful with my vitamins...but really, I felt great over there. It was wonderful.

Q. Now what happened when you...how long were you there?

A. I was there for 7 days.

Q. Okay. What happened when you came back?

A. I, well...of course coming back, you know, we were on the plane, what 8 hours, and this was during the night also, you know, so you expect to be tired when you get back; but I was in bed for 3 days. I could not get out of bed. I don't know, I came back to Houston and it was right back to the old cyanide bit. You...you know, you really have this tired, heavy feeling. You hurt in your arms. You have the headaches. Dr. Oesch had called me; he knew when I was getting back and he had called me and I...my daughter told him that I wasn't available because she knew that I was so extremely tired...but she was having problems too...but he said that he wanted me to call just right away, whenever I could, you know: it was very, very important. He even gave me his home number and it was something like 7:00, 7:30 that evening before I finally called him back, and only because my daughter insisted that he said it was important that I call back, and that's when I found out the test results.

Q. And what were those results?

A. I had a 51.8.

Q. On the urine thiocyanate?

A. Yes, and he was really very concerned, and at that time I didn't realize the danger point that I was at.

Q. What did you do?

A. Well, he asked me if there was somebody that could drive me to his home because he wanted to give me the antidote...because the store, there was only one drugstore here that handled that, and they were closed.

Q. What is that antidote?

A. It's a sodium thiosulfate.

Q. And did you go over there?

A. Yes. My husband took me over there, and as soon as I got there he had me take it right away. Within an hour, really, he said within an hour I'd feel better. I think it was about 45 minutes I started feeling a difference.

Q. And that helped those symptoms?

A. Yes.

Q. Do you know Dr. Hitt?

A. Yes, I know Dr. Hitt.

Q. Are you being treated by him right now?

A. Yes.

Q. What is...can you describe that for me.

A. Well, Dr. Hitt had worked in California on...I don't know the treatment that you call this, but it's where they take a concentrate of your urine, they remove the solids and sterilize it, and inject it back into you; and this is supposed to help build up your immunity against...like he does it for like food allergies; and this was just experimental which he told me it would be, that maybe it would help build up my immunity against the cyanide because you cannot be injected with cyanide, it would kill you. And so he asked me if I wanted to go through this, because I wasn't living. I was just existing. And I told him I would try it because he felt like, you know, it wouldn't harm me. It may not do any good, but it wouldn't harm me, and so I took...it was a series of shots, one a week for eight weeks which I went, I think it was 12 weeks I went on, and after the first couple of shots I really felt bad the next day because I had these shots in the evening, but then after that when I'd get my shot I got better and better. Then we had...it was more or less...I started these shots at the onset of winter which, you know, Houston, we don't have much of a winter but the air does get better, and I began feeling better, and then during the winter I felt good. [The boiling point of cyanogen chloride is 55 degrees Fahrenheit, and the boiling point of hydrogen cyanide is

79 degrees Fahrenheit. This is not to say that these poisons will not be released into the atmosphere from liquids below the boiling points of the poisons, and there are other factors such a pH involved, but certainly once the boiling point of cyanogen chloride or hydrogen cyanide is exceeded, then you can expect a rapid volatilization (escape into the air) of the poison.] I did not feel like I did during the summer; but after…at the beginning of this summer I've had a lot of spells and, well, I've been real sick and had to have emergency treatment.

Q. What sort of treatment?
A. Well, it's the sodium thiosulfate plus the alphaREDISOL: that's the name brand. It's called something else but it's like a B12 shot.
Q. Who is giving it to you?
A. My husband is giving the shots to me.
Q. Is he a physician?
A. No. He's not a physician.
Q. But, I mean this is under a doctor's recommendation?
A. Yes.
Q. Who is the doctor?
A. Dr. Oesch is the one.
Q. And those things, do they help?
A. Yes. Like, oh, it was the Friday before Good Friday: I had a real bad spell that day. I had tremendous headaches and when I have these headaches I have to take like 4 to 6 Excedrin to get rid of it and they make me a nervous wreck. I don't really like to do that but my husband had come home early and we went out to the dairy, he even helped me to get out but as I got out, oh, the air was awful and got worse and worse, and by the time we got back home he had to help me in the house.
Q. What sort of day was it? Was the day humid and the air not moving?
A. No. That was the funniest part was it was kind of cool and there was a breeze blowing, so I couldn't understand why cyanide should be affecting me, you know, that day.
Q. Was the breeze coming from the direction of that plant? Do you know?
A. Well, later on that night we found out that there was a truck that dumped chemicals along the highway and of course the city says they couldn't find the driver. The owner of the truck didn't know a thing about it and the city did not know what kind of chemical it was and I

think that's a bunch of bull: I know it is. You know, they just didn't want to say, but the winds were coming from that direction so I just assume this is what happened to me that day; and my daughter was affected too, you know, so it's not just me.

Q. What sort of symptoms does your daughter show?
A. The same thing I have.
Q. The headaches and the memory?
A. This has hampered her and her school work. She started her first year of college this year and she's going to San Jacinto which is in Pasadena. Of course Pasadena is nothing but industry and it has really hampered her learning ability. [Remember, there are many sources of airborne cyanide other than electroplating. Once an individual becomes sensitive to cyanide exposure in one location, that individual may certainly experience symptoms of cyanide intoxication in another location.]
Q. Does Dr. Hitt think you're allergic, you have an allergy to cyanide?
A. It's a 3 point plus allergy to cyanide, yes. [I think that Dr. Hitt graded immunological reaction to cyanide on a scale of 1 to 4.]
Q. And you are still seeing him?
A. Yes.
Q. All right. I think that's all the questions I need to ask you, Mrs. Black, this morning.
A. You're welcome.

[*Back at that point in time, I do not think that I had ever heard the word 'fibromyalgia.' Obviously, Mrs. Black had symptoms consistent with what would now be diagnosed as fibromyalgia, and I now consider airborne cyanide to be the world's leading cause of fibromyalgia. I have had very good response in treating fibromyalgia with antidotes for cyanide, as with 0.5 cc of Vital B12 daily, preferably supplemented with other antidotes. Vital B12 is a compounded form of vitamin B12 containing 25mg/cc of vitamin B12 as 12.5mg hydroxocobalamin/12.5mg methylcobalamin per cc. What is interesting about Dr. Hitt's work is that he was apparently working with patients to reduce their immunological reaction to cyanide. My approach in treating cyanide sensitivity is simply to reduce levels of cyanide in the body, whereas Dr. Hitt was targeting the body's* immunological response to cyanide as pertains to cyanide acting as a partial antigen or hapten. Since an individual can suffer from cyanide intoxication without any immunological response to cyanide, I definitely recommend antidotes to cyanide; but nonetheless, I would certainly like to see some present-day research in regard to fibromyalgia in light of Dr. Hitt's findings and treatment.]

Counsel For The Member: Let me identify myself. My name is Lieutenant O'Hanlan and this is a deposition taken by telephone on 14 June 1983, and could you state your name, please?
Witness: This is Eileen Bland.
Q. And your address, please, Mrs. Bland?
A. 4250 West 34th, Apartment 147, Houston, Texas.
Q. And what is your occupation?
A. I'm a teacher at Gulf Coast Bible College.
Q. What do you teach?
A. I teach pre-nursing science and biological science, science education.
Q. Are you a nurse yourself?
A. I am an R.N., yes.
Q. I am going to ask you to swear that, affirm that everything you say here is the truth, please?
A. Yes. What I am about to tell you in regard to all of this is the truth as far as I know it.
Q. Thank you, Mrs. Bland. How long have you worked at Gulf Coast Bible College?
A. About 10 years.
Q. Do you know Dr. Timothy Oesch?
A. Yes, I do know Dr. Timothy Oesch.
Q. How do you know him?
A. All right: I worked with him when he was the college physician, and he both helped me in teaching and also I referred students to him for medical problems because many times students would tell me things. Even though we had other counselors and so forth, we also have an advisee load of around 20 students per faculty member, and so a lot of my advisees would come to me and I would refer them to Dr. Oesch.
Q. So you are familiar with all the controversy about the cyanide poisoning issue in Houston?

A. Yes, I am.

Q. Do you feel that there was a problem in Houston; that there is?

A. Yes. I felt that there definitely was a problem. I'm not sure whether it has been cleared up or whether it is still existing.

Q. Did this affect you and your husband?

A. Yes. We, at that time, were living in the Heights where our college is. We lived down the street from the campus about, well, it was almost a block away from the building where I taught and about a block and a half from the administration building where the blood tests were drawn by the Houston Health Department in that part of the investigation of the cyanide poisoning that Dr. Timothy Oesch had detected.

Q. What does your husband do?

A. My husband teaches English at Gulf Coast Bible College.

Q. Did you and your husband suffer what you would think are symptoms of cyanide intoxication?

A. Yes. My husband walked, well, he still does, early in the morning hours around 4:00, 5:00 a.m. each morning. At that time he was walking 5 to 6 miles each morning and in the fall he became very ill, spiked a temp, and had, was diagnosed with pneumonia and was on antibiotic and so forth, and he is generally an extremely healthy man in that he seldom misses work. He had not missed any for several years. I don't remember the exact number of years, but I know it was five or six and last year when he had this pneumonia he missed a couple of days.

Q. Did he have it once or twice?

A. He had it twice.

Q. In how long a period of time?

A. Within 4 to 6 months. I don't remember exactly but it was all in the same semester.

Q. Did you notice any other symptoms?

A. In my husband?

Q. Yes, ma'am, or your own, that are generally associated with…

A. I don't recall his having any other physical symptoms except his mentioning: 'I can't remember as well as I used to, and I'm really getting concerned about it because I seem to start teaching something and I can't recall what author wrote it or what was said.' And I was noticing the same thing, plus I was having severe headaches.

Q. You were having severe headaches?
A. Yes.
Q. How old were you and your husband?
A. At that time we were 49. We're 50 now.
Q. And did you ever notice that on leaving Houston for any length of time that these symptoms sort of cleared up? That you didn't have the headaches?
A. Yes.
Q. Felt clearer?
A. Yes. Our daughter and son-in-law live in Oklahoma City and my husband's parents live in Guthrie, 30 miles from Oklahoma City, and when we would go up to see them I always felt considerably better, but thinking maybe that this was just vacation and I was relaxing, thought perhaps this might be why this was happening. But then I also was in school at East Texas State University at Commerce, Texas, and I was working on my doctors and was in some high pressure classes and I continued to feel better there whenever I would be away from Houston in school. For example, last summer I was a full-time student there, and last fall I also was. However, in the summer we, my husband and I, both lived there all summer and we both felt much better. It's a little rural farming community with the university there and in the fall I commuted back and forth. On weekends I would be at home and I didn't have a severe headache. I had more energy, just felt tremendously better.
Q. So how would you relate the workload and pressure of being in school to teaching? I mean, you wouldn't call that a relaxed environment like Oklahoma, like you were talking about?
A. No. There is definite pressure because we do carry a very heavy teaching load but I would say that I was under more pressure as a student on that side of the desk than I have as a teacher.
Q. Mrs. Bland, now I want to ask you if you ever have seen any of these symptoms clinically, like with Dr. Oesch?
A. Yes. The day that the Public Health Department came out to draw the blood from different ones of us who had had symptoms of this cyanide intoxication, I drew Dr. Tim's blood because he wanted a sample to send to a laboratory at the same time that the Public Health would send a sample to see if they got the same results, sort of as a control, and I drew his blood. However, Dr. Tim had been running all over campus and when I say running I mean literally running because

that's the way he always went at everything, full speed ahead, and I drew his blood and it was very bright red. Now this was not because I had drawn it with a syringe and it was open to the air but because it was drawn, I mean but because we felt that it was cyanide perhaps because it was drawn with a vacutainer in which it went directly from the bloodstream into the vacuum tube.

Q. And this is venous blood?

A. This is venous blood, right.

Q. Do you recall any of the results that came back from the tests?

A. Yes. My husband had somewhere in the 20's. I don't remember exactly.

Q. And this was a blood ---

A. ---blood test, right. And Dr. Tim's was high 20's. [Actually, my blood cyanide that day from blood drawn in the college administration building was 21 mcg/dl. The blood drawn by Mrs. Bland, on that same day, had a blood cyanide level of 104 mcg/dl. I have no doubt that Mrs. Bland was answering Lieutenant O'Hanlan to the best of her memory, because I have no doubt regarding her Christian faith and honesty.] I'm not sure whether it was 27, 28. I don't remember exactly but I know that it was high. High 20's.

Q. Okay. When was this? This was in December?

A. Yes.

Q. Of '81?

A. Yes.

Q. And do you remember what your test results were?

A. They were lower than my husband. I think mine was 20 and my husband's was 21 but I don't really remember for sure.

Q. Are you or your husband smokers?

A. Neither my husband nor I smoke. In fact none of the faculty of staff or administration at GBC smoke. GBC is Gulf Coast Bible College.

Q. What sort of environment were you in just prior to this blood test being done?

A. All right. I and my husband were sitting waiting in the administration building where it's air conditioned and we had probably been there at least 30 minutes and I would say more likely an hour and also this was during the time when my husband was ill, and in fact I had had to take him by car and this is not like my husband. He's a very independent person. From our house which is about a block and a half from the administration building because he was unable to walk, still having the illness, the symptoms of pneumonia.

Q. Was the building air conditioned?

A. Yes, and we did not have a central air home. Ours was just a wall unit but the administration building is air conditioned and centrally air conditioned and we had been sitting there for 30 minutes to an hour. The reason I know this and remember it so strongly is because my husband was so ill and I was so concerned about him and I wanted to get him home.

Q. Get him back home. All right. Was there anything, any other tests run? Did you go down to Baylor University?

A. Yes, Later, sometime during the spring and I don't recall whether it was March or April but as I recall it was sometime during the latter part of the school year, we were asked by our president to go down to Baylor Medical School because they were cooperating with the Public Health Department in regards to this investigation of cyanide, and we were examined, given thorough physical examinations and blood tests. When Dr. Wilson gave me, Dr. Howard Wilson, he was in charge of the investigation and in charge of working together with all the other doctors, and when he gave me my physical examination we talked in regard to this and he asked me if I thought it was cyanide poisoning ---

Q. –he knew you were a nurse and a science teacher?

A. Yes. He did know I was a registered nurse, and I said well, from the symptoms and from the way that the people have been sick and we've had more sickness this year and more sickness like what you would expect from something like a cyanide intoxication, then yes, it probably is cyanide poisoning but we haven't proven it and he said, I asked him if he thought that they would find out from their investigation, he said I doubt it, and I said why not, and he said because we are not running a 24 hour urinalysis on each individual, and I said why aren't you, and he said that it was because it often came in not done properly. People wouldn't void at the beginning and save the last specimen and I said but they could have been instructed and taught, and he said but it's too big a hassle and we thought this would be sufficient to satisfy what the public health wanted us to do.

Q. But he said that even if it was there what they were doing probably wouldn't find it?

A. That's correct.

Q. Did you notice any effect of this on the students you were teaching that year?

A. Yes. I did notice it considerably.

Q. Exactly what sort of effect?

A. I had a number of students complain to me that they would study and they couldn't remember the facts for their exams and these would be students that had never had this problem before.

Q. Generally good students?

A. I had a number of very good students that complained of this.

Q. Was this reflected in their grades? Did they do poorly?

A. They didn't do as well as they had been doing. It wasn't so significant that anyone failed or anything like this, but it was significant enough that we noticed it, you know, several points.

Q. Like a letter grade difference and things like that?

A. Yes.

Q. Yes, ma'am. When you were tested down at Baylor – where is Baylor in relation to the Heights area?

A. All right. I believe it's about 5 miles from here and it's on South Main Vanen (sic), and we are in the northwest part, so it would be not across town but it would be in a totally different direction.

Q. What sort of environment was it? Was it an air-conditioned building?

A. Very definitely an air-conditioned building and again as you nearly always do, you sit and wait.

Q. How long had you been waiting – how long had you been away from the Heights area when you were tested that day?

A. Well, of course we drove over there and we filled out some forms and they were pretty lengthy history forms and so some of the people had finished. I hadn't quite finished mine when we were called for our blood to be drawn so I would estimate around 30 minutes because it was fairly lengthy. That is 30 minutes after we arrived at the Baylor Medical Center.

Q. So would it be say an hour after you left the Heights?

A. Yes. Somewhere close to that.

Q. *And do you think that makes a difference? I mean the fact that you're in an air-conditioned building and away from ---*

A. *—definitely because with this your body can metabolize it and the liver can take care of it, and if you're out of the area it may not show up in the bloodstream in a significant quantity, that is.*

Q. *Are you all also living in the Heights?*

A. *Not now.*

Q. *Where do you live?*

A. *Last January we moved to the northwest, I mean farther northwest. We are about 4 miles north and west of our college now.*

Q. *Do you think that's made a difference?*

A. *I have definitely felt better. We here in this apartment have central air and heat and I've definitely felt better and I think my husband has also. All I know is that he seems to be back to his normal stride.*

Q. *He hasn't had any more pneumonia or anything like that?*

A. *No. No more. He's never had pneumonia and he's not had any symptoms of it since and he didn't have a cold or anything. The other time it just all of a sudden he became very, very ill.*

Q. *I see. Mrs. Bland, you've been real helpful. Thank you.*

A. *Thank you. Goodbye.*

Counsel For The Member: *Good morning, Mr. Thompson. My name is Lieutenant O'Hanlan. This is a deposition by telephone taken on 15 June 1983. Can you state your name, please?*

Witness: *My name is David L. Thompson.*

Q. *And your occupation, sir?*

A. *Owner of Spring Branch Medical Clinic.*

Q. *Are you a physician?*

A. *No, sir, I am not.*

Q. *And what is the address of the clinic?*

A. *1721 Pech, Suite 104, Houston, Texas 77055.*

Q. *Now, Mr. Thompson, do you swear that everything you will say in this conversation today is the truth, the whole truth and nothing but the truth, so help you God?*

A. *I do.*

Q. *Thank you, sir. Mr. Thompson, do you know Dr. Timothy Oesch?*

A. *Yes, sir, I do.*

Q. How do you know him, please?
A. He was an employee here at the clinic as a staff physician.
Q. When was this?
A. It was last year up until the time he went into the United States Navy.
Q. Up until he went in the Navy?
A. Yes, sir.
Q. Was he just in general medicine?
A. Yes, sir.
Q. What sort of work does the clinic do?
A. I would venture to say that 60% of our business is industrial medicine and 40% would be private patients.
Q. And industrial medicine involves a little bit of what?
A. Well, it involves pre-employment physicals for industrial companies and handling their injured employees when they need it in the line of work and for injuries. It could be back injuries, cuts, lacerations which would require sutures. Broken bones. Any number of occupational hazard injuries.
Q. Does occupational hazard, does that also mean some environmental work, too?
A. Yes, sir, it does.
Q. How many people, how many physicians do you have working at the clinic?
A. We have two physicians in the clinic. We have 36 physicians who are associated with us – which is a specialist in each field of medicine.
Q. In the work that the clinic did, did you ever have occasion to come in contact with the question in Houston about whether or not there was cyanide intoxication?
A. Yes, sir, I have.
Q. And what is your, can you give me some – talk about background or your opinion of that issue?
A. It's definitely here. It's all around us. I don't know how to start this, so bear with me.
Q. No, please, I'm right here.
A. Dr. Oesch, I knew of his involvement in the cyanide situation prior to his coming to work for us. Now, he was doing tests on patients of his prior to coming to work with us. Now, after coming to work with

us at the clinic, the Spring Branch Clinic, I kind of, well, I knew there was something there but there was a doubt in your mind – you know what I mean?

Q. Yes, sir.

A. We ran specimens on patients through three separate laboratories in three different locations in the United States. One was in California, one was in St. Louis and I think the other one was in New Jersey.

Q. Yes, sir.

A. And no laboratory, not one of the three, knew that we were sending specimens to another laboratory.

Q. Yes, sir.

A. And the same specimen from the same patient that went to these three different laboratories would come back, had the same test or same readings so to speak on all three, so it couldn't be lab error, and when you get confirmation like that, that wipes the doubt out of your mind automatically.

Q. And you did have patients who were tested – was this the urine thiocyanate?

A. As well as the blood levels.

Q. Blood levels, and they did come back that there was ---

A. –definitely high dosage. High exposure rate I should say.

Q. Were these people from the Heights that Dr. Oesch was –

A. –some of them were from the Heights and some were from the Spring Branch area. Now, Dr. Oesch did a tremendous amount of research into this thing. He called the Weather Bureau daily to see which way the wind blew the day before and the wind, I believe it was out of the east flowing west, that day we would have numerous patients in here affected with cyanide because the wind was blowing from this plant that was emitting it into the area and the people would have high exposure.

Q. And what sort of plant is that?

A. It's a metal plating or coating plant or something where you plate metals or some kind of, I forget what they, electro-plating I believe they call it.

Q. Electro-plating, and on days that the wind would blow from that plant, on days that the wind had blown the day before from that plant, then you would have more patients?

A. Yes, sir.

Q. Do you have any idea of the number of patients who were treated for this?

A. Off the top of my head in round figures I would say 40 or 50. No less than 40, and it may have gone more than 50. I, of course, being the owner and administrator, I don't keep up with each individual patient.

Q. Yes, sir, I understand. Was there one doctor, one physician in the clinic that handled most of these patients?

A. Yes, sir.

Q. Who was that?

A. Dr. Timothy Oesch.

Q. That was Dr. Oesch. What is the current status of that problem in Houston?

A. Well, the City Health Department said it wasn't there. Now, they tested the sewer water. They tested water in ditches. They tested water in the bayous nearby and they said there was nothing to it. The health division dissected a dog. The blood was sent in and the dog was, I think the blood level was at a lethal point. The dog did die from cyanide. There have been numerous pets that died that have been dissected and autopsies run on them and showed that they died from cyanide and I've seen people or patients that come in here with all kinds of symptoms. Depression, headaches. I know a man came in one day, his wife had to bring him in. He couldn't hardly walk or hold himself up. Crying like a baby, shakes, and he gave him the sulphate, salt and an injection of alphaREDISOL and in ten minutes that man walked out as happy as if nothing had happened to him.

Q. So the people visibly responded to that antidote?

A. Yes, sir.

Q. Mr. Thompson, is your clinic still treating patients for this problem?

A. No, sir. We are referring them to Dr. Hitt.

Q. To Dr. William Hitt?

A. Yes, sir. He's an allergist---

Q. ---yes, sir. I've spoken to Dr. Hitt---

A. ---and I don't know how his results are coming out cause I haven't been in contact with him personally recently but he was doing something that built up these peoples' resistance.

Q. Do you know if the City of Houston is being sued by any of these people?
A. That I don't know. I did hear of a class action suit being filed and I've got the attorney's name here somewhere. If you need it, I can get it for you.
Q. Would that be Brenda Jenkins?
A. That's it.
Q. But there's been no more – did the EPA come in and investigate or the Occupational Safety and Health Administration?
A. Well, I'll tell you about the EPA. I was told that they were here and I was told that they confirmed his findings. Now I never heard any more about it. There was nothing in the papers, nothing on TV. I don't know if they had to sit back and stay quiet because they were stirring up a hornets' nest or what. I don't know.
Q. How long a period of time did you observe Dr. Oesch?
A. I don't think I – what time did I have, what now?
Q. To know Dr. Oesch?
A. It was approximately a year.
Q. And what is your opinion of him?
A. I think he was a very intelligent doctor. He knows what the hell he is doing.
Q. What was the opinion of the people who, the other physicians with whom he was working?
A. They thought very highly of him. The reason – he was the one that handled the cyanide for the simple reason he was the only one who knew anything about it. He was the only one who had done the research on it, and he has done a tremendous amount of research.
Q. Was he, had he suffered some of the symptoms himself?
A. He definitely had and so had his wife.
Q. Had he moved away from the Heights at the time he came to work for you?
A. Yes, sir.
Q. So he wasn't suffering at the time but he was aware of it?
A. Well, I don't know. I remember him saying something about he was bothered with it in the Heights and that's why he moved out of that area. There were times when he came on duty in the morning that his eyes would be, his face would be red, well, I don't know how to explain it. He told me he was having problems with this cyanide at night, couldn't sleep, this sort of thing.

Q. So he was respected by the medical community down there?
A. He definitely was.
Q. He wasn't considered a maverick or an eccentric?
A. No, sir.
Q. That's the problem, Mr. Thompson, that according to the City of Houston this thing didn't exist.
A. Well, I don't care what the City of Houston says or what they think. It was definitely there. You are not going to find it unless you go to the right place to find it. Now, the run-off water from this plant, Dr. Oesch himself ran samples on the run-off water in the ditch in this plant and it was highly contaminated and I think he gave samples on the lawn or grass from the plant and it was highly toxic and of course if the City of Houston doesn't go to the source, you're not going to find it.
Q. Yes, sir.
A. Now this plant that is emitting is GE. Well, you know how big GE is. Virtually a lot of weight.
Q. Yes.
A. And GE does just about what GE wants if you want to know the truth and the City of Houston, they just said it was nothing there. Baylor College of Medicine, I think it was Baylor ---
Q. –yes, sir, ---
A. ---did some research on their own at random on individuals. Now these individuals from what I understand had those symptoms and they just took them at random. I don't remember, I think it was 13 or less than 20 people, I know that, and they said there was really nothing to it but that's not sufficient. You have to have people with symptoms. You can't just take Joe Blow off the street and his problems may be at the point he can tolerate anything.
Q. Now some of these patients that were treated at Spring Branch Clinic, when they would leave town or go away for a period of time, did they say that they got better?
A. Definitely. In fact, he advised them to get out of town, just a few miles, just to get out of, to get away from it.
Q. Your clinic would still have records of these patients, wouldn't they?
A. Yes, sir.

Q. Is there any way we could get hold of some of the test results that were done?
A. Sure.
(END OF CONVERSATION)

There was a fourth deposition acquired by Lieutenant O'Hanlan of which I have no copy. Jules Grant, M.D., testified to the fact that he found patients suffering from cyanide intoxication during the course of his medical practice in Houston. He also acknowledged having a positive laboratory test for cyanide exposure himself. This physician's office was located in Spring Branch, not far from Spring Branch Medical Clinic. His courage and concern were outstanding in the face of menacing political resistance by the Houston Health Department.

The day before my second hearing in Philadelphia [*note: this is an error—although the hearing pertained to happenings in Philadelphia, the hearing, itself, took place in Bethesda, Maryland*], I decided to call OSHA, the Occupational Safety and Health Administration. One of my naval associates had warned me not to call OSHA earlier, indicating that OSHA was sympathetic to the naval base and would merely report my action to the Commanding Officer. By June 27th, however, I suspected that the tip I received was misleading. My naval associate claimed that he was strictly forbidden to involve himself with the cyanide situation by a threat on his life. This may have been intended to intimidate me, I thought; I called OSHA on June 27th.

Chapter 19

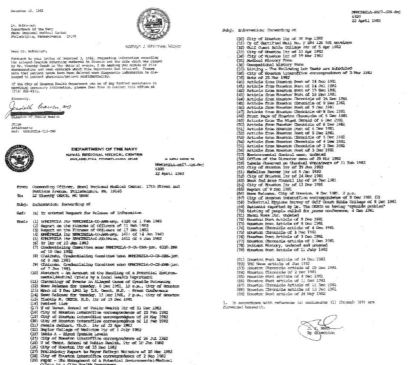

Second Hearing

Lieutenant O'Hanlan informed me that my wife was welcome to attend the second hearing on June 28th. She willingly obliged. I was optimistically hopeful that my psychiatric diagnosis would be overturned in light of the preponderant evidence gathered on my behalf. Lieutenant O'Hanlan elected not to inform me about the papers he found written by Captain Wilson which indicated that it was predetermined that the Board's decision would go against me. As he conveyed to my wife and me, his *faith in the system* was dependent upon the outcome of my case.

My hearing was again the first hearing of the morning. The same individuals were present in the same positions as during the first hearing, with the addition of my wife who sat in a chair about six feet behind me:

"Let the record show that this is a continuation of the hearing of Lieutenant Timothy Oesch," began Colonel Clark. "Lieutenant Oesch and Counselor, I would remind you that you are still under oath or affirmation and we will not repeat such. Let the record show that Mrs. Oesch is here and if she testifies later we will swear her in at a later time. Counsel for the Board may proceed."

"I offer into evidence Exhibit B for the Medical Board, papers pertaining to this case, the member and counsel for the member have had the opportunity to examine them," stated Lieutenant Reynolds. The papers she referred to was the information provided by the Houston Health Department.

"Subject to any objections they are accepted into evidence," returned Colonel Clark.

"No objection, sir," voiced Lieutenant O'Hanlan. This did not mean that he agreed with the information forwarded by the Houston Health Department. It simply meant that he did not object to allowing the information to be accepted by the Board as evidence.

"Counsel?" queried Colonel Clark, addressing Lieutenant O'Hanlan.

"I would like to offer into evidence further exhibits for the member, Exhibits *O* through *W*, responded Lieutenant O'Hanlan.

"Accepted."

"I would like to make a brief statement, an addendum to Exhibit *N* in the record, which is the statement from Brenda Jenkins, lawyer, in Houston. A suit has been filed against the Houston Health Department by Werner & Rusk."

"Are you sure that wasn't the plant?" I inserted. Brenda had informed me that a lawsuit might be filed against the Houston Health Department following the one against General Electric, but I certainly expected General Electric to receive the first lawsuit. Furthermore, the lawsuit against General Electric was not officially filed until June 29th, the day after the hearing—but the confusion of dates and lawsuit recipients was an honest mistake on the part of Lieutenant O'Hanlan.

"I guess the plant and the Houston Health Department," rejoined Lieutenant O'Hanlan, "and the named plaintiffs are Lieutenant Oesch and forty other people, it's a class-action suit. A copy of the complaint is being sent here and will be put in the record as soon as we receive it."

"Exhibit N is a telephone conversation, dated 18 May 1983, between Lieutenant O'Hanlan and Brenda Jenkins, is that what we are referring to?" inquired Colonel Clark.

"Yes, sir," affirmed Lieutenant O'Hanlan, "that suit has now been filed."

"Okay" the Colonel accepted. He did not seem very impressed, nor very interested.

"May I proceed with the questioning?" asked Lieutenant O'Hanlan.

"Yes," granted Colonel Clark.

Lieutenant O'Hanlan faced me and commenced with his examination. "Lieutenant Oesch, I draw your attention to your Medical Board, dated 10 January 1983, do you know Captain Galasyn?"

"I know him, not very well, but I do know him, yes," I replied.

"Have you ever worked for him?"

"Not directly."

"Was he your commanding officer?"

"Not that I know of."

"Was he your treating physician?"

"Not that I know of."

"Was he the Commanding Officer of the dispensary at Philadelphia?"

"Not that I know of."

"He never examined you or treated you?"

"No, he did not."

"How do you know him?"

"I know that he is the head of the Environmental Department. The first time that I met him, he came by the dispensary one day, and he knew that I had been involved with environmental work in Houston, and he talked to me about the possibility of doing a residency in environmental medicine and then using that education in the Navy."

"Tell us the entire extent of your dealing with him."

"The next time I remember speaking to him was on the 24th of November. At that time I was testing people for thiocyanate. I received a knock on my door and was told to go up to the Senior Medical Officer's office and that I would meet with Captain Galasyn there."

"Was he the Senior Medical Officer?"

"No, Doctor DeJesus was the Senior Medical Officer, but Captain Galasyn came over to the dispensary. There, he told me not to run one more test for thiocyanate, or I would be put in a psychiatric hospital. He also told me that he had already talked to Doctor Gilmore, and that she had agreed to cooperate with him. Also, I was going to give a lecture on chronic cyanide intoxication because Commander DeJesus had decided to have a lecture once every two weeks, and I was the first one picked to give a lecture, and it was agreed that I would lecture on chronic cyanide intoxication. After Captain Galasyn came, the lecture was cancelled. Whether he did it himself, or had Commander DeJesus do it, I don't remember for sure, but I know that he was responsible for the lecture being cancelled. All of that occurred on the 24th."

"Have you had anything to do with Captain Galasyn since then?"

"No, I don't recall having any more to do...oh yes I have, too. He came to my office on at least two occasions after that, and on one occasion he told me that I should quit taking antidote for cyanide intoxication. I explained to him that I became ill if I quit taking it. He told me that he did not believe that, and told me to quit taking it. He also told me two other things: he told me that patients might not want to go to a doctor who was treating himself, which I suppose was a threat on my future medical practice, and he told me that to be involved in such a thing as the cyanide problem at the base could be *very dangerous*."

"Dangerous to whom?"

"He just said it could be *very dangerous*."

"And that is the sum of your dealings with Captain Galasyn?"

"Correct."

"When he told you to stop taking your antidote, had he examined you or treated you?"

"No, he had not."

Lieutenant O'Hanlan turned to the Board members. "I would like to enter in the record right now, a challenge to the Medical Board just on the basis that the alternate member and senior person (Dr. Galasyn) signing it was neither Lieutenant Oesch's Commanding Officer of the Unit he was attached to, nor was he the chairman of any department that examined Doctor Oesch. I don't quite understand in what capacity he signed this Medical Board at all. From what I understand, the alternate member is supposed to be the Chairman of the Department or the Commanding Officer of the Unit at the hospital, and this man obviously is neither. I think that it is improper, especially given Doctor Oesch's testimony which reveals Captain Galasyn's obvious bias in the matter, for Captain Galasyn's signature to be on this Board. In fact, I think that this casts enough doubt on the Board that…"

"The mere presence of Doctor Galasyn's signature on the Board, though it means he agrees with the Board, does not mean that he wrote it," asserted Captain Wilson. "If I'm not mistaken, Doctor Gilmore wrote it."

"He didn't write it, Doctor Jacobs and Doctor Gilmore wrote it," conceded Lieutenant O'Hanlan, who had never claimed that Captain Galasyn wrote any part of the Medical Board, anyway. It seemed that Captain Wilson was purposely attempting to undermine Lieutenant O'Hanlan's strategy. "Doctor Gilmore being the internist and Doctor Jacobs the psychiatrist, but, as the reviewing authority…"

"Doctor Galasyn is the reviewing authority on it or is he the third signature on the Board?" rejoined Captain Wilson.

"Sir?" said Lieutenant O'Hanlan after the interruption. He had already plainly stated that Captain Galasyn was the *alternate member* on the Medical Board, which is the third signature.

"Doctor Galasyn is the reviewing authority or the third signature on the Board?"

"He is the third signature on the Board."

"All right, that is not the same as the reviewing authority," badgered Captain Wilson, exploiting Lieutenant O'Hanlan's technical error in terms. [*Technical error in his use of terms.*] "Who is the reviewing authority?"

"That is stated at the bottom of the first endorsement, that would be the Commanding Officer, Martinson," returned Lieutenant O'Hanlan, revealing that he did know the technical difference between the two terms.

"So what is your objection, Counsel?" berated Captain Wilson.

Lieutenant O'Hanlan was not so easily buffaloed. His objection was not erased by the defining of terms. "My objection is to Captain Galasyn's participation in this Board when it is obviously shown that there is bias or a purpose other than the objective evaluation of Doctor Oesch's medical condition."

"In what way bias?" questioned Captain Wilson.

"From what Doctor Oesch said, Captain Galasyn is the one that first ordered him to stop doing thiocyanate testing, and he was not his Commanding Officer or his departmental officer."

I decided Lieutenant O'Hanlan could use a little aid at that particular point. "In point, this was before any of the results were back from the tests," I added.

"I note your objection," declared Colonel Clark, snubbing any additional comment. The fact that Captain Galasyn ordered a halt to the tests before even receiving one result was apparently not a point the Board wished to dwell upon.

Lieutenant O'Hanlan resumed questioning me. "Doctor Oesch, let's go back before you came to the Navy. When you were growing up, did you ever have any interest in cyanide?"

"No."

"When you were in high school, in your chemistry class, did you ever take any interest in cyanide?"

"No."

"What was your major in college?"

"I majored in chemistry and biology, double major."

"Did you have any interest or knowledge about cyanide in any of those courses?"

"No."

"When you were in medical school, did you run across any cases of cyanide poisoning, or was it ever of any particular interest to you?"

"No."

"It wasn't the object of any courses or any professors doing research in it?"

"No."

"When was the first time that you ever considered cyanide intoxication?"

"I never seriously considered it until after obtaining an objective, positive test for cyanide. After seeing a patient who worked at an electroplating plant, and running a bunch of tests on him that all turned up negative, I asked him to bring me a list of the things he was exposed to at work. Then, I tested him for the ones that seemed most likely to cause his symptoms."

"What did the patient come to you for?"

"He had severe pain and paresthesia in his hands and feet, he also had headaches and tiredness. He had been to other physicians and had a gamut of tests performed, but he was still lacking a diagnosis. He came to me hoping that I could find out what was wrong with him."

"Why did he come to you? Did he know you were a specialist in cyanide?"

"No."

"Did you have any expertise in cyanide when this man came to you?"

"No."

"It was just as you said, all the way through high school and college and no expertise in this subject at all?"

"That's correct."

"What made you suspect it?"

"I didn't suspect it, at first. What I suspected, after running numerous tests, was that he might have been affected by some sort of industrial exposure, though I had no idea what kind. That is why I had him bring a list of everything that he was exposed to at work. I tested him for several things that appeared most likely to cause his symptoms, but the only test that turned out positive was the test for cyanide."

"What were some of the other tests?"

"Lead and copper were the only things that appeared at all likely besides cyanide."

Captain Wilson inserted a terse question. "Was carbon monoxide one of them?"

"No," I responded, somewhat startled by the question. Carbon monoxide seemed to be one of the Houston Health Department's pet scapegoats in attempting to clear cyanide of guilt. When Dr. Judith Craven described John's symptoms in her abstract, she mentioned only his depression, fatigue, headaches, dizziness, and nausea, symptoms which may appear in carbon monoxide poisoning [*she did not mention John's pain and paresthesia in his hands and feet*]. In John's case, though, I did not note any *reddish* or *pinkish* coloration to his venous blood [*as might be found in carbon monoxide poisoning*]. The red color in cyanide poisoning occurs only in more severe cases where little oxygen is absorbed from the bloodstream by the tissues. With carbon monoxide poisoning, on the other hand, the pink color is actually caused by the carbon monoxide itself bound to hemoglobin in the blood. Furthermore, John responded to treatment with amyl nitrite and sodium thiosulfate, which would not be helpful in carbon monoxide poisoning. He also had several positive laboratory tests for elevated blood cyanide.

Remarkably, the record of the second hearing does not even disclose that Captain Wilson was the one who asked me about carbon monoxide. Considering the previous omission of his erroneous statement that Captain Galasyn was my Commanding Officer [*in the First Hearing*], I cannot help but wonder how much *doctoring* of the record occurred before I received a copy.

"So then what did you do?" resumed Lieutenant O'Hanlan.

"For about a month to six weeks following that, I ran numerous tests on this patient, including complete blood counts and follow-up cyanide tests. I noticed that his cyanide levels increased after his visits to the plant, and that his hemoglobin levels would increase following an increase in his cyanide level. Also, his hemoglobin levels would go down following a decrease in his cyanide level. All of this is completely consistent with literature on cyanide poisoning. Of course, the literature on cyanide which I had then was very sparse compared to what I have now.

"After about four to six weeks, he came to me saying that his lawyer requested that his wife receive a test for cyanide to prove that they were not poisoning each other at home. I did not think that they were poisoning each other, but I agreed to do the test anyway since he wanted me to. When I tested his wife, she came out positive for cyanide. I questioned her as to whether she ever went down to the plant where her husband worked, but she said that she never went down there. So then I began wondering just what the source of cyanide might be, and I had another patient tested who was a neighbor to this one, and who was also a neighbor to myself. The neighbor turned out positive for cyanide too. That was what initiated my interest and investigation into the cyanide problem: positive, objective laboratory tests."

"When did you find it in yourself?"

"December."

"Relative to this patient?"

"He was first found to have elevated cyanide in September. I had been ill for several weeks before I tested myself, but I did not suspect that I had cyanide poisoning myself until discovering that he and the neighbor had cyanide poisoning."

"Did you live in the neighborhood?"

"Yes, I did."

"Before that time, I mean, cyanide was not even a passing interest to you?"

"No, it was not."

"Had you felt the symptoms yourself before then?"

"No."

"And you were active athletically all through high school, and college, and medical school?"

"Yes."

"Have you seen the tests that Doctor DeJesus submitted to the board?"

Along with the information from the Houston Health Department, NRMC in Philadelphia forwarded a few test results from civilians tested at the shipyard. Notably, this occurred after I presented copies of all the test results in the first hearing, and thus provided no new information. [*Note: I was eventually able to include two additional results from nonsmokers tested at the shipyard that resulted in a somewhat higher average urine thiocyanate level among the nonsmokers, but I am uncertain as to when this occurred.*] Nonetheless, perhaps Commander DeJesus was courageously attempting to help me by supplying the documents."

"Yes, I have."

"How would you interpret these tests?"

"Definitely positive, both according to the National Institute of Occupational Safety and Health, and according to all up-to-date literature giving reference values for urine thiocyanate."

Lieutenant O'Hanlan addressed the Board: "You may refer to Exhibit *I* to see the up-to-date reference values for urine thiocyanate levels which are given in scientific literature on the subject."

I addressed the Board also: "If you look on that paper, the National Institute of Occupational Safety and Health gives an average urine thiocyanate level for individuals with known industrial exposure to hydrogen cyanide gas, and the average they give is 6 to 13 mg/L (equivalent to 6 to 13 mcg/ml). The average among the workers at the Philadelphia Naval Shipyard was about 9 mg/L."

"You mean for smokers?" posed Captain Wilson.

At a time such as this, I was sincerely grateful for all the effort and cooperation which culminated in my possession of the data regarding the thiocyanate testing at the shipyard. "The average for smokers was about 8.9 mg/L, and the average for nonsmokers as about 9.1 mg/L, slightly higher than that for the smokers. This is very significant. The fact that the average level in the nonsmokers was higher than that in the smokers indicates that the environmental exposure to cyanide was great enough to override the normally higher level seen in smokers. Furthermore, the actual levels themselves were high. The level listed by National Medical Services of *up to 20 mcg/ml* includes smokers. I have actual, taped conversations with National Medical Services which I have with me if the Board would like to listen to them. On those tapes, toxicologists from that laboratory made such statements as that the normal level for urine thiocyanate is 1 to 4 mcg/ml, that the testing they do is not really sensitive enough to test for chronic cyanide poisoning, and that they normally use the test to monitor patients who are on nitroprusside therapy. Thus, the fact that they were able to detect the levels of thiocyanate present in the urine of the shipyard workers means that those levels were even higher than would be necessary to indicate chronic cyanide poisoning. Furthermore, a toxicologist indicated that they were going to lower their reference values."

"So what you are saying is that the levels cited on that Medical Board are not the recognized levels in the field today?" construed Lieutenant O'Hanlan.

"Definitely not. In fact, they are far too high," I affirmed.

"I think you can see further evidence for this," expounded Lieutenant O'Hanlan, turning to the Board members, "by looking at the transcript of the first hearing…ah…that the same information was given to me over the telephone and I read it into the record. It is in the transcript."

"Noted," was Colonel Clark's response. There was no request to listen to my tapes.

"So even National Medical Services themselves do not go by the reference values stated in the Medical Board," proclaimed Lieutenant O'Hanlan.

"I need to ask a question regarding Exhibit *V*," announced Captain Wilson, downplaying Lieutenant O'Hanlan's proclamation with a stark change of subject. "I need to know who wrote this? At the top it says: *Variability in Metabolism of Cyanide*."

"I wrote that," I replied.

"You wrote it?" Captain Wilson reiterated emphatically.

"I wrote it using three references," I clarified, sensing Captain Wilson's intention to discredit the data by insinuating that I fabricated the article un-fitly.

"Then in that case the only quotation from Sunderman and Sunderman is the one sentence: *There is a great variation in resistance of different individuals to cyanide intoxication*?"

"True," I acknowledged.

"The rest is yours?" coaxed Captain Wilson.

I had already stated that I used three references. "No, the rest is not mine. NIOSH gave the varying rate for detoxification of cyanide in the blood, and there is another reference below which says that those who develop symptoms from chronic exposure to cyanide should no longer be exposed."

"But the remaining business, the examples of variations and rate are yours?" persisted Captain Wilson. He seemed determined to make me claim responsibility for an article which I purposely based solidly upon other references.

"No, those are mostly from NIOSH," I replied. The specific numbers which I used in my examples, namely 0.6 mg/min and 1.8 mg/min, were centered around the average rate of 1.2 mg/min given by NIOSH, and they illustrated a threefold variation as stated by NIOSH."

"The second paragraph?"

"The difference in detoxification rate of 20 minutes to one hour, and also the average of 1.2 milligrams of cyanide per minute, those are all from NIOSH," I maintained, thinking that the derivation of the rest of my calculations from these values was obvious.

"The second paragraph, is that your own?" rejoined Captain Wilson.

"Yes, those are my mathematic calculations, but they use data given by NIOSH."

Captain Wilson made no mention of the third reference, *Industrial Toxicology*, Hamilton and Hardy, Third Edition, Publishing Sciences Group, Inc., 1974. Instead, he buffeted my article from a new angle. "You don't recall the edition of Sunderman that you are quoting, do you?"

In the case of this particular reference, I forgot to write down the publication date. There was no indication of edition number, which means it was probably the only or first edition, but I certainly did not remember that. "The edition?"

"Yes."

"No, I don't recall."

"The year it was published?"

"No, I don't recall." As it turned out, the book was published in 1970, so I was not trying to deceive anyone by using ancient Egyptian scripts. I did not like Captain Wilson's implications, nor did I like the way he sidestepped the evidence that tests on the shipyard workers were positive for cyanide exposure. "One thing I forgot to mention about National Medical Services," I interjected, "is that they do not give a reference value for urine thiocyanate in nonsmokers."

Lieutenant O'Hanlan picked up on my cue. "Do all the other labs that test for urine thiocyanate give a reference value for nonsmokers?"

"Yes. Of course, I think there are only three laboratories that do testing for urine thiocyanate: Bio-Science Laboratories, Metpath Laboratories, and National Medical Services. Most other laboratories you send such tests to end up sending them on to one of these three. Bio-Science Laboratories and Metpath Laboratories both agree that nonsmokers should normally have urine thiocyanate levels of two milligrams per liter or less."

"Was the test that was run by National Medical Services for urine thiocyanate specifically?" continued Lieutenant O'Hanlan.

"Yes."

"Do they normally run the test in checking for chronic cyanide intoxication, or do they normally run it for some other reason?"

"I was told that they usually run the test on patients taking nitroprusside, a drug that has the side effect of producing cyanide in the body. For such a purpose, their detection limit of five micrograms per milliliter is good enough. It's not really good enough for detecting chronic cyanide intoxication, though, which a toxicologist from National Medical Services related to me over the phone. However, several of the levels found in nonsmokers working at the Naval shipyard were higher than 5 mcg/ml anyway."

"So, based on that information and what you know about chronic cyanide intoxication and the practices by the other labs, do you think National Medical Services' testing is as reliable as that of Metpath Laboratories or Bio-Science Laboratories?"

"I believe that the results they obtained, when the urine thiocyanate levels were greater than 5 mcg/ml, were reliable. When the levels are high enough for National Medical Services to detect them, then they do measure true thiocyanate levels, which was affirmed to me by telephone, and that is what both Bio-Science Laboratories and Metpath

Laboratories measure also: true thiocyanate levels. This means that the results of the tests are not falsely elevated by the type of testing done."

Finally, Lieutenant O'Hanlan and I managed to convey the information about the tests performed at the naval shipyard which we wanted to convey: the test results were conclusively positive. "That is all the questions that I have," said Lieutenant O'Hanlan.

"Doctor Wilson?" directed Colonel Clark.

Captain Wilson then took his turn at questions and answers: "Lieutenant O'Hanlan has indicated during the previous hearing that perhaps it was in the best interest of the Houston Health Department, from their point of view and other powers, that your suspicions be downplayed or denied. Do you feel that government or other officials in Houston and Philadelphia have conspired to suppress our allegations or findings?"

"I don't know. I know that there has been communication between the Houston Health Department and the naval hospital in Philadelphia. I also know that an employee at the plant in Houston told me that some big shots came down to Houston from the plant's headquarters in Connecticut, and that they met with officials from the Houston Health Department. I do not know whether or not there was a payoff, but there has been a lot of investigation going on down there. They have not told me hardly anything about what they have found in the investigation, or about what's going on now."

"You have seen the material that was forwarded to us from Philadelphia?"

"From Hou…"

"The exhausted material from the Houston Health Department?" Captain Wilson inserted sternly.

"Well, I think it would be sensible to think that the Houston Health Department would like me to be found psychologically off, considering that they may have a lawsuit filed against them. So, one should expect their material to be rather prejudiced," I responded. It was blatantly obvious that Captain Wilson was setting me up with questions that would either force me to lie or give answers that might be misconstrued as signs of paranoia. I was not going to lie.

"Do you feel that they are in possession of truth, that there is a significant level of cyanide—significant incident of cyanide intoxication in certain areas of Houston, and that they have deliberately denied this in their reports?"

"Well, I was given the name of someone in the Texas Department of Water Resources by a friend of mine. I called the State official, and he told me that the State found cyanide in the discharge water from the electroplating plant. I would think that the Houston Health Department has access to information from the State, so it seems likely that the Houston Health Department would have some proof of positive testing."

"I have no other questions," stated Captain Wilson.

"Commander Wyvill?" directed Colonel Clark.

"No questions," returned Commander Wyvill, participating as actively as during the first hearing.

Colonel Clark then played his own hand, though he may have been tutored by Captain Wilson. "Referring to Exhibit O, *Addendum To Psychological Evaluation*, this is, as I understand, an evaluation by two civilians or civilian organizations, is that correct?"

Actually, the addendum was just an additional test result reported by Edward G. Daniels and cosigned by Doctor Botbyl. Lieutenant O'Hanlan spoke up first:

"Exhibit *B* is the first, is the psychiatric report by Doctor Sanfacon. Exhibit *C* is the psychological and psychometric report, and this is an extension of that report."

"There were three, actually," I added, referring to the number of professionals who signed the reports. Doctor Sanfacon signed the first report, Exhibit *B*, and both Doctor Botbyl and Edward G. Daniels signed the second reports, Exhibits *C* and *O*.

"It's a civilian organization?" pressed Colonel Clark.

"Civilian psychiatrist and psychologist," answered Lieutenant O'Hanlan.

"Doctor Oesch, if you would, just give me your opinion as to this statement: *He tends to blame others and demonstrates less efficient introspection.* What does that mean? First, is that a fair analysis?"

If nothing else, the Board certainly was predictable. I decided to give a response that was clearly introspective. "It may be, in a way. I'm a preacher's son, and when it comes to things like smoking, drinking, and such as that, I would tend to blame those who do those things. I have pretty high moral standards; in fact, I'm a preacher myself. I guess I'm a little condemnatory when I see immorality, and things like that might come out on a test like that one: a test of personality."

Colonel Clark did not press the issue any further. "Lieutenant O'Hanlan, do you have anything else to add?"

"Yes, sir, I have a brief argument."

"Please proceed."

"I will try to avoid repeating what I argued at the first day of this hearing. Note Exhibits O through W. The Board continued the hearing so that they could find out more information about Houston, and all of this additional information received in support of the Medical Board was forwarded from Houston. If you look at Exhibits O through W, you have depositions from persons who were treated either by Doctor Oesch or Doctor Hitt or Doctor Grant, Exhibit S, who ordered these same tests done and they were found to be positive. These Exhibits corroborate the same symptoms occurring in the patients: the same fatigue, the same forgetfulness, anxiety, and all of that. These are Exhibits P through S.

"Then you have Exhibits T and U that are affidavits from nurses in Philadelphia who state that Doctor Oesch did not have any focus on cyanide in his clinical treatment of people."

"We have read the exhibits," stated Colonel Clark.

Lieutenant O'Hanlan continued unabashed. "You have exhibit W, which is an affidavit showing that laboratory tests were withheld from patient charts in Philadelphia. Exhibit W was added just to show that there is further irregularity in the way that the Command in Philadelphia handled these tests.

"Now, I have here, and I didn't introduce it as an exhibit because I didn't want to belabor our copying machine or the Board's patience, but I would like you to look at these." Lieutenant O'Hanlan presented an additional stack of papers; they were medical notes and test results forwarded by David Thompson. [*David Thompson was the owner of Spring Branch Medical Clinic in Houston.*]

Colonel Clark was first to rejoin. "Either enter them as exhibits or…"

"I want to enter them as exhibits but I didn't enter them earlier because I didn't want to make three copies," explained Lieutenant O'Hanlan.

"Well, I really don't worry about the copying machine," remarked Colonel Clark.

"I want you to look at these as you deliberate," proceeded Lieutenant O'Hanlan. "We will make copies of them and have them included in the record."

"You wish all of them entered as exhibits?" inquired Captain Wilson.

"As Exhibit X," confirmed Lieutenant O'Hanlan.

"The entire thing as Exhibit X?" queried Colonel Clark. "It will be marked as such?"

"Yes, sir, I will," maintained Lieutenant O'Hanlan.

"I will accept that as Exhibit X," conceded Colonel Clark.

"These are notes, Doctor Oesch's clinical notes, and tests and thiocyanate tests done on patients that he saw in Houston at the Spring Branch Medical Clinic, from which you have the deposition, Exhibit P, from David Thompson," disclosed Lieutenant O'Hanlan.

"What was your relationship with the Spring Branch Medical Clinic, which I assume is an organization in Houston?" Colonel Clark inquired of me.

"I was a physician there," I replied.

"Moonlighting?"

"No, at the time I was there, the clinic had only one physician, and I was that physician."

"Were you in the Navy at the time?"

"Yes, I was."

"Were you moonlighting?"

Colonel Clark was apparently very unfamiliar with my military background. "No," I restated, "the Navy postponed me for two years."

"You lived in Houston, civilian Reservist?"

"Right." Actually, looking back, I'm not sure whether *civilian Reservist* properly defined my position or not. I had signed up for active duty, and was simply put on hold.

"And then you worked for Spring Branch Medical Clinic?"

"Right."

"I understand," proclaimed Colonel Clark.

Lieutenant O'Hanlan returned to the subject at hand. "Those are tests, thiocyanate tests that were ordered by Dr. Oesch and performed by Metpath Laboratories, which is one of the national laboratories that do these tests."

"There are results from three laboratories," I pointed out.

"Some of them are by Bio-Science Laboratories and some of them by National Medical Services as well," expounded Lieutenant

O'Hanlan. "These show tremendously high thiocyanate levels in these people's urine. The question was raised as to whether or not there was proof of cyanide contamination in Houston, and I think this proves beyond any doubt that there was such a situation in Houston—whether it came from this particular plant, or whatever, we are not in any position to prove. These tests show that these people did have cyanide poisoning. The clinical notes with each case show some of the symptoms that were exhibited, the same ones that we have gone over in this hearing. The thiocyanate levels in these tests are far greater than any others this Board has seen.

"Even more important, if you look at the notes you will see a little bit of Doctor Oesch's clinical approach. He does not have a focus on cyanide. He was very deliberate and very open-minded in his approach to an individual's medical problems. You will see tests in there, I wish you would look through them, because you will find tests that aren't as high as others, and you will see his notes. Some of the high ones say: *very high, notify patient*. Some of them say: *inconclusive, this man smokes and has taken aspirin*. Some of them say: *negative test*; you know, no cyanide intoxication."

"I assure you we will look at them in depth," voiced Colonel Clark. "Just to help the Board along, what is the total number of people?"

"I think there were forty some," replied Lieutenant O'Hanlan.

"So each of these sheets is a different patient?"

"Different patient."

"You are talking about a community of forty people?"

I do not know what induced Colonel Clark to ask the preceding question. It was already stated that Spring Branch was located in Houston, a city of millions.

"These are all patients that he saw at Spring Branch Medical Clinic," responded Lieutenant O'Hanlan, perhaps not perceiving the implication of Colonel Clark's question. Exhibit X represented only a fraction of the patients I saw at Spring Branch Medical Clinic. "Now," continued Lieutenant O'Hanlan, "the Medical Board states that Lieutenant Oesch has paranoia and a specific delusion of cyanide intoxication. The definition of a delusion is a belief that is held even in the face of overwhelming facts and evidence to the contrary. I think if you look at this man's approach, the highly positive tests, and the affidavits that are given, it is obvious that his beliefs about cyanide intoxication are not held with evidence to the contrary. The fact that he is willing to have these tests done by objective laboratories, and to not do them himself, shows that he is interested in establishing the truth, and that there is not some boogieman in his mind about this.

"There is realistic evidence of cyanide intoxication in his own Medical Board; it shows both signs and symptoms of cyanide intoxication which he experienced himself. I can run down a whole list of them: the bright red venous blood, tachycardia, blue lips and fingernails with cyanosis, weight loss of ten pounds in ten days which is found in his medical records from his hospitalization in Philadelphia, vertigo, and even more importantly—the blood testing that was done: the lowered gammaglobulin, the elevated thiocyanate; and he also had a vision loss in the last year. None of these were explained or even admitted as unexplainable by the physicians in Philadelphia who compiled the Medical Board, they were just mentioned and then passed over.

"The Medical Board standards are clear that before you diagnose someone with a psychiatric illness you should rule out the possibility that the illness is physiologic in origin. Slurred speech, memory loss, those things are organic in origin, they are not psychologically caused. All of these are recorded in his Medical Board and unexplained. The Board is flawed, the psychiatric tests were done at a time when he was complaining of cyanide intoxication and no attempt was made either to take him out of the environment or to insure that environmental factors were not causing his illness. Add to that Captain Galasyn; we do not know what effect he had on the Medical Board, but his signing of the Board casts further doubt on it. All of that, I think, thoroughly discredits this Board. This man's career it at stake. If he is discharged from the Navy with a diagnosis of paranoia, he will lose his medical license, and the Navy will lose a doctor."

"How do you know that?" posed Colonel Clark. He did not seem so surprised by the content of the statement as by Lieutenant O'Hanlan's delivering it.

"Because if you read the Medical Board recommendations, it says, *contact the States that he is licensed in and recommend withdrawal of the license*," disclosed Lieutenant O'Hanlan.

This recommendation in the Medical Board is curious when coupled with a previous statement in the Medical Board: *The Houston Health Department, believing patients were being misdiagnosed and mistreated, is said to have initiated actions at that time toward removal of his Texas Medical License.* None of the information that I received from Philadelphia, which was forwarded to Philadelphia from Houston, revealed the intended action of the Houston Health Department to revoke my Medical License. This indicates that there was additional communication between the Houston Health Department and the naval hospital in Philadelphia, either written or otherwise, that was withheld from me. Considering that a legally binding request was made to the naval hospital for all information about me, such withholding of information was illegal. [*And another thing that was probably highly illegal, I know now, was turning on water hoses and using them to overflow fluids from plating tanks in building number forty-one at the Philadelphia Naval Shipyard. This water, to the best of my memory, ran over the concrete floor and into the storm sewer. The storm sewer, it would be my guess, likely ended up flowing into the Delaware River. I remember Captain Galasyn telling me that what I was doing could end up leading to a congressional investigation, a statement that he made in connection with his ordering me to stop testing patients for cyanide exposure, and in connection with his making several threats. It would be no wonder, then, in consideration of the Clean Water Act (CWA) passed in 1972, an amendment to the Federal Water Pollution Control Act of 1948, that the Captain of the Environmental Department did not want what was going on in building forty-one to be found out.*]

Lieutenant O'Hanlan continued. "All we are asking is that this Board be conducted properly. To find him fit for duty is not going to send him back to work. It will not put him back in medical practice, it will just send him back to his command. If they think he is in need of further evaluation, then they can order it. If they think he should practice medicine, then they can order it."

"We understand that," stated Colonel Clark.

"He has put significant time and effort into achieving what he has today, and the Navy has a lot to gain from his experience and background. So, before he is cavalierly dismissed as a paranoiac, the Navy should properly carry out this hearing. The Medical Board, in the way it is worded and considering the circumstances of this whole situation, is reminiscent of some Soviet approach to the problem. Namely, when someone rocks the boat, give him a mental diagnosis. It smacks impropriety. In the Houston situation, the suit has been filed.

It's just like the situation with the V.A. and Agent Orange in Vietnam; clearly there is a problem, clearly people are suffering from something, but until they decide to what extent the government is going to assume liability and to what extent they are going to take care of these people, the door is shut, they are denying everything. The Houston Health Department is forced to take the stand they are taking because they are facing a multi-million dollar liability. You are talking about the city's health, so you are talking about the future of the city as far as moving in and moving out, the whole thing; the Houston Health Department is taking the only approach that they can take until the legal questions are solved. That colors the entire report from the Houston Health Department, and that is the only report which this Board has about the situation.

"What else can Lieutenant Oesch do? How do you prove a negative? You are behind the eight ball from the very start to prove a negative. He has a psychiatric evaluation and psychometric testing saying that he is fine. That is directly opposing the Navy evaluation. If you think that because a Navy doctor has evaluated him as a paranoiac, that the Navy's imprimatur means that it deserves more credibility than anything else, there is no point in even having these hearings."

"Lieutenant O'Hanlan, I chalk it up to your lack of expertise in this area, but there is nothing inconsistent in the diagnosis of paranoia and those psychometric evaluations," denounced Captain Wilson.

Considering that one characteristic of paranoia is lack of insight, and that my psychometric testing revealed two of my three strongest points to be social insight (judgment, discernment, and insight being equivalent in this case) and analytic reasoning, Captain Wilson's remark was obtrusively false.

"But he also had a psychiatric evaluation," contested Lieutenant O'Hanlan.

"I realize that, but they are not inconsistent," maintained Captain Wilson. "The nature of the examination by both the civilian psychiatrist and psychometric psychologists are of such a nature that it would not necessarily be elicited of psychopathology and the nature of…"

"I do not purport to know how to interpret psychometric testing," interjected Lieutenant O'Hanlan, "but I can see that what you have here are two completely opposing views of this man, and I think the doubt should be resolved in his favor. He has considerably more to lose from a negative decision than the Navy has to lose by allowing him to go back for further evaluation."

I was somewhat stunned by Captain Wilson's denunciation of my civilian, psychiatric report. A complete psychiatric evaluation was requested, screening for any type of psychiatric abnormality whatsoever. Doctor Sanfacon plainly stated that there was *no evidence of a thought disorder*. She stated that I had *no ideas of reference or influence*, and that I was *friendly, warm, and cooperative*, both statements directly confronting the diagnosis of paranoia.

"I might add, that paranoia was considered by the civilian psychiatrist among other things," I inserted.

Captain Wilson faced me with a look of contentious suspicion. "I do want to ask you, were both the psychiatrist and the psychologist aware of your situation?"

This, perhaps, was one of the most revealing questions of the entire hearing. Captain Wilson superseded clear, conspicuous information by raising the question at all. My civilian psychiatric evaluation included the following reason for referral:

Dr. Oesch is a 28 year old white married male who presented to the clinic for psychiatric and psychological evaluation. The evaluation was requested by his attorney who is representing him in a hearing concerning his dismissal from his duties as a Navy physician at Philadelphia. He relates that the dismissal resulted from his presenting his concerns about a potential environmental problem.

Also, my civilian psychological evaluation included the following reason for referral:

Mr. Oesch is a medical doctor, presently in the Navy and assigned to the Philadelphia Naval Hospital. Due to his concern and questioning of a potential environmental problem, Dr. Oesch was dismissed from his duties pending a hearing. The Navy is questioning his sanity, and, therefore, psychiatric and psychological evaluations are requested of Dr. Oesch's attorney. Dr. Oesch is married and is originally from Oklahoma. He has been in the Navy since 1978 and is presently a lieutenant. Dr. Oesch attended the University of Texas Medical School in Galveston.

Thus, Captain Wilson displayed either a faulty memory, a slack unawareness, or a careless compulsion to finagle a negative verdict.

"Right," I replied to Captain Wilson. "If you read the opening statements by the psychiatrist and psychologists, I think you can see that they were aware of my situation."

Interestingly, the way the record of the hearing transcribes my above reply is: "If you read the opening statement I made I think that…" Those eleven words followed by a couple of dashes are not only an abridgement, they are misleading. They indicate that I was directing Captain Wilson to something I wrote rather than to what the psychiatrist and psychologists wrote. The record definitely seems to have received some editing.

"So," remonstrated Lieutenant O'Hanlan, "I think that this clear-cut evidence deserves this Board's taking into consideration everything that has been presented. And I would ask, what else could possibly be done to disprove this Medical Board? If this Medical Board is ironclad, then there is no point in having his hearing. We have met the Board at every level with either some kind of flaw in the Board itself or with evidence directly opposing it. It is clear that this Board has been handled improperly. There are circumstances which are unexplained and unaccounted for, including medical factors that should be accounted for and which normally are accounted for. So I would urge this Board to find Lieutenant Oesch fit for duty and let the Command back in Philadelphia send him back for more evaluation or let him go back to duty. This thing has been going on for over six months now, and this cloud should be removed from over this man's head once and for all."

"Anything else to add?" asked Colonel Clark.

"No," replied Lieutenant O'Hanlan.

"Lieutenant Oesch, do you feel that you have received both in this continuation and your original hearing before the Board a full and fair hearing?"

"Yes, sir," I answered. Lieutenant O'Hanlan had done a very good job. Despite the obvious prejudice of the Board, I could not see how they could decide against such overwhelming evidence. Perhaps I was still just a little naïve.

"Do you have anything you would like to add?"

"No, sir."

"This Board will close for deliberations."

At the close of the record of the hearing is a section entitled *RATIONALE*. It was a summary of the Board's final decision, and read as follows:

The nature of the member's disorder precludes further service as a Naval Medical Officer. It clearly antedates entrance on active duty. The evaluation by the civilian psychiatrist and psychologist are not inconsistent with the diagnosis. The documentation of the Houston Health Department investigation (Exhibit B for the Board) is well summarized in Doctor Judith Craven's abstract. In general, there is no material evidence to substantiate the member's allegations and competent evidence to the contrary. His rationalization of causes and pathogenesis are hypothetical and unsubstantiated. Exhibits entered by member's counsel are either not supportive of the member's contentions, contrary, anecdotal, or, in the case of Exhibit X, offers several instances of a diagnosis of cyanide intoxication in spite of low cyanide levels, on the basis of symptomatology, which the member admits is not characteristic of cyanide intoxication alone, but also of an almost limitless range of other ailments. Doctor Galasyn's signature on the Medical Board is regarded as both satisfying the requirement for three physicians' certification of competence, and as indicating the inclusion of that physician's knowledge of the case.

Despite Lieutenant O'Hanlan's advance tip on the Board's decision, namely the papers he found written by Captain Wilson after the first hearing, he was still morally astounded by the impudent verdict. The next step was another written rebuttal, this time to the Physical Review Council. Lieutenant O'Hanlan elected to write the rebuttal himself. It was completed and dated July 26, 1983: a very excellent and conclusive exposition. As of October 20, 1983, I have not received any response to it. [*While looking through papers today, the date being 3/8/2020, I found an official form marked as REBUTTAL CONSIDERED, dated 9 NOV 1983, and also marked as CONCUR IN THE FINDINGS OF THE PEB. PEB is the abbreviation for PHYSICAL EVALUATION BOARD. The DISPOSITION is given as MEDICAL DISCHARGE (NO DISABILITY BENEFITS). The authenticating members are listed as J. P. MC WILLIAMS, COL, USMC, PRESIDENT; J. M. KRATT, CAPT,*

USNR, NON-MEDICAL MEMBER; O. B. EMERINE, CAPT, MC,USN, MEDICAL MEMBER; AND W. C. BYERLY, LT, USN, RECORDER.]

Chapter 20

```
         RECOMMENDED FINDINGS (Indicate applicable statements)
☐   THE MEMBER IS FIT FOR DUTY
☒ 1 THE MEMBER IS UNFIT BECAUSE OF PHYSICAL DISABILITY;          DISABILITY RATING
          DIAGNOSES (ICD 9 Codes Required)          V.A. CODES   PERCENT

Paranoia, chronic, severe, unchanged, #29710 .

    EXISTED PRIOR TO ENTRY, NOT AGGRAVATED,
    NOT RATABLE
```

Present Status

It was miserably hot in Washington, D.C. on June 28, 1983 with the air conditioner malfunctioning in our car. My wife finally crawled into the back seat and lay down as we crept through city traffic toward the House Office Building. The air conditioner was repaired in Greeneville, Tennessee only days before, but the mechanic forgot to put any oil into the compressor. Considering that he specifically charged us for the oil, perhaps the mechanic's forgetfulness resulted from his proximity to the penny, electroplating plant. That may sound farfetched, but I have seen the effects of cyanide intoxication enough to know that it is only too probable.

After the Regional Physical Evaluation Board delivered their verdict, Lieutenant O'Hanlan suggested that I contact my congressman and senator. The senator's office asked that I contact a military representative in Houston, but Congressman Bill Archer's office told me to come on over. That was easier said than done; my wife and I arrived at about 2:30 p.m. We met with Congressman Archer's caseworker. The caseworker listened to my wife and me with perceiving interest, and made copies of the material that I did not already have copies to give her.

About two days later, back at our apartment near Cherry Hill, I received a response from OSHA. They had decided to review the matter, and that encouraged me. When I initially called OSHA on June 27th, I was told that they could not do anything about my problem because I was military. After I explained that most of my patients were civilians, however, their response totally changed. I hoped, as of

September 15, 1983 when I first penned the preceding sentences, to receive a report of their findings. I now doubt that I ever will.

Toward twilight on June 30th, I received a phone call from Barbara Preskin:

"Oesch's residence, Tim speaking," I said after picking up the receiver.

"Doctor Oesch, this is Barbara..."

"Barbara! Hi!"

"Well, what did they decide?" posed Barbara. She was one of the persons who agreed to give Lieutenant O'Hanlan a phone deposition.

I told Barbara about the hearing.

"I knew it. A kangaroo court, that's all it was. I could have told you that would happen in the first place."

Barbara was very seasoned politically and she definitely took a personal interest in my predicament. "Yea, I guess you're right."

"Sure I'm right," affirmed Barbara. "Now listen, Doctor Oesch, I'm going to give you some good advice, okay?"

"Okay," I obliged, not that I had much choice. Barbara had called me a few days earlier in Greeneville and advised that I get copies of all my information to someone else. She expressed a great deal of relief when I told her I had already done that. It was a good suggestion, though.

"Doctor Oesch, don't test anyone else for cyanide, don't go public with anything, don't make any waves, just get yourself an honorable discharge out of the Navy and get back to Houston," directed Barbara.

Despite her civic sophistication, Barbara still seemed to have a mother's instinct. "Well, the Navy's trying to tag me with a psychiatric diagnosis right now. If I want to practice any medicine when I get out, then I'd better try and stop it."

"The important thing now, Doctor Oesch, is just to get out of there. You aren't going to be able to help anybody if you're dead, are you?"

"Well..."

"There's no way to win, Doctor Oesch. The people you're up against are just too big. They have big guns, Doctor Oesch—missiles! I paid my own money to hire a lawyer to give advice for you, Doctor Oesch, and he said this problem could involve billions of dollars, even trillions."

"Well, with God's help..."

"I know, Doctor Oesch, but can't God work with you down here in Houston?"

Barbara talked with persuasive urgency. I could not help laughing, not at Barbara or what she said, but at the contrast between Barbara's open frankness and the guarded, subversive denial that I faced in Philadelphia. "Honey," I called to Melody, knowing that Barbara could hear me over the line, "Barbara thinks I should get out of the Navy. Do you think I should get out of the Navy?"

Sometimes Melody does not know when to take me seriously. Her feelings about the Navy, at that point, were no shrouded secret. "Yes, I wanted that a long time ago," she asserted.

"Melody wants me out of the Navy too," I said larkishly.

"Good for her," praised Barbara. "Now listen to your wife."

"I appreciate your concern, Barbara," I confided, "and I assure you that I'm not trying to get myself killed. This is very important, though. There are a lot of other people's lives to think about. Someday this problem will be recognized…"

"Of course it will, Doctor Oesch, but it's going to take time, and there's no use in your getting burned at the stake in the meantime," persisted Barbara.

I appreciated Barbara very much; I also knew she was very stubborn. My commission regarding the cyanide situation was something I respected as a godsend. [*Or, in more proper English in regard to my intended meaning, a commission from God.*] There was no way I could guarantee Barbara that I would carry out her requests. At the same time, though, I was beholden to her concern and efforts on my behalf.

"I'll keep what you said in mind," I remarked.

"All right, Doctor Oesch, and let me know what happens up there."

"Okay."

About a week later, on Thursday evening, July 7th, I approached our preacher after choir practice at church in Marlton. The church was not located as close to Cherry Hill as was our apartment.

"Pastor Glyndale," I said.

The Pastor turned around and shook my hand. "Why, good evening Brother Tim, what can I do for you?"

My wife and I grew quickly and deeply attached to the Church in Marlton, so I knew it would not be easy to tell the Pastor that we would have to move. "Well, you know my wife and I had to move here from

Pitman because we were experiencing cyanide intoxication in Pitman and found out we were only about one and one half miles from an electroplating plant," I began.

"Yes," acknowledged Pastor Glyndale, his countenance growing quite sober.

"Now we are experiencing illness here in our apartment when winds come out of the west. There's a lot of industry over toward Philadelphia, and…"

"Don't you live in the Shadyrest Apartments [*fictitious name*] over off Woodhollow Drive?" inquired Pastor Glyndale. His voice played portentously upon my ears.

"Yes."

"Do you know there's an industrial park about one mile west of you?"

Once in college, in December, some classmates drenched me with a bucket of ice water after tricking me into chasing one of them outside in my underwear. I was stunned. An industrial park one mile west of our apartment! "No…"

"That's right. Come into my office and I'll draw you a map."

Pastor Glyndale drew me a map, and I brought the news home to my wife. She was almost used to it, but the whole thing was still sickening. The next day we borrowed a local phone book, since we still did not have one, and checked the yellow pages for electroplating plants. There was one about two miles west of us which was separate from the industrial park. We drove about the industrial park and discovered an etching company that electroplated. That pinpointed potential sources to our problem one and two miles to our west.

My wife and I drove to the electroplating plant two miles to our west. We both entered the front door, planning to ask some questions, then turned around and walked out. No one was in the front room, but large vats were visible through an open hallway. Music was playing in the next room. We both grew dizzy simply standing there…it seemed wisest just to leave.

The next day, Saturday, I drove back to the industrial park alone. There was very little going on. Driving behind some large buildings, I spotted two workers wearing dust masks and emptying debris into garbage vats. I stopped my car, stepped out, and approached them. One of them proved to be quite talkative.

Quickie Plating [*fictitious name*], the plant where my wife and I grew dizzy, was the chief suspect according to my informant in the industrial park. He said the pollution control was very poor there, and that they probably dumped waste into the East Branch Creek. There was also the matter of his friend's wife, whom his friend had to move to the country for her health's sake. I gave my informant some information on chronic cyanide intoxication, and he said he would pass the information on to his friend. It did not seem right that American citizens lived in such ignorance.

With the probable sources of cyanide contamination in our apartment near Cherry Hill pinpointed, my wife and I decided to simply move a few miles to the east. That way we could still attend the same church, which was about three and one-half miles east of the aforementioned electroplating plants. Pastor Glyndale assured me that industry was sparse farther east, and he even suggested a particular apartment complex, the Sherwoodsville [*fictitious name*] Apartments. My wife wanted to look before we decided where to move, and we spent the better part of a Saturday doing so. After finally locating the apartments that suited us best, and apartments were rare in that direction, we discovered that we had selected the Sherwoodsville Apartments, the same one Pastor Glyndale suggested in the first place.

On July 11th, I wrote the following letter to my landlord:

Dear Mr. Merril:

My wife and I have been sick for several months now—and it has reached the point where we again must move. I had hoped the summer winds would change mostly to southeast winds, but they apparently remain primarily westerly here. We are very obviously ill when winds come from the west, and we feel much better when they are from the east. My wife has had a positive laboratory test indicating cyanide exposure—which along with the wind direction and the fact that there is an electroplating plant two miles west of us, is conclusive for cyanide intoxication. There is also electroplating done at the industrial park one mile west of us, but from what little investigation I have done, the plant two miles west of us seems the most likely polluter.

We like your apartment very much and regret that we must move. (Besides the inconvenience, it is quite expensive to move as often as we have in the past two years.) I notified Vickie Winkler on July 10th—and informed her that we plan to move on August 15th. I will mail a check as usual for August which covers the latter fifteen days of my thirty day notice.

Sincerely,
Timothy Oesch, M.D.

Vickie Winkler was my landlord's financial manager. She met with us when we originally rented the apartment, and agreed to return our deposit if my wife suffered cyanide intoxication at that location. In return, I agreed to give her a thirty-day notice if such occurred. Having found a new apartment farther east, my wife and I decided to escape the cyanide intoxication until shortly before we moved. We packed a couple suitcases and left for my in-laws' in Iowa on July 19th.

Prior to that, on July 13th, I was very pleased to receive correspondence from Congressman Archer. Included were two letters, a cover letter addressed to me, and a copy of a letter to the Secretary of the Navy. The cover letter read as follows:

Congress of the United States
House of Representatives
Washington, D.C. 20515

Dear Timothy:

I understand that you have been in touch with a member of my Washington staff, Linda Figura, concerning the Navy's intention to process you for a medical discharge.

As you know, we have been in contact with your attorney, Lt. Edward O'Hanlan, and have today written to the Secretary of the Navy in support of your rebuttal to the Physical Review Council. Enclosed is a copy of my letter to the Secretary for your files.

We'll be sure to continue to keep in close touch with Lt. O'Hanlan and you on any developments on your case.

Thank you for this opportunity to be of service to you, Timothy. With best wishes, I am

Sincerely

Bill Archer

Bill Archer

Timothy Swiss

Member of Congress

The copy of the other letter, to the Secretary of the Navy, read as follows:

Dear Mr. Secretary:
I have been contacted by my constituent, Timothy Oesch, a former resident of Houston now on active duty with the U.S. Navy as a Lieutenant in the Medical Corps.
Lt. Oesch has informed me that he is being processed for a medical discharge from the Navy. He has been diagnosed as having 'paranoia, chronic, severe.' The Navy physicians who treated him expressed their opinion that the specific delusion underlying the paranoia is his concern with chronic cyanide intoxication in industrial environments. The 'delusion' purportedly has its origin in Lt. Oesch's activities as a physician in Houston, Texas prior to his entry on active duty. In 1982, while stationed at the Philadelphia Naval Station he began to complain of symptoms similar to those several of his patients had exhibited, and began to test for cyanide intoxication. This was followed by his own hospitalization, and psychiatric evaluation.
Seeking to disprove the Navy diagnosis and to show his fitness for duty, Lt. Oesch appeared before the Regional Physical Evaluation Board at the Naval Bethesda Hospital on May 19, 1983 and June 28, 1983. That Board's concurrence with the diagnosis of paranoia has prompted me to write to you.
Enclosed please find transcripts of the hearing and various pieces of evidence presented by Lt. Oesch to the Regional Physical Evaluation Board. There is a psychiatric evaluation stating that Lt. Oesch suffers from no mental disease. There are affidavits and medical notes on Lt. Oesch showing symptoms he has exhibited during his hospitalization in December, 1982 that were either omitted or simply glossed over in the Navy medical board report.
As for the issue of cyanide intoxication, the R.P.E.B. demanded proof and Lt. Oesch presented affidavits and test results from physicians and patients in Philadelphia and in Houston attesting to the existence of such a problem. The navy introduced evidence of the publicity the issue had attracted in Houston in 1981 and reports from a toxicologist and the Houston Health Department disagreeing with

Lt. Oesch's theory. I do not pretend to possess the expertise to even begin to weigh the evidence on this question. I have been informed, however, that a lawsuit was filed on June 29, 1983 in Harris County Texas District Court brought by alleged victims of cyanide intoxication against a major industry in Houston.

The provisions for the evaluation of a service member's fitness for duty are set out in the Disability Evaluation Manual (SECNAVINST1850.4A, 30 March, 1982). Foremost among these is a presumption of fitness for duty which can be overcome only by clear and convincing evidence of the member's unfitness. Based on the definition of this standard in the Manual and from the use elsewhere of the evidentiary standard of a preponderance of the evidence, I must presume that these phrases carry their full legal meaning. I question how the Navy diagnosis of Lt. Oesch was found by the R.P.E.B. to have met this high standard of evidence when so many points were in conflict.

Lt. Oesch's future, not just as a naval officer but also as a physician, is at stake. The decision is not simply one of fitness or unfitness, the Manual clearly empowers the Boards to delay decisions in order to seek better evaluation or to resolve conflicts or questions. The Manual sets out an objective of evaluation under its provisions as "the equitable consideration of the interests of the Government and the individual service members." Therefore, I strongly urge a most scrupulous review of this case by your office and the Physical Review Council.

Thank you very much, and I look forward to hearing from you at your earliest convenience as to any further action taken on this case.

With best wishes, I am

Sincerely,

Bill Archer

Bill Archer
Member of Congress

Honorable John F. Lehman, Jr.
Secretary of the Navy
Department of the Navy
The Pentagon
Washington, D.C. 20350

Before my wife and I departed, I informed Lieutenant O'Hanlan of my in-laws' address and phone number in Iowa. I also purchased a telephone answering machine that could be operated by remote control from Iowa. Inexperienced in operating the machine, I failed to detect my grandmother's attempts to call me until toward the end of our three-week visit. Fortunately, my dad called my in-laws, and then informed my grandmother of my whereabouts. She was aware of my political embroilment, and her inability to contact me worried her tremendously.

After arriving back at our home near Cherry Hill on about August 11th, my wife and I packed to move for the sixth time in two years. We were more than glad to do it in order to escape the pains of cyanide intoxication. The effects of cyanide intoxication can be devastatingly depressing; when we moved from our Shadyrest Apartment there was still paper taped on the windows, and pictures leaning against the walls rather than hanging, after five-and-a-half months of residence. In contrast, within our first month at our Sherwoodsville Apartment, we had curtains hemmed and hanging, all the pictures up, new furniture purchased and assembled, touchup painting completed, plus my wife and I both resumed exercising. I was not running any world-class times, but the feel of my legs striding beneath by body again was graciously heartening.

My wife, with improved health, decided to get a job. She was soon accepted by Plymouth Retirement Home as a nurse's aide. The retirement home was situated next to our church, about three miles west of our new apartment, and about three and one-half miles east of the electroplating plants that we moved to escape. Doctor Chowsky, the physician I spoke to who worked with the New Jersey State Department of Health, claimed that cyanide gas would not travel very far on the wind and affect people's health. He made other statements, though, that I knew were untrue.

Using a little physics and record keeping, I was soon able to ascertain that cyanide is not only stable on the wind, but is able to cause illness for a breadth of miles. My wife soon had to quit her work; her stool and urine turned green, she was fatigued, and sores appeared in her mouth. She managed okay as I recorded winds shifting around from the southeast and southwest, but as soon as we experienced a steady flow of air from the west, she was wracked. That was not all. When winds blew steadily from the west, perhaps slightly from the northwest, at about ten miles per hour, my wife and I both experienced cyanide intoxication at our Sherwoodsville Apartment. In this instance, atmosphere in the region of the industrial plants moved to our new apartment in about thirty minutes of time.

The preceding paragraph is one of my bravest. [*I know, now, that there may be cyanide produced as far away as China entering the lungs of persons in New York, and vice versa.*] I was strongly impressed in Houston that winds carried hydrogen cyanide gas and caused illness over spans of miles. Still, how could I be sure that cyanide compounds were not first dispersed across miles in waterways? After two years of experience and study, noting that hydrogen cyanide is almost exactly equivalent to nitrogen gas in weight, and studying wind direction and cyanide symptoms at varying distances from a contaminated region; I believe that cyanide is a potential offender for several miles from any significant source. This is important, indicating that the number of people in the United States who suffer varying degrees of cyanide intoxication is probably astronomical.

Around August 20th, I received my first correspondence from the office of Senator John Tower. Unlike the correspondence I received from Congressman Archer, it did not appear that Senator Tower was personally involved with my case. The letter I received read as follows:

Dear Lieutenant Oesch:
In reference to our previous correspondence, I am enclosing a copy of an interim report received in your behalf.
As soon as any additional reports are received, I will be back in touch with you.
Best regards.

Sincerely yours,

John Tower

The interim report came from A.C. Wilson, Head of the Congressional Correspondence Branch for the Department of the Navy. It read as follows:

Dear Senator Tower:
This is in response to your inquiry of July 8, 1983, on behalf of Lieutenant Timothy Oesch, Medical Corps, United States Naval Reserve.
I have been advised that the Commander of the Naval Medical Command has had to obtain additional information on this matter. You will be provided a complete report as soon as the requested information has been received.

Sincerely,

A. C. Wilson

A. C. Wilson

Just a few days later, I received additional correspondence from Senator Tower's office. Again, the correspondence seemed to be perfunctory and did not seem to indicate personal involvement on the part of Senator Tower. The letter read as follows:

Dear Lieutenant Oesch:
Upon receiving your recent communication, I contacted the appropriate authorities and requested background information on your situation.
The enclosed copy is self-explanatory. I hope that this response provides sufficient information to answer the questions you raised.
If I can be of any further assistance, please feel free to call on me. Best regards.

Sincerely yours,

John Tower

John Tower

The enclosed copy was a letter from Captain S. M. Strieber, Deputy Chief of the Department of the Navy. It read as follows:

Dear Senator Tower:

A Breath of Cyanide

    This is in further response to your inquiry of July 8, 1983, on behalf of Lieutenant Timothy Oesch, Medical Corps, United States Naval Reserve.

    The Commander of the Naval Medical Command has informed me that Lieutenant Oesch was hospitalized at the U.S. Naval Hospital, Philadelphia, Pennsylvania, on December 7, 1982, (this was an error in date; actually it was December 2, 1982) for evaluation of purported environmental cyanide intoxification. (He means intoxication.) Laboratory data was essentially negative for cyanide intoxification and a psychiatric consultation was obtained. He was discharged from the hospital on December 17, 1982, to convalescent leave pending review by a board of medical officers. The medical board convened on January 10, 1983, and found Lieutenant Oesch to be severely impaired and unfit for duty. The final diagnosis was chronic paranoia, severe. It was the opinion of the medical board that Lieutenant Oesch's disability existed prior to his entry into the naval service and recommended that he be discharged. The findings of the medical board have been affirmed by the Central Physical Evaluation Board and the Regional Physical Evaluation Board. Lieutenant Oesch's case has been forwarded to the Physical Review Council for further review. Therefore, we have requested an additional report from the Director of the Naval Council of Personnel Boards. As soon as that information is received, you will be promptly notified.

    I am advised that Lieutenant Oesch's allegations that an environmental problem concerning cyanide contamination exists at the Philadelphia Naval Shipyard have been investigated by the Environmental Health Service Branch, Naval Hospital, Philadelphia. Air samples were taken from the plating shop identified by Lieutenant Oesch as a likely source of cyanide contamination. Air and water samples were also taken from various other locations, including the dispensary where Lieutenant Oesch had been working. The results of these tests show that cyanide levels are well within acceptable, safe limits. A level of 10 ppm requires action to reduce concentration levels of cyanide. Results of the aforementioned tests reflect values of .08 ppm or below.

Sincerely,

Timothy Swiss

S. M. Strieber

S. M. Strieber
Captain U.S. Navy
Deputy Chief

I was far from satisfied with issuing a complaint against the Navy, and then having the Navy reply that the Navy was guiltless. Somehow, there seemed to be a serious loophole in the procedure. I wrote the following letter in response, dated August 31, 1983:

Dear Senator Tower:
I recently received a letter from you disclosing the information forwarded to you by the Department of the Navy, Office of Legislative Affairs, Washington, D.C. 20350. In reading your response, that the letter was self-explanatory, I was not certain whether or not you noted that the letter presented blatant lies and omitted important data. You then stated that you hoped this response provided sufficient information to answer the questions I raised. The question I am raising is this: are you willing to take concern about a problem which has affected many voting citizens in your own state, and for which a resident of your state is now being unjustly 'framed' as a 'psychiatric case' because he attempted to reveal the problem in another state. I believe the seriousness and widespread existence of chronic cyanide intoxication behooves you to search out the facts, not just accept additional lies from the very individuals who I claimed were lying in the first place.

The Navy claimed that my evaluation in the Naval hospital was essentially negative for cyanide intoxication. Blood drawn from my arm on 11DEC82 was found to have a serum thiocyanate level of 1.8 mg/dl (milligrams per deciliter), and I am a nonsmoker. You have a copy of this test. This finding is definitely positive for cyanide exposure, not essentially negative. Please consult the poison control center in Atlanta, and check with any and every published article on reference values for serum thiocyanate in nonsmokers, and you will find that what I am claiming is true. The level is so highly positive, in fact, that the claim that it is negative very likely stems from purposeful falsification. This falsification may be traced to such politically embroiled sources as the Naval Environmental Department in Philadelphia, and to their laboratory consultant situated in proximity to a Naval Air Station, namely Dr. Jason Mills.

My positive serum thiocyanate test, though conclusively high, is only a drop in an ocean of evidence to the fact that many people are grimly suffering from a basically undisclosed environmental plague. You have received my article entitled 'Chronic Cyanide Intoxication at the Philadelphia Naval Shipyard.' According to 'Br J In Med' 32(3):215-9 Aug. '75, the level of urine thiocyanate in the nonsmokers tested in that study revealed an average workday exposure to approximately 16.4 ppm cyanide. Also, be aware that many people living in the Heights, Timbergrove, and Spring Branch areas of Houston were found to have even higher levels of urine thiocyanate.

The problem of cyanide intoxication is very real and gravely serious. An attempt to stop revelation of the problem is an assault upon the lives and health of American citizens. Indolence on the part of informed political leaders, such as yourself, could contribute to extended ignorance and suffering among the American populace. On the other hand, a willingness to assert yourself prior to it simply becoming a matter of 'jumping onto the bandwagon' may help bring direly needed education and enlightenment. You could help at this time by making the necessary effort to find out that the Naval claims are false, namely by consulting published literature and the National Poison Control Center, and then by informing S. M. Strieber, Captain U.S. Navy, Deputy Chief, Department of the Navy, Office of Legislative Affairs, Washington, D.C. 20350 that the Navy has been found to be in error according to published literature and the National Poison Control Center by your office. Also, when you call the poison control center in Atlanta, you may wish to ask whether or not my blood cyanide level of 104 mcg/dl (micrograms per deciliter), found in Houston, was indicative of cyanide exposure rather than psychological disturbance. The phone number to the poison control center is XXX-XXX-XXXX. [The phone number has changed.]

Sincerely,
Timothy Oesch, M.D.

Copy to: Bill Archer, Member of Congress

In reading the preceding letter, one may gain the impression that I was beginning to get a little aggravated. Perhaps this is true. Knowing what one day in the life of an individual afflicted with cyanide intoxication is like, I was hardly impressed by self-serving subterfuge of a problem which belabors human life. It was in such a frame of mind that I received a copy of the Naval Medical Command's response to my Article 138 Complaint. Their response was mailed to the Secretary of the Navy, and read as follows:

> *From: Commander, Naval Medical Command*
> *To: Secretary of the Navy (Judge Advocate General, Code 13)*
> *Subj: Request for Redress of Complaint of Wrong Under Article 138, UCMJ*
> *Ref: (e) JAGMAN, Chapter 11*
>   *(f) Article 0727, Navy Regulations*
>   *(g) MANMED, Chapter 18*
>   *(h) 37 U.S.C. 602*
>   *Encl: (86) COMNAVMEDCOM 1tr MEDCOM-00D3-1-DJM of 9 Aug 1983*
> *1. Readdressed and forwarded*
> *2. The basic correspondence alleges a complaint of wrong was submitted by Lieutenant Oesch to his commanding officer and, having received no action, is now seeking redress under reference (a). (I assume reference (a) to be 'Article 138, UCMJ). The decision to forward the basic correspondence notwithstanding Lieutenant Oesch's failure to comply with the requirements of references (a) and (e) as noted in paragraph 1 of the First Endorsement is concurred in. (This is again a claim that the 'Request for Redress of Grievances' which I hand-delivered to the Commanding Officer's secretary on 29March 83 was not received.)*
> *3. The basic correspondence does not specifically indicate what alleged wrong was committed by Lieutenant Oesch's commanding officer. Lieutenant Oesch requests revocation of a medical board report which concludes with a final diagnosis of 'Paranoia, chronic, severe, unchanged #29710, EPTE.' Lieutenant Oesch further requests 'affirmation of diagnosis of chronic cyanide intoxication.' The alleged wrong, therefore, is interpreted as being the commanding officer's decision to convene a medical board and the commanding officer's*

subsequent endorsement of the medical board's report. For the reasons discussed below, it has been concluded that the complaint is without merit and the request is denied.

4. As officer exercising general court-martial jurisdiction over the respondent within the respondent's chain of command, and in accordance with section 1108 of reference (e), the Commander, Naval Medical Command inquired into the facts and circumstances surrounding the complaint. The inquiry has disclosed that the decision of the Commanding Officer, Naval Hospital, Philadelphia, Pennsylvania, to convene a medical board and to endorse the report of that board was in no way arbitrary, capricious, or otherwise unjust. Reference (f) requires a commanding officer to ensure a satisfactory state of health and physical fitness of personnel under his or her command. Under references (d) and (g), the commanding officer of a naval hospital has the authority to convene medical boards and report upon the state of health of members of the naval service. The medical board was properly constituted as required by reference (h) and its report is thorough and complete. The medical board found Lieutenant Oesch to be unfit and recommended that he be discharged from the service. The commanding officer reviewed the report for completeness and accuracy and forwarded the report as required by regulation. The decision to convene a medical board is fully supported by the medical board's report. There is simply no evidence to support a complaint that the commanding officer acted without basis in an unfair, arbitrary, or capricious manner.

5. As noted in paragraph 5 of the First Endorsement, Lieutenant Oesch retains numerous opportunities to rebut the substantive question of his physical/mental evaluation and fitness for duty within the disability evaluation system. The relief requested by Lieutenant Oesch is properly within the cognizance of that system. It is administratively noted that as of the date of this endorsement, the findings of the medical board have been affirmed by the Regional Physical Evaluation Board, Naval Medical Command Bethesda Hospital.

6. In view of the foregoing, it is considered that Lieutenant Oesch's complaint of wrong under article 138, UCMJ is without merit and his request for relief is denied.

Commander, Naval Medical Command

Regarding the claim in number 2 above that I did not turn in the memorandum that I hand-carried to Captain Martinson's secretary on March 29, 1983, Lieutenant Norris told me that she could vouch for receiving a copy of the memorandum. Besides that, the fact that my authorization for *home subsistence* is dated March 30, 1983, and the fact that Captain Martinson's recommendation for termination of my special pay came on April 1, 1983, is evident indication that Captain Martinson received something on March 29th that did not please her. At any rate, I responded to the Naval Medical Command's report without even mentioning the March 29th memorandum. There were other factors more brazenly erroneous and serious. My letter, dated September 3, 1983, read as follows:

From: LT Timothy Oesch, MC, USNR
  [*My address at that time was placed here.*]
To: Commander, Naval Medical Command
   Department of the Navy
   Washington, D.C.
Subj: Request For Redress of Complaint of Wrong Under Article 138, UCMJ
Ref: (a) LT Timothy Oesch, MC, USNR, 1tr of 12 Apr 1983
1. In response to reference (a), the Naval Medical Command interpreted the alleged wrong to be 'Captain Martinson's decision to convene a medical board and her subsequent endorsement of that board's report'. This interpretation is in gross error. The alleged wrong was clearly defined under number 4 on the first page of reference (a) as: 'a. Attempted subterfuge of industrial cyanide pollution. b. Misdiagnosis, mistreatment, and potential, negligent homicide.'
2. To prevent further misinterpretation, I will break down the alleged wrongs and define each component more clearly.
b.1. 'Misdiagnosis'—In the face of definite symptoms of cyanide intoxication, and absolutely conclusive serum thiocyanate level of 1.8 mg/dl (I am a nonsmoker), the specific finding of bright red venous blood, and my willingness to explain how these entities definitely disclose cyanide intoxication—Captain Martinson still elected to attribute my physical symptoms solely to a psychiatric problem. This was a clear misdiagnosis.

b.2. 'Mistreatment'—In the face of serious symptoms of cyanide intoxication, and despite my specific request for alphaREDISOL, a harmless antidote for cyanide intoxication, the antidote was made unavailable to me. This was despite my communicating that the antidote had relieved my symptoms of cyanide intoxication in the past.
b.3. 'Potential, negligent homicide'—As a result of my misdiagnosis and mistreatment, I suffered probable cardiogenic shock with cyanosis (affirmed by affidavit) and blood pressure as low as 80/40. My antidote was still withheld during these times.
a.1. 'Attempted subterfuge of industrial cyanide pollution'—Urine thiocyanate test results were withheld from the charts of eleven civilian employees who submitted urine for testing on November 22nd, 23rd, and 24th, 1982. This is affirmed by a legal affidavit. Seven of these employees were nonsmokers, and the average urine thiocyanate level among these seven men revealed an average, workday exposure to air containing approximately 16.4 ppm cyanide. This can be deduced by consulting industrial literature comparing urine thiocyanate levels to ambient, atmospheric levels of cyanide, namely 'Br J Ind Med' 32(3):215-9 Aug. '75. On one occasion, I attempted explaining how I thought cyanide compounds were being mishandled and dispersed into the environment, after which they break down and produce cyanide gas, to Captain Martinson. This was after I actually visited an electroplating plant on the base and witnessed the industrial operation firsthand. Captain Martinson would not listen; in fact, she walked away from me.
3. In light of the above clarification, I request that the Naval Medical Command completely reconsider reference (a) taking the correct complaints into consideration.

Sincerely,
LT Timothy Oesch, MC, USNR

Copies to: Bill Archer, Member of Congress
         The Honorable John Tower,
           United States Senator
         Honorable John F. Lehman, Jr.,
           Secretary of the Navy

I hardly had the preceding letter in the mail when, on September 6th, I received a copy of the following document which was signed by the

Deputy Commander for Personnel Management of the Naval Medical Command.

> From: Commander
> To: Lieutenant Timothy Oesch, MC, USNR
> Via: (1) Commander, Naval Medical Command, Northeast Region, Central North Lakes
> (2) Commanding Officer, Naval Hospital, Philadelphia
> Subj: Special Pays for Medical Corps Officers Review Board; recommendations of
> Ref: (a) SECNAVINST 7220.75A
> (b) Your Medical Additional Special Pay Agreement of 20 July 1982
> (c) CO, NRMCPHILA-SA07-JJN-dmj 7220, Ser: 0206 of 04 April 1983 with enclosures

1. Under reference (a) the subject board was recently convened to develop and forward a recommendation to the Director, Naval Medicine/Surgeon General concerning your entitlement to Medical Additional Special Pay. Reference (b) constituted your agreement to remain on active duty for twelve months for, upon approval of same, a concomitant entitlement to Medical Additional Special Pay as authorized by reference (a). By reference (c) your Commanding Officer has recommended your entitlement to Medical Additional Special Pay be terminated effective 30 March 1983 based upon deliberation and due consideration of your record and performance.

2. Under reference (a), based upon a thorough review of your official personnel record, and after due deliberation, you are hereby advised that the subject Board has recommended to the Director, Naval Medicine/Surgeon General that in the Board member's professional judgment your entitlement to Medical Additional Special Pay be terminated effective 07 January 1983, date of suspension of privileges to practice medicine. The reason for this recommendation is that your demonstrated performance does not warrant such pay. Specifically, the available records reveal unsatisfactory to marginal performance with less than minimal acceptance of responsibilities commensurate with those required within the parameters of sound and prudent medicine.

3. *Pursuant to reference (a) you are privileged to submit a rebuttal to the Director, Naval Medicine/Surgeon General concerning the Board's recommendation within 15 days of receipt of this notification. The Director, Naval Medicine/Surgeon General, accordingly, shall render a final determination upon the Board's report, and, if applicable your rebuttal.*

Stewart P. Hodgkin
Deputy Commander for
Personnel Management

In response, I issued the following cover letter to both Congressman Archer and Senator Tower. Congressman Archer's name is used for illustration:

From: Timothy Oesch, M.D.
    [*My address was placed here.*]
To: Congressman Archer
Subj: Political harassment by those attempting to conceal a serious environmental problem
Encl: Special Pays For Medical Corps Officers Review Board; Rebuttal to
Dear Congressman Archer:
I am deeply thankful for your concern and attention to the vital issue of industrial cyanide contamination in our nation, and for your help in resisting unjust castigation by individuals who seemingly esteem financial and political advancement more significant than human life and health.

Naval administrators are now seeking to drastically reduce my pay effective January 7, 1983. This predated cut in pay would potentially enable them to present me with a bill threatening bankruptcy. This action is underway despite the unresolved status of my Medical Board.

If you have any further questions, please feel free to call [*my phone number was written here*].

Thank you for your help and concern.

Very Sincerely,
Timothy Oesch,

M.D.

The letter enclosed with the preceding one which I wrote to rebut the predated termination of my special pay read as follows:

From: LT Timothy Oesch, MC, USNR
   [My address was placed here.]
To: Director, Naval Medicine/Surgeon General
Via: Stewart P. Hodgkin, Deputy Commander For Personnel Management, Department of the Navy, Naval Medical Command, Washington D.C. 20372
   Subj: Special Pays For Medical Corps Officers Review Board; Rebuttal to
1. Due to an administrative move against me, my Command elected to suspend me from duty. This was not my decision, and was not based upon an inability to perform my work as claimed. I have legal affidavits from nurses verifying my medical abilities and testifying to the fact that I had no problem with my daily workload. I did not miss a single day of work between my first hospitalization on November first and my second hospitalization on December second, during which time I took an antidote for exposure to an environmental contaminant. My second hospitalization occurred because of an administrative disagreement that was mischanneled via a Medical Board. I am now in the process of attempting to have that Medical Board overturned.
2. Until such a time as the question of my Medical Board is resolved, a question which addresses any and all claims against me by my Command, there should be no other or subsequent administrative actions taken against me. Specifically, the status of my special pay should remain unaltered until the Medical Board is resolved. I received a politically-based, administrative threat on November 24, 1982. Any and all evaluations by my Command following that date should be considered tainted by that issue. My Medical Board rebuttals address the aforementioned threat, and provide tangible proof for my claims.
                                                    Sincerely,
                                           LT Timothy Oesch, MC, USNR
Copies to: Bill Archer, Member of Congress
         The Honorable John Tower, United States Senator

The day before I mailed the preceding letter, my wife had an interesting conversation with an employment agent named Jack Green. Her health again improved once she began staying on the far-east side of Marlton, and she decided to seek employment farther east yet. Mr. Green happened to live on the far-east side of Marlton just as my wife and me, and he told my wife that he moved in order to get away from industry. Furthermore, he disclosed that in addition to Quickie Plating and the industrial park that were situated near the western border of Marlton, there was also a government plating plant farther west.

Mrs. Marie Black called me after my move to the Sherwoodsville Apartment. She was still experiencing cyanide intoxication, and she was having difficulty acquiring additional sodium thiosulfate. Henry Armstrong left his practice at Northwest Pharmacy, and the pharmacist who replaced him refused to refill Mrs. Black's prescription for sodium thiosulfate; in fact, he told her that it was poisonous. This seemed rather bizarre considering that sodium thiosulfate comes in food grade as well as pharmaceutical grade, and that it is not any more a prescription agent than aspirin or vitamins. Furthermore, I was advising my patients not to use over two grams or two cubic centimeters of sodium thiosulfate crystals daily.

I wondered where Henry Armstrong went and why he left his practice—as of today I still do not know. Mrs. Black seemed surprised to learn that sodium thiosulfate did not require a prescription, but she still did not think the new pharmacist at Northwest Pharmacy would let her have any. Just in case she could not acquire any in Houston, I gave her Catherine Lawton's phone number in Pitman, New Jersey. Mrs. Lawton purchased a pound or two of sodium thiosulfate and was selling it in smaller quantities at a little profit. I acquired sodium thiosulfate from Mrs. Lawton myself.

On Friday, September sixteenth, I talked to a civilian employee from the Philadelphia Naval Shipyard by phone; he was home at the time. The employee told me that a couple people from OSHA had talked to him; at least one of them actually approached him at the shipyard. This seemed encouraging until the employee went on to say that the OSHA representatives were, in his opinion, against me. He said they belittled his definitely positive laboratory test for cyanide exposure, and that they referred to me as some sort of troublemaker. Thus, I found myself repenting of any misgivings toward my Naval associate who warned me not to call OSHA, expressing that his life had been threatened after he did so, and also sharing that his baby had mysteriously died while sleeping. [*He felt that his baby may have died from the airborne cyanide pollution. One cause of death in acute cyanide intoxication is the cessation of respiration. Smoking while breast feeding appears to negate the apparent protection from SIDS which breast feeding otherwise bestows, and cigarette smoke contains cyanide. I agree with my Naval associate, his baby may have died from SIDS, and airborne cyanide may be a major cause of SIDS.*]

It is not unreasonable or unfeasible to estimate that the number of individuals in some way affected by cyanide exposure in the United States reaches the millions. Some of these people spend day after day in tormenting agony, not even aware that their health could be otherwise. Others die. The lawsuit in Houston goes on, my embroiled battle with the Naval hierarchy goes on, and meanwhile a plague of ignorant suffering goes on. This is not good, it is horrendous; hopefully this book will step out from the ranks of political stalemate and let American citizens know the present status of their environment.

Take the time to check your yellow pages under *plating*; are there electroplating plants near you? [*At the time I wrote this book, I still had a lot to learn. There are very major sources of airborne cyanide other than electroplating facilities.*] Do you suffer symptoms from time to time such as those described in this book? If so, keep track of wind direction to see if the symptoms arise when winds blow from a particular direction and abate when winds come from the opposite direction. Take heed if you decide to be tested for thiocyanate that the laboratory utilized is capable of detecting and measuring levels of [*urine*] thiocyanate as low as two milligrams per liter or two micrograms per milliliter. [*I now recommend utilizing a laboratory that will report levels of urine thiocyanate as low as one microgram per milliliter, which is the same as one milligram per liter.*] Also, be sure to acquire the numerical results of such tests, not just subjective comments. [*Thiocyanate is excreted variably. It is fine to test for it, but a trial of treatment with agents such as sodium thiosulfate pentahydrate, alpha ketoglutaric acid, and hydroxocobalamin appears to be superior to any presently available laboratory testing in determining whether or not an individual suffers from airborne cyanide sensitivity.*]

Perhaps, in the future, some doctors will have to relocate because poison-infested communities are suddenly relieved of a devastating pollutant masquerading as chronic viral infections, migraine headaches, irritable bowel syndrome, psychiatric problems, arthritis, heart disease, and many other diverse and intriguing ailments; but that is okay, the world can do with fewer doctors if there is less disease. Some industries may have to develop procedures using elements or compounds other than a potent poison, but that is okay too, they should have never so carelessly proliferated sufficient cyanide to annihilate the entire population of our nation daily, with more cyanide to spare than would be required in the process, nor should they have ever so indifferently discarded their cyanide wastes into our neighborhoods, our homes, and our bodies.

How many viruses did you contract last year? If you live in a city, or within a few miles of an industry where cyanide is utilized, they may not have been viruses. Do you have trouble with recurrent sore throats, pneumonia, or urinary tract infections? So did too many of my patients, patients whose cells probably died and sloughed from body organs because they were asphyxiated by poison and then served as decaying breeding grounds for pathogenic bacteria. It is not pretty to see suffering people cry from relentless pain, and it is not pretty to see the heartlessness of those who would allow that suffering to continue for money's sake. I know there is a just God in heaven, and I believe, too, that there are still red-blooded, God-fearing Americans with enough moral fortitude to set priorities straight, and to rid this land of a foe that destroys our bodies from within. Are you one?

* * * * * * * * * *

Note: that concludes the pages I penned in the 1980s, and the rules for placing any added material within brackets, using italics, no longer applies to the remainder of this book. Anything written hereafter is being written now, in 2020, and I will no longer be using any fictitious names whatsoever, other than to disclose the real names of some persons who were given fictitious names previously in this book. The next chapter will summarize what took place with me and my wife after my discharge from the Navy, bringing the reader up to my present status. The Navy went ahead and discharged me with the diagnosis of *Paranoia, Chronic, Severe, Unchanged, EPTE*. The lawsuit in Houston was eventually dropped by the law firm handling the case, an event which was initiated in 1986—apparently the law firm claimed that it was no longer economically feasible to continue with the case.

One may question, of course, whether or not the perpetration of a trumped-up diagnosis of paranoia by the Navy had anything to do with the Attorney of Record for the suit against GE, namely Brenda S. Jenkins of the Werner and Rusk law firm, informing plaintiffs that the case was being dropped. The discharge from the Navy with a diagnosis of paranoia took place in 1984, and Brenda wrote my wife and me a letter in July of 1986 informing us that if we would not sign her Motion and Order to Withdraw as Attorney of Record, then she would file it with the Court without our signatures and let the Judge make a decision on the Motion. My and I refused to sign the Motion unless Brenda helped us acquire another attorney, which did not happen, and so we never signed the Motion. Nonetheless, the Court apparently permitted the Werner and Rusk law firm to Withdraw.

In a letter to me from Brenda, dated May 23, 1989, Brenda wrote the following:

Your (I think she meant "You") *further asked me to address the issue of whether or not the action taken by the Navy contributed to or caused the loss of your legal representation. I feel as though, and I at least hope, that I made it clear in the past that I chose not to proceed with your case because your case was not getting the attention that it needed in my office, nor did I have the financial resources to adequately prepare it. The fact that the Navy had made statements concerning your psychiatric condition could have seriously limited your credibility had it been admitted at the time of trial as a witness in that case. It further being the case that you may have ultimately been the sole medical witness on behalf of the plaintiffs. The damage to the case, would have been, or potentially could have been, devastating.*

A tremendous, extensive, and valiant effort to keep the lawsuit in court was carried out on a pro bono basis by an attorney by the name of Alan Lawrence Schechter, of Schechter & Eisenman law firm, who issued a MOTION FOR NEW TRIAL dated March 31, 1988. In the PROCEDURAL POSTURE he wrote as follows:

A Breath of Cyanide

This lawsuit was filed on June 29, 1983. The Defendant filed a Motion for Summary Judgment in the litigation on or about February 5, 1988. Plaintiffs did not file a response to that Motion although many of the Plaintiffs appeared at the hearing on the Motion for Summary Judgment. The hearing on the Motion for Summary Judgment was heard on February 29, 1988. The Court granted Defendant's Motion for Summary Judgment and signed the Order on March3, 1988.

This Motion for New Trial is brought within the time allotted for the plenary jurisdiction of the Court pursuant to Rule 329b of the Texas Rules of Civil Procedure in that this filing is prior to thirty (30) days after the time of the signing of the Judgment by the District Court. Therefore, the Court retains jurisdiction over this proceeding for forty-six (46) additional days as of the time of the filing of this Motion for New Trial.

Following is a paragraph from that MOTION, filed in the District Court of Harris County, Texas, 269th Judicial District:

The Court should grant Plaintiffs a new trial for five (5) reasons. The reasons the Court should grant a new trial are: (1) there are material issues of substantial disagreement about the existence of toxic poisoning in Houston, Texas by Defendant, GENERAL ELECTRIC COMPANY: (2) THERE WAS A LACK OF DUE PROCESS THROUGH Defendant's failure to serve timely notice to all Plaintiffs; (3) Plaintiffs lacked adequate counsel even though they made continuous efforts to find counsel to represent them; (4) Plaintiffs can now guarantee future representation in the course of this litigation should the Court grant this Motion; (5) the Defendant GENERAL ELECTRIC COMPANY will not be prejudiced by the granting of this motion for a new trial; and (6) the public interest in truthfulness, the right of the public to know, and the Court's interest in equity and justice merits the Court's action. (Note: I will mention, also, that a written statement by Attorney Schechter, in an affidavit, was as follows: *I am representing the Plaintiffs in this litigation solely for the purpose of filing a Motion for New Trial to preserve the trial Court's plenary jurisdiction over this litigation so that it may consider all of the facts in an orderly fashion as provided by the Texas Rules of*

Civil Procedure. This one-time representation is <u>pro bono</u>, for the good and well-being of our community.)

In addition to this one-time representation, an AFFIDAVIT by a plaintiff named Bobbie J. Crawford stated that she had acquired commitment for future representation from another counsel and that she would assist in all good faith with the prosecution of the claim.

By 1988 I was living in Oak Ridge, TN, as the next chapter will disclose. The family of Marie Black was kind enough to provide housing for me as I revisited Houston for the purpose of aiding the attempt to achieve a successful MOTION FOR NEW TRIAL. The material, exhibits (*A* through *M*), and affidavits that were provided to the Court on behalf of this MOTION are rather voluminous, and much of the data would be repetitious to what has already been provided in this book, so I will not transcribe everything provided for this MOTION. I will, however, include a few things. First, from *Exhibit A*, *Plaintiff's Exhibit "B"*, three paragraphs written by me:

First, there was a breach of the letter of the law. I, Timothy R. Oesch, M.D., did not receive notice regarding the summary judgment which took place on February 29, 1988. My most recent address, as stated above, had been on file in the 269th Judicial Court for over four months prior to the stated date of February 29, 1988. In addition, as the attached copy of my phone bill verifies, I made personal contact with the law office of Mr. McFall, attorney for General Electric Company, on the date of 9/9/87. I requested that Mr. McFall call me collect, and I gave my home phone number, but Mr. McFall never returned the call. Furthermore, Marie Black, whose address is (omitted), *and whose phone number is* (omitted), *personally called the office of Mr. McFall on the following date: <u>fall of '87, local call</u>: and gave that office my present address as stated above. She still has the letter which I sent her instructing her to give my address directly to Mr. McFall's office. Thus, Mr. McFall was given my present address and phone number, plus my current address was on file at the court, and yet I was not issued any notice.*
Prior to the actual hearing on February 29, 1988, Marie Black, one of the plaintiffs, got word to me concerning the notice she had

received regarding the summary judgment. I did not feel that she nor any of the other plaintiffs had much chance without my evidence and witness, and I assembled pertinent data regarding the case and flew to Houston in time for the hearing. My pertinent data was not accepted as material toward the summary judgment on the grounds that I had been issued proper notice of the hearing and had not properly responded. As previously stated, this was false. I appeal, on behalf of (names omitted), *that there was not proper grounds on which to reject my pertinent data regarding the case since I was legally still an active plaintiff and I had not been issued notice of the hearing. This pertinent data was directly applicable to each of their cases.*

Sometime after the February 29th hearing, and after I proved that my most recent address was on file, the attorney for the defendant produced a certified mail receipt signed by M. Zamarripa which Judge David West apparently interpreted as grounds that I had been served proper notice of the summary hearing. Mary Ann Zamarripa was a resident of Austin, Texas, and she did not know where I was, nor did she know my address or phone number, and she did not forward the certified letter to me. To this date, I still have not received that certified letter. At the time M. Zamarripa signed the receipt, I was living here in Oak Ridge, TN. Thereafter, about two months prior to the summary hearing on February 29, 1988, another certified letter was delivered to the same medical facility in Austin, Texas where Mary Ann Zamarripa signed the first one. Doctor Roberto Miranda started to sign and accept the second letter, but then he noticed that my name, rather than his, was on the letter. Dr. Miranda then returned the letter to the carrier, and informed the carrier that he did not know where I was. By this time my actual, current address was on file at the court, and I had made a personal phone call to Mr. McFall's office giving them my phone number—plus Marie Black called Mr. McFall's office and gave them my current address on the previously stated date. Legally speaking, I was not served proper notice; and ethically speaking, it is apparent that the attorney for the defendant willfully chose not to serve any notice to my correct address. Therefore, summary judgment against me was without legal basis; and rejection of the pertinent data I prepared on behalf of all the plaintiffs was without legal basis since I was still an active plaintiff and had not received proper notice of the summary hearing.

Second, from *Exhibit F, Plaintiff's Exhibit G*, is the following brief letter from *James E. Cone, MD, MPH, Assistant Clinical Professor and Chief, Occupational Health Clinic, University of California, San Francisco...A Health Sciences Campus*:

Dear Dr. Oesch,

Thank you for your letter of 2/24/88 requesting that I review the blood and urine tests which you kindly provided.

Cyanide, as you know, is found in low levels in non-occupationally and non-environmentally exposed people due to metabolism of cyanogenic foods and cigarette smoking. Whole blood cyanide levels in 10 non-smokers was found to average 1.6 micrograms/deciliter (Ballantyne B, In vitro production of cyanide in normal human blood and the influence of thiocyanate and storage temperature. Clin Tox 1977;11: 173-193.)

This compares with your populations' mean whole blood cyanide level among non-smokers of 12.8 micrograms/deciliter, with a range of 2-104 micrograms/deciliter. This represents a much higher level (the mean value itself is 8 times normal) than would be expected in a non-exposed population.

The normal urinary thiocyanate concentrations range from 1-4 mg/liter in non-smokers, and 7-17 mg/liter in smokers (Maliszewski TF, Bass DE. "True" and "apparent" thiocyanate in body fluids of smokers and nonsmokers. J Appl Physiol 1955;8:289-291). This contrasts with your much higher population findings among non-smokers (average of 17.8 mg/liter, range of 0 -51.8 mg/liter), and smokers (average of 25.7 mg/liter, range of 0 to 49.9 mg/liter).

Serum thiocyanate levels were similarly elevated in the smaller number tested.

These levels are certainly consistent with the history of exposure to excessive environmental sources of cyanide, if dietary and other potential confounding exposures are excluded.

I enclose a brief reference which you may find useful. Thank you again for the opportunity to review this data.

Sincerely yours,
James E Cone
James E. Cone, MD, MPH
Assistant Clinical Professor

A Breath of Cyanide

and Chief, Occupational Health Clinic

The enclosure referred to by Dr. Cone consisted of a few pages from a book entitled: Biological Monitoring Methods for Industrial Chemicals, Randall C. Baselt, Ph.D., Biomedical Publications, Copyright 1980. Following next, third, is the major content of *Exhibit D, Plaintiff's Exhibit E*. It is comprised of a letter I wrote to Doctor Francis W. Weir, Director of Environmental Safety, University of Texas Health Science Center, P.O. Box 20036, Houston, Texas 77225. Note that this letter was written after I received data that was gathered and sent to me through the efforts of Walter Davis. Mr. Walter Davis went to the effort to acquire boxes of data from the legal office that dropped the suit against GE in 1986, and then he shipped these boxes of data to me. If not for the heroic efforts of this gentleman, the finding of cyanogen chloride in discharge water being released into the public sewer system in Houston, Texas would likely have never been made known to me. The letter to Dr. Weir is dated March 17, 1988:

Dear Dr. Weir:
Greetings from East Tennessee.
Mrs. Marie Black provided me with a copy of your affidavit which was written in support of General Electric Company's claim that no cyanide poisoning problem existed in Houston in 1981 and 1982. It appears that you were only served a very limited and select sampling of information regarding the pollution and poisoning, and I would like you to have the opportunity to see more of the test results which were obtained, and also to have opportunity to recant the statement that no evidence of cyanide intoxication existed in the patients tested in Houston.

To begin with, a copy of the City of Houston's blood cyanide results from December 2, 1981, is enclosed. This report reveals that the Harris County Medical Examiners Toxicology Laboratory found 61% of the persons tested to have blood cyanide levels of 15 mcg/dl or greater, with a high blood cyanide in a nonsmoker of 36 mcg/dl. I realize there could have been some degree of error in the results, but the results could have been low as well as high. Only two persons were tested in an outside air (non-centrally air-conditioned) environment on Dec. 2, '81, and these two persons yielded blood cyanide levels of 55 mcg/dl and 104 mcg/dl. Both of these tests were performed by Severance and Associates Laboratories, San Antonio, Texas. I was the one with a blood cyanide level of 104 mcg/dl, and my venous blood which was drawn at that time was bright red in color like arterial blood—a fact which one of the Houston Health Department physicians affirmed.

You are probably aware that HCN (hydrogen cyanide gas) is about the same weight as nitrogen gas, and would disperse vertically as well as horizontally in the outdoor environment. The much more potent and threatening outdoor pollutant which is converted to cyanide inside the human body is CNCl (cyanogen chloride). Since outdoor air was pointed out as the source of poisoning, this "toxic war gas" (CNCl) should be considered the chief suspect—especially the complaints of burning eyes, bronchitis, pneumonia, irritated mucous membranes, and tight chest which were evident among my poisoned patients. I have not seen the results of any air testing done to detect the presence of CNCl—have you?

You are probably also aware that blood cyanide levels are useful in testing for acute cyanide poisoning, but that chronic poisoning from CNCl (see enclosed material which verifies the entity of chronic poisoning) should be investigated by testing for thiocyanate levels in victims. I saw no thiocyanate levels given in the affidavit on behalf of GE, nor in the attached material from the Houston Health Department. Enclosed are copies of many thiocyanate tests revealing levels of thiocyanate as much as twenty-five times higher than the upper limit of normal listed by the laboratory doing the testing. Also enclosed, as a helpful reference, is information sent to me by James E. Cone, M.D., M.P.H., who is Chief of Occupational Medicine, Univ. of CA at San Francisco. This information reveals the average blood cyanide, blood thiocyanate, and urine thiocyanate levels in persons exposed to airborne cyanide who developed symptoms of cyanide poisoning. Blood thiocyanate levels may be converted to serum thiocyanate levels by dividing the result by 0.55, or by multiplying the result by 1.8. (Note: to explain the preceding sentence: since thiocyanate is primarily found in the serum of blood, rather than within the red blood cells, one would multiply the blood thiocyanate level by 1.8 to acquire a serum thiocyanate level, or divide a serum thiocyanate level by 1.8 to acquire a blood thiocyanate level.) *A* statement by Doctor Cone is enclosed as well, as are some blood cyanide findings.

After examining the enclosed laboratory findings from Houston patients and the information supplied by Doctor Cone, I hope you will decide to recant the denial that evidence of cyanide intoxication was found in Houston. In order for such recantations to be helpful, they should be received by Ray Hardy, District Clerk, and by me as soon as possible—definitely by March 31, 1988. Pre-addressed, stamped envelopes are provided for that purpose, and the one to Ray Hardy contains a cover sheet.

The process of converting chlorinatable cyanides to NaCN using NaOH, and NaCN to CNCl by exposure to free chlorine supplied by NaOCl in cold water, may be fairly common in industries across the United States. Likewise, alkali metal cyanides may be brought into contact with chlorine in cold water by other means also. Thus, environment pollution with CNCl may be one of the most serious and widespread pollutant problems in our nation. It would be a crime against humanity to delay recognition and solution of such a problem. I beseech you, in the face of the laboratory results furnished herein, to recant your affidavit; I will dearly appreciate your cooperation in this matter.

Sincerely,
Timothy R. Oesch, M.D.

Sadly, despite extreme and prolonged efforts, the victims of cyanide intoxication in Houston, Texas, 1981-1982, were never afforded the legal privilege of a jury trial. This contrasts rather starkly with an individual employee in East Tennessee who acquired positive testing for cyanide exposure while suffering symptoms of cyanide intoxication, and who was accused of paranoia, and who then won a $600,000.00 lawsuit through trial by jury—but I'll get to that in the next chapter. Given the derogatory (and false) information about me that was sent to Philadelphia by the Houston Health Department, as well as the mistreatment and misdiagnosis I received from the United States Navy, I educated myself in regard to legal proceedings and filed lawsuits against the City of Houston and against the United States Navy. Both lawsuits were dismissed without the benefit of trial by jury. As in the case of the Motion for New Trial, it would be rather lengthy and somewhat redundant to provide everything that was produced in regard to these lawsuits, but in regard to the lawsuit against the City of Houston, I would like to include some material that was written for *THE UNITED STATES DISTRICT COURT FOR THE EASTERN DISTRICT OF TENNESSEE* and the *UNITED STATES COURT OF APPEALS FOR THE SIXTH CIRCUIT*. First is some material written for *THE UNITED STATES DISTRICT COURT FOR THE EASTERN DISTRICT OF TENNESSEE*:

TO THE HONORABLE JUDGE OF SAID COURT:
COMES NOW, TIMOTHY R. OESCH, M.D., Plaintiff, arguing against dismissal of Case No. 3-90-409, and would respectfully show the Court the following:

I.

Plaintiff herein would respectfully show the Court that an <u>official</u>, <u>Court</u> <u>copy</u> of the PLAINTIFF'S ORIGINAL PETITION, and an <u>official</u>, <u>Court</u> <u>copy</u> of Summons, both for Case No. 3-90-409, were delivered together upon the City of Houston on July 23, 1990. This service was accomplished by an official Process Server, acting in his official capacity, who delivered a copy of the Summons and of the Complaint upon the chief executive officer of the City of Houston, namely Kathryn J. Whitmire, by delivering such at the official office of Kathryn J. Whitmire, and obtaining signature upon an Original Summons directed to CITY OF HOUSTON, Kathryn J. Whitmire, Mayor. The present, street address of the office of the Mayor of Houston was stated on the reverse side of the Original Summons, namely 901 Bagby, Houston, Texas. The Original Summons, dated July 23, 1990, is now on file at the Court as Docket Entry No. 12. This stated Service of Complaint and Summons fulfills the demands of FED. R. CIV. P. 4(3)(6) for service upon a municipal corporation.

II.

Plaintiff herein would further show the Court, in addition to his MOTION TO DENY DEFENDANT'S MOTION TO DISMISS, the relevance of Exhibit AB which follows. (Bear in mind that the Defendant withheld from the citizens of Houston, as well as from the Plaintiff, the finding that a toxic war gas, cyanogen chloride, was released upon the environment in public sewage water within the city limits of Houston, and that this war gas readily escapes into the atmosphere from typical, city sewage waters.) Exhibit AB consists of *ten pages numbered 90 through 98, and also page 109 which follows page 98—all of which pages are numbered in the upper, right-hand corner. Page 90 of Exhibit AB shows that tests for "cyanide" can be negative—even when cyanogen chloride is present. Pages 91 and 93 of Exhibit AB show that an effort to obtain information about cyanogen chloride occurred. Page 92 reveals that, after the presence of cyanogen chloride was brought up by Howard Kaye, Ph.D., limited sampling for cyanogen chloride was approved. Pages 94 and 95 of Exhibit AB show that <u>positive</u>, <u>environmental</u> tests for a <u>toxic war gas</u> did, in fact occur; and page 109 shows that this war gas, CNCl, causes <u>cyanide poisoning</u> in humans. Pages 97 and 98 of Exhibit AB show that patient testing directed by the Houston Health Department revealed <u>positive results</u> for blood cyanide in citizens of Houston. Therefore, material sent to Philadelphia by the Houston Health Department, material which denied the presence of cyanide pollution in Houston and of widespread cyanide poisoning among citizens of Houston, was very misleading. The Navy used this unjustly biased material which was received from the Houston Health Department as evidence to ascribe the diagnosis of severe paranoia against the Plaintiff.*

III.

Plaintiff herein would further show the Court that Exhibit AC, following, which consists of two pages numbered 37 and 38 in the upper, right-hand corners, provides highly-qualified, professional ascertainment of the presence of cyanide poisoning among the Plaintiff's personal patients in Houston, Texas. The Plaintiff had at least <u>eighty</u> patients who were positively diagnosed with cyanide poisoning by objective, laboratory testing; and he obtained <u>over one-hundred</u>, <u>positive</u> laboratory tests for cyanide poisoning using several different laboratories. <u>Actual copies</u> of these laboratory test results were provided to Dr. Cone for interpretation, and the Plaintiff has legal custody of all of these laboratory test results and/or copies thereof.

IV.

Plaintiff herein would further show the Court that, given the facts stated in Sections II and III above, the City of Houston demonstrated wrongful, conspiratorial bias against the class of Houston citizens upon whom environmental poison was released, with favorable bias toward the polluter—namely General Electric Company; and bear in mind that General Electric Company operated under a permit granted by the City of Houston. This bias was profoundly demonstrated through wrongful, conspiratorial disparaging of the chief medical witness in a suit against General Electric Company, Namely the Plaintiff, Timothy R. Oesch, M.D.

Respectfully submitted,
Timothy R. Oesch, M.D.
Timothy R. Oesch, M.D.

And then, I have included some excerpts from the *UNITED STATES COURT OF APPEALS FOR THE SIXTH CIRCUIT*. Sadly, none of the court cases filed against either General Electric Company or the City of Houston were ever granted the right of trial by jury:

(2) Did the District Court incorrectly decide the facts? **Yes**
If so, what facts?
District Court was wrong in claiming that the Plaintiff did not allege a class-based invidiously discriminatory animus. The conspiracy between the CITY OF HOUSTON and the UNITED STATES NAVY that is named in the PLAINTIFF'S ORIGINAL PEITION, Section II, is plainly expounded in the Plaintiff's ARGUMENT AGAINST DISMISSAL OF CASE NO. 3-90-409, Section IV, as wrongful, conspiratorial bias against a class of Houston citizens. This wording was meant to make it clear that the Plaintiff is, in fact, alleging a class-based invidiously discriminatory animus. This Case, therefore, falls under jurisdiction of Federal Courts according to 28 U.S.C. 1343a as a violation of 42 U.S.C. 1985(2).

(4) Do you feel that there are any other reasons why the District Court's judgment was wrong? **Yes** *If so, what are they?*
The Plaintiff made it clear that the City of Houston sent at least eighty items of information to the United States Navy in Philadelphia, as plainly stated in his MOTION TO DENY DEFENDANT'S MOTION TO DISMISS. Yet the District Court implied that any communications between the City of Houston and the United States Navy occurred only in Houston, Texas—if at all. Thus, judgment was based upon a false premise: Timothy R. Oesch, M.D. was discharged from active duty in Philadelphia, Pennsylvania—not Houston, Texas.

(5) What action to you want the Court to take in this case?

The Plaintiff pleads that the COURT OF APPEALS <u>annul</u> the order by JUDGE JAMES H. JARVIS to Dismiss Case No. 3-90-409 in the UNITED STATES DISTRICT COURT FOR THE EASTERN DISTRICT OF TENNESSEE, and to allow Case No. 3-90-409 to continue toward Trial By Jury.

*(6) Do you think that this Court should hear oral argument in this case? <u>**Yes**</u> If so, why do you think so?*

In the event that his Court would rule against ordering the annulling of dismissal of the Case, then this Court should hear oral argument. The widespread, serious entity of environmental cyanide pollution likely affects many thousands, or even millions of persons in the United Sates and across the world—and yet is mostly unrecognized. The dismissal of this Case would be damaging to the future recognition and hopeful solutions to this problem—and would thereby constitute a cruel crime against humanity.

And then, after failing to receive a favorable response from the judge in the United States Court of Appeals for the Sixth Circuit, I wrote an appeal to that response. The appeal, which was also unsuccessful, was worded as follows:

No. <u>3-90-409</u>

TIMOTHY R. OESCH, M.D.	IN THE UNITED STATES COURT
VS	OF APPEALS FOR THE SIXTH
CITY OF HOUSTON	CIRCUIT

<u>APPEAL TO ANNUL ORDER ON CASE NO. 3-90-409</u>

TO THE HONORABLE JUDGE OF SAID COURT:

COMES NOW, TIMOTHY R. OESCH, M.D., Plaintiff, and files this his APPEAL TO ANNUL ORDER ON CASE NO. 3-90-409 which ORDER was made by James H. Jarvis in the UNITED STATES DISTRICT COURT FOR THE EASTERN DISTRICT OF TENNESSEE on October 3, 1990, and for cause of action would respectfully show the Court the following:

I.

Plaintiff herein would respectfully show the Court that James H. Jarvis is wrong in claiming that the Plaintiff has cited no violation of any civil right. In the PLAINTIFF'S ORIGINAL PETITION, Section III, the Plaintiff plainly claimed a violation of the Civil Right of Trial By Jury. This violation, which finally occurred in 1988 in Houston, Texas, was accomplished unjustly. Also, the Plaintiff is prepared to show that this violation caused the loss of a SIX MILLION FIVE THOUSAND AND NO/100 DOLLAR lawsuit in which he was a plaintiff. Furthermore, this violation falls under jurisdiction of Federal Courts according to 28 U.S.C. 1331, which was already pointed out in the Plaintiff's MOTION TO DENY DEFENDANT'S AMENDED MOTION TO DISMISS, Section I—sixth sentence.

II.

Plaintiff herein would respectfully further show the Court that James H. Jarvis is wrong in claiming that the Plaintiff did not allege a class-based invidiously discriminatory animus. The conspiracy between the CITY OF HOUSTON and the UNITED STATES NAVY which is named in the PLAINTIFF'S ORIGINAL PETITION, Section II, is plainly expounded in the Plaintiff's ARGUMENT AGAINST DISMISSAL OF CASE NO. 3-90-409, Section IV, as wrongful, conspiratorial bias against a class of Houston citizens. This wording was meant to make it clear that the Plaintiff is, in fact, alleging a class-based invidiously discriminatory animus. This Case, therefore, falls under jurisdiction of Federal Courts according to 28 U.S.C. 1343a as a violation of 42 U.S.C. 1985(2).

III.

Plaintiff herein would respectfully further show the Court that James H. Jarvis is wrong in stating that the Plaintiff did not allege communication between the CITY OF HOUSTON and the UNITED STATES NAVY which occurred outside of Houston, Texas. In the PLAINTIFF'S ORIGINAL PETITION, the Plaintiff plainly stated that the CITY OF HOUSTON conspired with the UNITED STATES NAVY in a manner causing the involuntary discharge of the Plaintiff from the Navy. In the Plaintiff's MOTION TO DENY DEFENDANT'S MOTION TO DISMISS, the Plaintiff made it clear that the CITY OF HOUSTON sent at least eighty items into the City of Philadelphia, Pennsylvania; and that the Plaintiff was stationed in Philadelphia, not

Houston, at that time. The "involuntary discharge from the Navy" was enacted in Philadelphia, Pennsylvania.

Thus, the CITY OF HOUSTON <u>has</u> <u>not</u> availed itself the privilege of conducting activities within the State of Texas, but has superseded those privileges by conducting harmful activity against the Plaintiff into the State of Pennsylvania. This occurred while the Plaintiff was employed in Pennsylvania and was living in New Jersey. Furthermore, this very action led to the forwarding of derogatory claims against the Plaintiff into the State of Tennessee, as pointed out in the Plaintiff's MOTION TO DENY DEFENDANT'S AMENDED MOTION TO DISMISS, Section III. The Plaintiff was a citizen of Tennessee in 1988 when the violation of his Civil Right of Trial By Jury occurred. He is still a citizen of the State of Tennessee.

IV.

Plaintiff herein would respectfully further show the Court that he recently read an article in JAMA (Journal of the American Medical Association) asking for help in diagnosing the illness of a patient in Oklahoma. The Plaintiff was able to recognize the Patient's symptoms as those of cyanide intoxication, and was able to help the author (a physician) diagnose the patient's illness. The patient, a nonsmoker, had a very positive test for cyanide exposure—namely a urine thiocyanate level of 28 mcg/ml. The <u>upper</u> <u>limit</u> of normal in a nonsmoker is less than 4 mcg/ml, so this patient was more than seven times higher than normal. This patient experienced illness at home.

I use this as an example to illustrate the fact that cyanide intoxication is a very widespread, yet mostly unrecognized cause of illness. I would estimate that many thousands, or even millions of persons across the United States and the world suffer from this malady. There may not be any other single type of pollution in the world that is causing so much frank illness. The cover-up of this problem in Houston and Philadelphia, conducted by the UNITED STATES NAVY and the CITY OF HOUSTON in conspiracy, amounted to no less than mayhem against the human race—by probably delaying widespread medical recognition of this problem by at least several years. I mention this to caution the Court against dismissing this Case offhand. Society may someday backtrack to find out how a devastating problem of illness-causing pollution was kept from public notice for ten or more years after its discovery.

V.

For all the reasons listed above, the Plaintiff prays that the Court grant this APPEAL TO ANNUL ORDER ON CASE NO. 3-90-409, and respectfully moves that the Court order the UNITED STATES DISTRICT COURT FOR THE EASTERN DISTRICT OF TENNESSEE to annul its order to dismiss Case no. 3-90-409, and to allow Case No. 3090-409 to continue toward TRIAL BY JURY.

Respectfully submitted.

Timothy R. Oesch, M.D.
Timothy R. Oesch, M.D.
Oak Ridge, TN
PLAINTIFF

Before moving on to the next chapter, I'll mention that I petitioned the Board for Correction of Naval Records after moving back to Texas from New Jersey. I remember thinking that my response from that Board made my petition seem as though I were petitioning a brick wall. I further produced a follow-up to that request, also unsuccessful, containing something that has not been previously addressed in this book—namely, some content from my naval entrance physical performed on June 8, 1982 in Houston, Texas prior to my active duty in Philadelphia. Contained in the follow-up request sent to the Board was the following information regarding my June 8, 1982 entrance physical:

Physical

My Naval physical, performed on 08JUN82, contains the following statement, "Most of the symptoms marked positive (basically all of them except hay fever and sneezing) are associated with chronic cyanide poisoning. I am much improved since moving to Katy (still working in Houston), and expect complete symptomatic (or at least substantial) recovery after leaving Houston. Note: Diagnosis verified with blood cyanide of 104 mcg/dl, serum thiocyanate of 0.9 mg/dl, etc."

A Breath of Cyanide

Symptoms recorded as positive on my physical included headache, tiredness, fatigability, weight loss, memory defect, and balance problems—all of which recurred when I again suffered cyanide intoxication in Philadelphia. Note that my physical also relates that I was taking antidote to cyanide exposure, namely alpha-Redisol and sodium thiosulfate, in order to maintain my health while working in Houston. These antidotes also enabled me to work and maintain health in Philadelphia, but were withheld from me during my second hospitalization. In short, the Navy affirmed that I had suffered from cyanide intoxication in Houston, and also affirmed that I was still psychologically normal and fit for active duty. The Navy is without excuse in failing to recognize the threat to my health in placing me near cyanide-utilizing industries, and the Navy is also without excuse in attributing my illness to paranoia simply because the illness recurred on one of their bases.

The Navy recognized my susceptibility to cyanide exposure and rated my psychological condition as normal—even when I was taking daily doses of antidote to cyanide in Houston. The Naval Captain who signed my physical on 08JUN82 accepted the objective findings of a blood cyanide level of 104mcg/dl and a serum thiocyanate level of 0.9 mg/dl as substantial proof of cyanide poisoning. Note that a serum thiocyanate level of 1.8 mg/dl, twice that found in Houston, was found in Philadelphia.

And one last item before moving on: I confronted the Board for Correction of Naval Records with a list of twelve simple questions that the Board <u>failed</u> to answer. The questions were as follows:

Question 1.) Is the Board aware that a blood cyanide level of 104 mcg/dl is highly positive for exposure to cyanide?
Yes ___ No ___
Question 2.) Is the Board aware that a serum thiocyanate level of 1.8 mg/dl is positive for exposure to cyanide in a nonsmoking individual who is not on nitroprusside therapy or other medications?
Yes ___ No ___
Question 3.) Is the Board aware that a urine thiocyanate level of 21 mcg/ml is positive for cyanide exposure in a nonsmoker suspected of environmental cyanide exposure?
Yes ___ No ___

Question 4.) Is the Board aware that Timothy R. Oesch, M.D., had a blood cyanide level of 104 mcg/dl, a serum thiocyanate level of 1.8 mg/dl, and a urine thiocyanate level of 21 mcg/ml?
Yes ___ No ___

Question 5.) Is the Board aware that cyanide is used industrially both in Houston and Philadelphia, as well as many other places?
Yes ___ No ___

Question 6.) Is the Board aware that more than eighty persons had positive, objective laboratory tests for exposure to cyanide in Houston, and that six different medical laboratories found positive levels?
Yes ___ No ___

Question 7.) Is the Board aware that doctors other than Timothy R. Oesch, M.D. identified persons suffering from cyanide intoxication in Houston, and that at least two such patients were referred to Dr. Oesch for treatment from two separate doctors?
Yes ___ No ___

Question 8.) Is the Board aware that materials used by the Board as evidence against the petition by Timothy R. Oesch, M.D. were supplied by the Houston Health Department?
Yes ___ No ___

Question 9.) Is the Board aware that a major lawsuit regarding cyanide pollution has been filed in Houston, and that the lawsuit had already been filed for some time before any communications occurred between the Naval establishment in Philadelphia and the Houston Health Department? (Note: this statement appears to be an error on my part. The suit against General Electric was apparently not officially filed until June of 1983, and communication between the Houston Health Department and the Navy began at least as early as the latter part of 1982.)
Yes ___ No ___

Question 10.) Insomuch as the denial of Dr. Oesch's petition is based upon the presupposition that no problem with cyanide pollution ever existed, would the Board approve Dr. Oesch's petitions if probable proof that cyanide pollution did exist were made evident?
Yes ___ No ___

Question 11.) If the answers to any of the preceding questions numbered 1 through 9 are answered "No" by the Board, would the

Board approve Dr. Oesch's petition if proof to the statements therein were provided?
Yes ___ No ___
Question 12.) Does the Board now choose to maintain denial of the request presented by Timothy R. Oesch, M.D.—docket number 1535-85?
Yes ___ No ___

Chapter 21

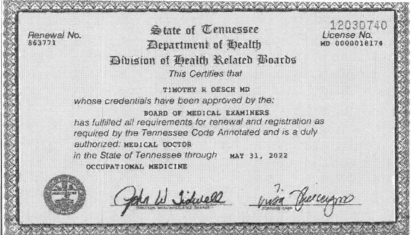

What Happened After That?

For a while, then, my wife and I escaped. We returned to Texas, but not to Houston. First we moved to Blanco, Texas where we purchased a mobile home and set it up on property owned by the doctor who took me in as a partner, namely a Christian doctor by the name of David Vause, M.D. I appreciate the work provided by Dr. David Vause, and working in a county with very few doctors was different and interesting (I think there were three doctors in the county, when they were all present). Dr. Vause kept chickens that provided us with eggs, and I acquired milk straight from a dairy. Filling in as the doctor to cover high school football games was quite an experience, and I can assure you that rural towns in Texas take high school football seriously.

The air in Blanco was sufficiently devoid of cyanide that my wife and I got along fine without any antidotes for airborne cyanide exposure. I worked with Dr. Vause from March to October of 1984, and then my wife and I moved our mobile home to Star Rt. 1B Box 84 W, Dripping Springs, Texas, 78620. Dripping Springs had been without a physician for over twenty-five years, and my wife and I opened a solo practice from scratch, similar to what we had done in Houston in 1981. Our practice took off and did very well (until the Oil Crash of 1986); and like in Blanco, our health was fine without taking any antidotes for cyanide. I did everything from delivering a baby to serving as coroner, made house calls, shot my own X-rays and developed them in a dip tank, applied casts to fractures, performed minor surgeries, and was on call twenty-four hours a day; and at least once, I accepted vegetables as payment. We got so busy with our medical practice that we hired someone to assist Melody. Melody worked up front as a receptionist and in the back as a medical assistant.

My wife and I acquired a gym membership and enjoyed exercising together, though we had to travel to the border of Austin in order to reach a gym—and we also drove quite a distance to reach a sizeable grocery store. My memories of Dripping Springs, at least prior to the Oil Crash, are happy memories. We attended a local church where I served as choir director and wrote the music and lyrics for songs. At church, we met Jeff and Deborah, a young couple who became two of the closest friends of our lifetimes. We began purchasing property at a beautiful swimming hole where Jeff and I would swing on a rope and drop into the water. A large snapping turtle lived at the bottom of that pool, but he never bothered us.

In addition to church music, I also wrote poems for the local newspaper. To the best of my knowledge, the newspaper was called the Harbinger. The poems were humorous compositions based upon true life experiences, and several of them are featured on the internet site www.silentwords.com per The Poets' Corner sponsored by Nan Crussell Computer Services, and you can find my poems by simply bringing up the first page of that site and clicking on my name, *Timothy R. Oesch*. The second and third poems in my collection both involve a roach, and they both also involve my wife. *Feelers* is based upon the event described in the first paragraph of Chapter 1 of this book, namely where my wife is in the bathtub; and *Roach Scare* involves my wife in quite a different manner.

For two summers, during the period of time that I attended college at Houston Baptist University, I served as a lifeguard at Stude Pool in Houston. My cousin, Richard Cantrell, was kind enough to let me share his upstairs apartment, located within walking distance to Stude Pool. I slept on a mattress on the floor, and my cousin slept in a twin bed. One night a large roach decided to visit my cousin in bed, and the poem

Roach Scare is based upon what occurred when my cousin became aware that he had company. So then, I decided to put *Roach Scare* to music, added a few dramatic stanzas to the poem, and then proceeded to produce a skit for a local talent show that was held where we attended church. The skit was hilarious and proved to be a smashing success, with my friend Jeff playing the part of my cousin, with me serving as narrator as I played the piano and sang, and with my wife taking on the role of the roach—her outfit was adorable, her antics were delightful, and I daresay that a cuter roach has never set foot upon the surface of the earth.

When the Oil Crash hit in 1986, our business in Dripping Springs suffered a major decline. In July of that year, we moved our mobile home to Rt. 1 1900 Pecan Box 57, Lot #57, Maxwell, Texas, 78656, and I started filling in at other physicians' offices in order to acquire financial income. I worked for a while under the employment of Dr. Roberto Mirando at an Emergiclinic in San Marcos, Texas, and then acquired additional work in the office of Dr. Nilon Tallant—Dr. Tallant's office was also situated in San Marcos. While working in Dr. Nilon Tallant's office, I spotted a magazine that advertised a job with Martin Marietta Energy Systems in Oak Ridge, Tennessee. Jeff and Deborah had announced, after taking a vacation to Tennessee, that they were going to move to Townsend, Tennessee, located not too far from Oak Ridge; and in addition to that, my dad was pastoring a church in Greeneville, Tennessee. To the best of my memory, the recruiter who answered the phone in Oak Ridge had the first name of Dan, and the conversation went something like this:

"Hello, this is Dan."

"Hi. This is Tim Oesch, I'm a doctor in Texas. I'm interested in the advertisement for a job with Martin Marietta Energy Systems in Oak Ridge."

"Advertisement? What advertisement?"

"Here in this magazine."

"Magazine?"

I paused and inspected the magazine. The magazine appeared new, but the date on the magazine was not December 1986; but rather, December 1985.

"Oh…I'm sorry," I said. "This magazine is a year old. Sorry to bother you, good-b…"

"No, wait!" interrupted Dan as I was about to hang up the phone.
"What?"
"We haven't advertised any physician jobs lately, but it just so happens that we have an opening."
"Really?"
"Yes. Tell me a little about yourself."

I talked to Dan; and before long, I took a trip to Tennessee for an interview. I think Jeff and Deborah traveled with us, all in the same car, and the interview was successful. I began working at the K-25 industrial plant in Oak Ridge, Tennessee in the early part of 1987. K-25 is one of the three industrial plants in Oak Ridge associated with the production of the first nuclear bomb during WWII. My wife and I choose where we would live carefully, checking maps and doing research to avoid notable proximity to plating plants or other likely sources of airborne cyanide.

At first my wife and I rented, moving into an apartment complex on the west side of Oak Ridge, in Roane County, south of the Oak Ridge Turnpike. Our health did okay, even with my working at K-25 and not taking any antidotes to cyanide exposure, and we then moved into a home situated north of our apartment. As in Texas, we were blessed with a very close friendship with a wonderful Christian couple, this time having the names of Scott and Chris. With Scott and Chris, we founded a small, local church in Oak Ridge, known as God's Church. Scott preached to adult services, and I preached in children's church; and pertaining to music, I played the piano and Scott played the harmonica. The doctrines we taught, striving to stay true to divine Scripture, are presented in a book entitled *Angelic Commission* by *Timothy Swiss*.

Martin Marietta hired me so quickly that I did not even possess a Tennessee medical license when I reported for work. Then came a shock. The Navy apparently disseminated negative propaganda to the state medical licensing boards in keeping with one of the threats I received from Captain Galasyn. The Texas State Board of Medical Examiners must have simply disregarded whatever negative report the Navy propagated, and I appreciate that. It was less likely, of course, that the Tennessee State Board of Medical Examiners would be familiar with me and with the history of my dealings with cyanide pollution in Houston. So then, I was required to take additional psychiatric testing and meet with the Tennessee State Board of Medical Examiners in person.

I met with the members of the Tennessee State Board of Medical Examiners in Nashville, Tennessee. There, I presented data showing that I had suffered from environmental cyanide intoxication, and they also had results from the psychiatric testing that they required. After everything I had gone through in Houston and Philadelphia, an enormous quantity of supportive evidence had been assimilated; and I also assume that my additional psychiatric testing granted further support to my claims, though I cannot remember if I actually received a copy of that testing. It was then and there that I received, in my opinion, one of the greatest compliments that I have ever received during my entire lifetime: one of the Board members faced the other members of the Board and said—*he walks to the beat of a different drummer*.

The Tennessee State Board of Medical Examiners granted my Tennessee Medical License with no restrictions. Furthermore, I received a request, from the Board, to serve as a counselor for their impaired physicians' program. I certainly felt honored by this request, but with having just started a new job, and with having found out that my wife was pregnant, I respectfully declined the request. Not long thereafter, I found myself in a small room with white walls and a tape recorder, answering questions in regard to my receiving Q clearance, a type of clearance utilized by the United States Department of Energy and the Nuclear Regulatory Commission—this is the highest level of clearance available with the Nuclear Regulatory Commission. As with the Tennessee State Board of Medical Examiners, I presented evidence supporting the claim that I had suffered from environmental cyanide intoxication and that I was not paranoid. My Q clearance was granted with no restrictions.

In 1987 my wife and I were blessed with a son; and in 1991, we were blessed with a daughter. Both children have grown into wonderful Christian adults, and we have now been further blessed with a wonderful Christian daughter-in-law. I enjoyed coaching soccer and track as my children grew up, and I certainly attended a large number of dance recitals in regard to my daughter. I think it was about 1991, or close to it, when something else occurred that would bring about dramatic changes: I think it was around this time when I finally accepted the fact that I was again experiencing significant symptoms of cyanide intoxication.

A large incinerator had been constructed at K-25 for the purpose of incinerating hazardous waste, referred to as a toxic waste incinerator. As I would later learn while seated with a group of scientists at the Oak Ridge National Laboratory, burning anything that contains carbon and nitrogen produces cyanide. My illness returned slowly after the incinerator was put into operation. As when living near Cherry Hill in New Jersey, I resisted acceptance of the fact that I was again suffering from cyanide intoxication. Over time, my health deteriorated further and further, until I again lost down to 135 pounds as I had done previously in Houston. Finally I faced facts—I was again suffering from environmental cyanide intoxication. I improved the day I started back on sodium thiosulfate pentahydrate. In fact, the antidote enabled me to quickly gain back my weight and return to my regular athletic pursuits.

Along with the awareness that I was suffering from cyanide intoxication while employed at K-25 came the realization that many of my patients at K-25 also suffered symptoms of cyanide intoxication. I was appreciative of my job, and I did not consider it a fault on the part of my employer that my employer hired a physician—perhaps the only physician in the world—who could readily identify symptoms of cyanide intoxication amongst the workforce. I also did not consider the large incinerator located on the premises of K-25 to be somehow peculiar or special when it came to producing cyanide—burning coal certainly produces cyanide. However, if the K-25 incinerator happened to produce higher levels of a heavier cyanide gas, namely acetonitrile (also named methyl cyanide), then one may hypothesize that persons in close proximity to the incinerator experienced higher exposures to cyanide than would occur with hydrogen cyanide gas. The molecular weight of hydrogen cyanide gas is 27.03 grams per mole, whereas the weight of acetonitrile is 41.05 grams per mole.

My feelings of sympathy on behalf of my employer did not change the fact that I could not simply ignore the suffering of patients. I knew that small doses of sodium thiosulfate pentahydrate, an inexpensive salt that can be acquired without a doctor's prescription, could proffer substantial improvement and relief. On the other hand, my sympathy on behalf of my employer did influence my choice of laboratory tests. I chose to solely conduct urine thiocyanate tests and to avoid performing any blood cyanide tests. The only exception to this choice pertained to a patient with symptoms of acute cyanide poisoning and bright red venous blood, but that incident is addressed later in this chapter by Sherrie Farver.

Urine thiocyanate tests are more sensitive for ascertaining the presence of airborne cyanide than blood cyanide tests, and therefore served the need to objectively show patients at K-25 that they were being exposed to cyanide. I will mention, however, that I've obtained positive urine thiocyanate tests on persons living various places in East Tennessee who do not work at any industrial facilities, and I would expect to be able to do the same in cities and towns around the world. Patients who tested positive for cyanide exposure at K-25 were introduced to sodium thiosulfate pentahydrate with remarkable results, just as I expected. One man told me that he was able to mow his lawn for the first time in a year, and one woman told me that she went dancing for the first time in a year. By avoiding tests for blood cyanide, I felt that I was taking my employer into consideration as well as my patients—the half-life of blood cyanide is twenty minutes to an hour, whereas the half-life of urine thiocyanate may be about two days. Thus, positive tests for blood cyanide would be much more conclusive in regard to recent, substantial exposure to cyanide, and I figured that such positive tests would put my employer in a much more difficult position when it came to potential lawsuits. I did not order a single test for cyanide exposure on myself.

As in Houston, someone in East Tennessee brought the matter of cyanide poisoning to the attention of the press. Articles in this regard can be found by doing a google search for *The Tennessean Archives* and then going into the archives and entering *Illness Among K-25 Workers Oak Ridge* in the search bar. Most or all of the articles pertinent to this issue can be found between the dates of 8/11/97 and 12/12/97. Although my medical supervisor instructed me not to perform further tests for cyanide exposure at K-25, no one at K-25 threatened my life, and I was not ordered to stop taking sodium thiosulfate pentahydrate salt crystals. By this time, I had fine-tuned the dosing of sodium thiosulfate, and my response to treatment was excellent. Furthermore, sometime during the 1990s, a scientist employed by Oak Ridge National Laboratory, namely James C. Norris, Ph.D., Diplomate of the American Board of Toxicology, and Eurotox Registered Toxicologist, introduced me to another antidote for cyanide intoxication that proved very beneficial, namely alpha-ketoglutaric acid. I was *downsized* from my job at K-25, with my last day of employment being 12/31/98, but I do not know whether or not my finding of cyanide intoxication among workers had much to do with my being downsized since there was quite a bit of downsizing in general going on at K-25. The toxic waste incinerator at K-25 was shut down in December of 2009.

Sometime after I was forbidden to test anyone else at K-25 for cyanide exposure, one young woman who was employed at K-25 learned about my cyanide findings from a friend and took matters into her own hands. Her name is Sherrie Farver. Sherrie was experiencing symptoms consistent with a rather severe case of environmental cyanide intoxication; and because of bureaucratic requirements related to her employment, she was eventually evaluated by a psychiatrist. The psychiatrist gave her a mental diagnosis despite physical symptoms of cyanide intoxication and despite obviously positive testing for cyanide exposure; and as a result, her security clearance under the U.S. Department of Energy was taken from her. Sherrie's experience was remarkably similar to what happened to me in Philadelphia, with the diagnoses given to her being *Paranoid Delusional Disorder (297.1) and Personality Disorder NOT* (not otherwise specified) *with hypochondriacal and Depressive features*. Her symptoms, which she had experienced for several years since the toxic waste incinerator was put into operation, included depression, nervous problems, severe fatigue, unrefreshing sleep, exhaustion, short-term memory problems, poor concentration ability, decreased learning ability, muscle/joint pain, and numbness in her hands and arms. In his report, the psychiatrist admitted that he had not reviewed Sherrie's medical records, but he went on to state that, from her account, it sounded like the findings had been quite minimal. Such was not the case.

On November 6, 1995, Sherrie had blood and urine tested for blood cyanide, serum thiocyanate, and urine thiocyanate by a highly-respected occupational physician in Oak Ridge whose medical office was several miles away from the K-25 Site. The blood and urine were collected at 9:21 a.m. on a Monday morning, rather than after a day at work, and she had been away from the K-25 industrial site all weekend. In this testing, she had a negative blood cyanide, a serum thiocyanate which was in the upper normal range at 0.3 mg/dl, and a highly positive urine thiocyanate at 17 mcg/ml. She has always been a nonsmoker. (Her first urine thiocyanate level, from urine collected by her primary care physician in Clinton, Tennessee on 10/12/95, was 16 mcg/ml.)

Then, on November 10, 1995, on a Friday afternoon following a full work week and after going directly from work to the same occupational physician's office in Oak Ridge, Sherrie received the same testing as before, but this time having blood and urine collected at 5:12 p.m. Her afternoon urine thiocyanate was positive at 11 mcg/ml, her afternoon serum thiocyanate was normal at less than 0.2 mg/dl, and her afternoon blood cyanide was highly positive at 40 mcg/dl.

Forty micrograms per deciliter (the same as 0.4 mcg/ml) is one of the highest blood cyanide levels resulting from environmental exposure to airborne cyanide that I have ever seen, with only two blood cyanide levels in Houston being higher. The high blood cyanide level of 0.4 mcg/ml with a normal serum thiocyanate level of 0.2 mg/dl is in keeping with the fact that elevated thiocyanate levels lag behind elevated blood cyanide levels. Cyanide flees the bloodstream rather rapidly, but thiocyanate can be detected thereafter for a period of days. The elevated urine thiocyanate level of 11 mcg/ml was indicative of prior exposures to cyanide, such as during the two or three days preceding the collection of urine.

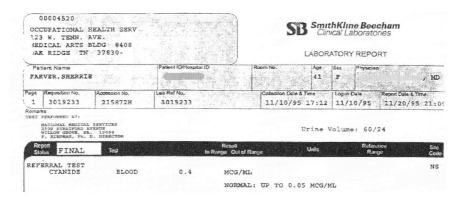

Sherrie obtained several additional tests for exposure to environmental cyanide. Her highest urine thiocyanate level was 28 mcg/ml, found in urine collected at 9:30 a.m. on 1/26/96, a Friday. One of her urine thiocyanate tests was performed through Emory University Hospital with testing per Roche Biomedical Labs rather than National Medical Services, yielding a urine thiocyanate level of 1.4 mg/dl which is equal to 14 mcg/ml, and this urine specimen was also collected on a Friday, namely 12/15/95.

Considering that she was a whistleblower in regard to the airborne cyanide pollution at K-25, Sherrie realized that her particular situation was important to the validation and consideration of many very ill workers who were employed at K-25. And in addition, with her background, education, and experience, she knew that it was also important to the health and well-being of persons living in communities outside the boundaries of the K-25 industrial complex. She decided to file a lawsuit for medical malpractice regarding her psychiatric diagnosis, a diagnosis that resulted in the suspension of her security clearance under the U.S. Department of Energy and the eventual loss of her employment with Lockheed Martin Energy Systems. I was called upon to appear before a judge and jury on her behalf and answer questions pertaining to environmental cyanide intoxication. When all was said and done, Sherrie won her case—she was awarded $600,000.00.

Sherrie knew that she suffered from cyanide intoxication. Her beliefs were in no way based on delusions or paranoia but on stark reality. The DOE consultant psychiatrist failed to seek any external corroboration whatsoever from Sherrie's doctors or her workplace to verify that what she was telling him was truthful. He assumed, concluded, and reported that he *"would be concerned about her in a security setting because of her poor common sense, logic and judgment, and because of her paranoid delusion symptoms."* His diagnosis was not only flawed but simply wrong.

In the following, scanned, court report, I have replaced the DOE consultant psychiatrist's name with *(Psychiatrist)*:

> " Farver v. (Psychiatrist), Anderson County, Tennessee Circuit Court Case No. 98LA0168, Tennessee Court of Appeals Case No. E1999-01840-COA-R3-CV, Transcript page number 323 (hereafter "Farver v. (Psychiatrist) Tr."), Jury Trial of Twelve, March 31, April 1 & 5, 1999: $600,000 compensatory damages for medical malpractice by DOE's consultant psychiatrist in attacking whistleblower's security clearance on the basis she was "paranoid, delusional and psychotic."

Sherrie had no choice in regard to who the psychiatrist would be who evaluated her; that choice was made by her employer. Following is an excerpt from that psychiatrist's testimony before a judge and jury in court:

Q: Sherrie told you that she had a lab report that she had that she was excreting thiocyanate and had toxic levels of cyanide; is that correct, sir?

A: Yes, she did.

Q: And she told you that the company and the plant would not put that report or those reports into her file; is that correct, sir?
A: Yes, she did.
Q: And you did nothing to confirm or deny that allegation; is that correct?
A: No, I did not.
Q: You thought it was paranoid?
A: I thought that was, yes.

And then, I want to include a couple of excerpts from my testimony at that same court proceeding:

Q: If Dr. (*Psychiatrist, name omitted*) had asked you about Miss Farver's physical health and possible toxic exposures, what would you have told him, sir?
A: I was certain that she did suffer from cyanide intoxication.
Q: Had Dr. (*Psychiatrist, name omitted*) called you, would you have encouraged him to take Sherrie's concerns about cyanide seriously?
A: Yes, sir.

Finally, in regard to Sherrie's court trial, I believe it is pertinent and appropriate to include excerpts from the testimony of Mr. Harry Williams, now deceased, who at that time was the President of the Coalition for a Healthy Environment:

Q: Have you ever observed Sherrie work as a member of a group?
A: Sure.
Q: And how does she work as a member of a group?
A: Sherrie is very outspoken, she is very honest and she gets along well with a group. Sherrie doesn't entertain fools well. She will take issue with you in a minute. But if she sees she is wrong, she'll stand down. And if she sees – if she thinks she is right, she will argue her point of view as an adult.
Q: Does she get along well with others?
A: Sure, she gets along great.
Q: Are you an officer in any organizations at the current time?
A: I am the president of the Coalition for a Healthy Environment.

Before proceeding, I want to include some specific texts from articles written by Sherrie Farver. Note that these texts are excerpts applicable to the subject matter of this book, and are not all-inclusive of the text in Sherrie's articles. The resourcefulness, concern, and diligence portrayed through her efforts and achievements are very noteworthy—perhaps she will someday write a book of her own. Her descriptions of the physical, emotional, social, psychological, and political realities that can devastate the lives of persons who are sensitive to airborne cyanide, realities that she has experienced firsthand, are exceptionally insightful and enlightening. I share the following texts with Sherrie's permission and approval, albeit with the understanding that she may have preferred that I did not replace some proper names with the descriptions of those persons' jobs:

Testimony of Sherrie Graham Farver
Ill Oak Ridge K-25 Site Former Worker

Submitted to the Senate Committee on Governmental Affairs
Senator Fred Thompson, Chair

March 29, 2000

To supplement the record of the 3/22/00 Washington D.C. Hearing by the Senate Committee on Governmental Affairs on Worker health issues at Department of Energy site in Oak Ridge, Tennessee and Piketon, Ohio

Brief Job History:

1985-86	Two health physics student internships at Oak Ridge National Laboratory
June 1986	Associate of Science, Health Physics Technology, Roane State Community College, Magna cum Laude
July 1986	Health Physics Tech, International Technology Corporation Provided job coverage at Oak Ridge National Laboratory
Oct. 1987	Health Physics Tech, Martin Marietta later to become Lockheed Martin

Oct. 1991	Earned certification from National Registry of Radiation Protection Technologists
Feb. 1996	Removal from K-25 Site due to cyanide concerns
Sept. 1996	Transferred to Oak Ridge Y-12 Nuclear Weapons Plant
April 1997	Began part-time schedule due to health
March 1999	Terminated due to "security reasons"
Today	Unemployed and unemployable in my field

I want you to revisit the year 1989 with me. That is the year that fatigue and depression came to live with me, and neither has left me since. That is also the year that the Toxic Substances Control Act Incinerator (TSCAI) came on line at K-25. To this day, it is categorized as "experimental," and it is the only incinerator in this country that is permitted to burn hazardous waste that is both chemically and radioactively contaminated in addition to polychlorinated Biphenyls (PCBs). Sadly, this incinerator is located near housing developments and communities of people. Monitoring of the incinerator stack is done for oxygen and carbon dioxide content to determine what degree of incineration has been achieved. There is no continuous or real time monitoring for contaminant emissions from the stack. DOE and LMES defend the incinerator by saying the emissions are within permitted guidelines. How do they know this? They rely on trial burn data and calculations that were done many years ago under ideal operating conditions. What happens when one figures in operator error, aging equipment malfunction, and the burning of unpermitted and even unknown contaminants? I think the answer lies in my body and the bodies of so many others. A route of emissions and subsequent exposures manifests itself in the air that the workers and nearby residents breathe. If you look at the list of emissions from hazardous waste incineration, you will see the same list as what is found in our bodies.

Many of the ill K-25 workers mention 1989 as being a critical year with their health. Former K-25 staff physician, Dr. Timothy Oesch, also noticed the flaring of symptoms around 1989. At first, I blamed my health problems on aging (I was 35 at the time). I realize now that people shouldn't feel like I do at my current age of 46, nor at 56, 66, or even 76. It's not normal. If you look at the harmful effects of chemical exposure to humans, some become readily apparent. This is not "rocket science" and it doesn't take a genius to understand what happens. Headaches, respiratory problems, numbness of the extremities, sinusitis, extreme fatigue, heart palpations, sweating, loss of sex drive, depression, blurred vision/loss of vision, depressed immune system, rapid heart rate, and muscle/joint pain are among the common symptoms. Most of us cannot point to an acute occupational exposure. In contrast, our poisoning was slow and chronic in nature. Yes the body can do a lot to repair itself but as the exposure continues, the body becomes "sensitized" to the point of reacting to smaller and smaller levels of exposure.

My health problems continued to intensify. In 1991, I was diagnosed as clinically depressed and I was suicidal. The combination of fatigue and depression was so severe that I felt as if I was in a long tunnel, crawling and clawing desperately to get out but never finding the end of it. I virtually ceased to live. Very little if anything brought me joy or pleasure. That's when I began treatment with Prozac. Within weeks the change in me was obvious to those around me. There was a bounce in my step and a twinkle in my eyes where none had been before, and life was once again precious and treasured. This time period saw me through an agonizing divorce. Just as I had tried to blame my health problems on aging, I found myself blaming them on the divorce. As time passed, I adjusted and my life became stable and secure. I remarried in 1994 after a two year courtship which was smooth and without upset. Why then, did my health problems (including the depression) keep worsening? Life was good again, why wasn't my health?

The fall of 1995 brought the answers to my questions. I worked in the same department with Ann Orick, the same Ann Orick who testified before you at the hearing on 3/22/00. Ann said that one of the doctors at K-25 (Dr. Oesch) had been noticing symptoms of cyanide poisoning in many of his patients. She had been tested and suggested that I might want to do the same. I acquired some literature about cyanide poisoning and was amazed to see my main complaints of depression, fatigue, and muscle/joint pain described as symptoms. At that very moment, I began to suspect that my debilitating problems had been caused by my workplace. I went to my private physician who sent a urine sample to the laboratory to be analyzed for thiocyanate, a metabolite of cyanide. A few days later, he called to say that my results were 16 mcg/ml and that normal results for a nonsmoker such as myself were only 0 – 4 mcg/ml. I hung up the telephone and for a split second, I smiled and told myself that this was wonderful because after all these years, I finally had an answer to what was wrong with me. The elation quickly eluded as the harsh reality of cyanide poisoning and levels that were four times greater than the highest range for normal set in. I was afraid, and I cried.

A few days later, I had the urine thiocyanate test repeated. This time, my husband who worked at Y-12 also left a urine sample. The results were staggering. My sample was even higher than the first one, and my husband's sample was "none detected." That was my turning point. There was absolutely no doubt in my mind that the cyanide poisoning was coming from my workplace, the K-25 Site.

I went to the K-25 Medical Department to provide a copy of my lab report just as we were expected to do with medical tests. I had also jotted down a page full of questions to ask Dr. Oesch. When the nurse asked the purpose of my visit, I told her that I had a lab report showing cyanide exposure for her to put with my plant medical records and that I wanted to talk to Dr. Oesch about it. She looked at the lab report and shoved it back into my hands as she told me that she could not put that report in my records. When I asked why, she said because Lockheed Martin Corporate had determined this to be a "controversial" and a "sensitive" issue. She proceeded to tell me that I could not see Dr. Oesch because he was not supposed to be "discussing or treating cyanide intoxication on the job." She even said that she was just "trying to keep both of you out of trouble." I was shocked and left with the lab report and questions in hand without seeing Dr. Oesch. Another turning point for me, what kind of company was this that I worked for? What was so wrong here that a physician was suppressed and medical data was ignored? Was a cover-up in progress? My fear of the cyanide and of my workplace continued to escalate.

Ann Orick and I consoled each other daily. We read everything on cyanide that we could get our hands on. We reported the actions of our medical department to local and corporate Lockheed Martin Ethics representatives. We called and met with K-25 industrial hygiene personnel and begged them to order urine tests for the other people who worked in our building. Their response was "no, we do not want to *alarm* anyone." We met with our division manager who was the site manager of health and safety. We went together to meet with Dr. (Supervisor, name omitted), the director of K-25 Health Services with our lab reports in hand. She was cold and rude to us as she quickly glanced over the reports and quipped, "I see nothing remarkable about these." A few days later, Ann and I returned to health services to file a medical incident report on cyanide. We spent most of the day there even to the point of staying after our shift had ended. The way we were treated there was traumatic to the point that both of us were terribly nervous and upset on our jobs the next day. Ann and I have the experiences described here well-documented and can readily make this documentation available if anyone from the committee requests it.

In fear for our health and for our jobs, Ann Orick and I continued our struggle. We realized that we had become "whistleblowers." Looking back, I don't know how either of us would have endured without the support of each other. I saw the rash of large sores that appeared on Ann's face and head. Dr. Oesch had told her that in his opinion it was a "cyanide rash." We had read about such a thing. I also had a mysterious rash all over my scalp that my doctor had no idea of what it was or what caused it. It did not respond to the ointment he prescribed and took many weeks to go away. I remember the day well that I sat in Ann's office with her and watched a heart monitor record "120" beats per minute while she sat in her chair. I also remember the day that I sat in the same office with her as she suffered chest pains. I begged her to let me call the site medical department or even let me drive her into Oak Ridge to the hospital. She refused as she explained to me that Dr. (Supervisor) had threatened to take her job if more medical events happened. Ann needed her job and did not want to risk losing it. Against my better judgment, we sat and waited and waited until finally the pain subsided.

I implore you, believe the testimony that you heard from Ann Orick. I have known her for many years and we have remained in close contact by telephone since both of us left K-25 in early 1996. Ann is telling you the truth. Her suffering and pain has been and remains immense coupled with the plight of her husband Mack, who was the first diagnosed case of chronic beryllium disease from K-25. Her courage and determination in the face of adversity is immeasurable. Whether these efforts will be recognized favorably in Ann and Mack's lifetime remains to be seen. Her ultimate concern is—do not allow these things to happen to anyone else. That sentiment was echoed by all four of the witnesses who testified before you in the hearing. I share that sentiment. Our health is sacred; no one or no establishment has the right to take it from us. For when you have lost your health, you have indeed lost almost everything.

Together Ann and I went to meet with our site manager, (name omitted), to ask him and to beg him to initiate a health hazard evaluation on cyanide by the National Institute of Occupational Safety and Health (NIOSH). We told him that if he did not initiate it, that we would. Both of us told him that it would "look better" on the site if he did it instead of us. He told us that we as workers could not request the evaluation from NIOSH, and he would have to discuss any action of requesting the evaluation with management. We returned to his office a few days later on a snowy morning in January as a follow-up. We were aware that one of our coworkers, Rhonda, had been seriously injured that morning in an automobile accident as she tried to report to work. After a short while in Mr. (Manager) office, he took the phone call with the news that Rhonda was dead. Ann and I fell to pieces and quickly left his office. I will never forget Ann and I standing outside in the cold and the snow as we held each other with tears streaming down our faces and saying over and over again, "it's just not worth this – none of this is worth it."

Ann, myself, and several other workers signed the petition to request a NIOSH health hazard evaluation. Mr. (Manager) was wrong. We did have the right and the power to request and to get the evaluation. Unfortunately, NIOSH failed miserably in their efforts. No blood, urine, or tissue samples were taken from any worker. Additionally, field sampling was only done for compounds of hydrogen cyanide. Many of us urged NIOSH to investigate for other compounds to include nitriles. Very important, a nitrile compound converts to cyanide after entering the body. Through our studies, we knew this. Through our own investigations, we also knew that mass quantities of acetonitrile had been stored and incinerated at K-25. Once again, this is not rocket science. NIOSH would not sample for nitrile compounds. We were left with the report that no source of cyanide exposure was found at K-25, knowing full well that their report was inaccurate and *inconclusive by design*. Ill workers petitioned NIOSH a second time to broaden the scope of their investigation to cover other heavy metals and contaminants. Our request was refused on the basis of it being such a large and costly investigation. NIOSH denied having the resources to take on this task.

I was totally convinced that Ann's condition and the continued exposure to cyanide had become life-threatening to her. Personally, I was experiencing major tingling and numbness of my hands and arms and was fearful of permanent nerve damage. How can DOE or LMES ethically put this type of risk on someone's life and health? This is not an acceptable risk, and the mere thought of such risk still is beyond my realm of understanding. I filed an "Employee Concerns Report" with DOE (see attachment I) only to receive no contact for several weeks. I also filed an "Employee Concern/Response Program" complaint with my employer, LMES (see attachment II). In this complaint I detailed my concerns for Ann and myself and provided possible solutions. I was thorough in detailing the problem and the solutions only to receive a short written response weeks later from LMES that was typed on a blank piece of paper with no date and no signature. Ann and I waited almost six weeks for the meager response. The mental strain and our fear was incredible.

Thankfully, Ann left K-25 on disability leave soon after the mishandling of our cyanide concerns. As for me, I continued to ask, and beg, and plead, and even demand to be removed from K-25 until it could be proven that I was not at any risk of being harmed from cyanide exposure. I met personally with (name of President) who was then the president of LMES and (name of Vice President), the then vice president of LMES. This was as high as I knew to go. I asked that they remove me from the site immediately. No, it did not happen again. I was removed within a couple of weeks later following these two events. First, I put it in writing to management that I suspected permanent nerve damage was occurring with my hands and arms and that I held management personally responsible for this damage. Second, confidentiality was violated by management as a frightened group of lab workers came to my building to meet with a nurse from NIOSH. I had contacted these workers to speak with the nurse and fully assured them that their confidentiality would be protected. It wasn't. The events and the fears of the past couple of months culminated, and I broke down into an uncontrollable crying spell that lasted close to two hours. Was it any wonder? I was and probably still am a strong-willed person, but there is only so much that a person can be expected to endure. My division manager was called. He transported me to medical where I sat in the office of the site psychologist until my tears were under control. After returning to my office the phone call came to say, "take what you can carry with you and go to Mitchell Road in Oak Ridge now." That is how I left K-25. My cyanide concerns began in October of 1995. I struggled and fought to be removed from K-25 until February of 1996 when I received that phone call. This was unacceptable. DOE nor LMES had no right to leave me in harm's way for weeks that evolved into months. Damn them both as well as their unethical, corrupt, and criminal actions.

I apologize for the emotions. Please, please understand that these memories are hard to relive. These memories not only anger me but hurt me very deeply. It's similar to what a rape victim must feel when remembering or telling of her rape. I was violated in many ways during the remainder of my employment.

A couple more things, before I finish telling my cyanide story. I am one of the few, perhaps the only worker, who has conclusive evidence of cyanide poisoning that implicates the K-25 Site. A local occupational physician drew blood from me on a Monday morning before I went to K-25 to work. The same test was repeated on the following Friday afternoon after I had been at work at K-25 all week. The Monday-morning sample showed "none detected" for cyanide in my blood. The Friday-afternoon sample showed "0.4 mcg/ml" of cyanide in my blood. The normal level for cyanide in the blood is "up to 0.05 mcg/ml." The toxic threshold is 0.5 mcg/ml which means that any person would be symptomatic. A level of 1 microgram/milliliter is considered to be "acutely toxic." As you can see, **my cyanide blood level on the Friday afternoon after leaving K-25 was 8 times the highest range for normal**. Very important, cyanide only stays in the blood with a half-life of 20 minutes. To detect cyanide in the blood indicates a recent exposure due to the relatively fast clearance from the blood. On that Friday afternoon, I went straight from work to get the blood drawn at the doctor's office in Oak Ridge. There may have been time elapsed of 30 minutes or so.

After I left K-25 in February of 1996, I spent the next 9 months off-site. During that time, I was given only one small job assignment that took less than 2 days to complete. The rest of the time, I sat idle as a full-time employee. I was isolated from coworkers and given no work to do. I volunteered to answer phones and do filing, but nothing was given to me. **This is classic treatment of a whistleblower**. There is a distinct pattern of isolating the employee, removing job duties, and then retaliating against the employee for being unproductive. Often the retaliation escalates into being singled out for a layoff or into a termination.

Incidentally, I repeated the urine thiocyanate test after the nine-month period of being away from the K-25 Site. As expected, that test showed "none detected" (see attachment III). I will stop my discussion of cyanide now other than to say that I know in my heart of hearts that I and others were being poisoned by a cyanide or a nitrile compound while at K-25. I have my laboratory reports, and I have the knowledge of what happened to my body. Can I ever prove this in a court of law? Maybe not, but I know with a full degree of certainty and others know. I believe with all my being that I and others were exposed to acetonitrile and that the TSCA Incinerator was the culprit. By the way, I failed to mention that **cyanide is a known by-product of incomplete combustion and that acetonitrile is one of the most difficult waste products to achieve complete combustion**. Once again, this doesn't take a genius to figure out and it's not rocket science. For all we know, the private sector who is now leasing land at the K-25 Site may be receiving chronic exposure to cyanide today. No one has taken blood or urine samples to find out. The industrial sector and those who strive for economic development and growth would probably rather just not know.

One last thing on cyanide though. I recently sat in a court of law and witnessed sworn testimony by former K-25 staff physician, Dr. Timothy Oesch. He testified that during the cyanide controversy, he was called to a special meeting with the LMES corporate medical director, (name omitted), and then K-25 health and safety manager, (name omitted), and given instructions on how he would be allowed to practice medicine at the site pertaining to cyanide intoxication. He was told, actually ordered, by (Medical Director and Health and Safety Manager) to not even let the word "cyanide" cross his lips when dealing with patients. He testified that the consequences of talking about cyanide to his patients at K-25 would impact his job. Dr. Oesch received a poor performance rating the following year and was eventually laid off from LMES. Dr. Oesch also testified that a patient was brought to K-25 medical and was convulsing. Blood drawn from the patient's vein was bright red in color. Once again, we're not dealing with rocket science here, it doesn't take a genius to research medical literature on cyanide poisoning to learn that bright red venous blood can be an indication of acute cyanide poisoning. Dr. Oesch testified that the then K-25 medical director, Dr. (name omitted), forbade him to have the blood analyzed for cyanide. The patient was transported to the hospital in Oak Ridge. With the passage of time and with the lack of knowledge of treating emergency-room physicians there, it is more likely than not that the patient was not checked for acute cyanide poisoning. **Medical malpractice? Cover-up? Criminal activity?** I will ask you these questions. Personally, I was labeled as "psychotic and paranoid delusional" by a DOE consultant psychiatrist by assuming such things. And yes, this did result in a competent and ethical radiation protection technician being fired from her job one year ago.

ON MONDAY, APRIL 6, 1999 (LESS THAN 2 WEEKS OF MY FIRING) AN ANDERSON COUNTY JURY CONVICTED DR. (Psychiatrist) OF MEDICAL MALPRACTICE AND AWARDED A $600,000 JUDGEMENT.

Thank you for your time and your attention. Thank you for considering my written testimony. Please contact me if further information or clarification is desired.

Respectfully Submitted to the Senate on Governmental Affiars, this 29th day of March, 2000.

Sherrie Graham Farver
Sherrie Graham Farver

Following, next, are the three attachments that Sherrie mentioned in her preceding written testimony:

Timothy Swiss

(Attachment I)

U. S. DEPARTMENT OF ENERGY   **OAK RIDGE OPERATIONS OFFICE**

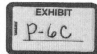

EXHIBIT P-6C

EMPLOYEE CONCERNS REPORTING FORM
HOTLINE NUMBER: 1-615-241-ECMS (1-615-241-3267)
or 1-800-ORO-ECMS (1-800-676-3267)

USE THIS FORM TO REPORT SAFETY, HEALTH, AND ENVIRONMENTAL CONCERNS
MAIL FORM TO: US DOE, SE-331, FEDERAL BUILDING, PO BOX 2001, OAK RIDGE, TN 37831
OR FAX FORM TO: 615-576-3725

DOE has established the Employee Concerns Management System (ECMS) for DOE Federal and contractor employees to help identify and resolve nuclear & nonnuclear safety, health, and environmental concerns relating to DOE programs. Your assistance in notifying us about such concerns is essential to the success of these programs. However, to give your employer an opportunity to respond to your concern, you should first report it to your supervisor. Contractor employees are also requested to first use your own organization's established Employee Concern or Complaint Reporting Procedure; if no resolution can be made, if you fear reprisal, or if you want to request confidentiality, you may use the DOE ECMS.

Please fill out this form as completely as possible and mail it to the address shown above, or call the 24-hour Hotline number. If you call, please be prepared to provide the same information as requested on this form. Your name will be kept confidential if you request. If you choose to remain ANONYMOUS, please insert any 3 letters of the alphabet below the signature line, so you can check its status later, and record the date and the 3 letters separately for your reference. After reporting a concern, you may check on its status by calling the ORO Employee Concerns Coordinator during normal working hours at 615-576-0832. Your report must not contain any classified information. Thank you for your cooperation.

Please fill in appropriate spaces and check ALL items below which apply to your concern.

THIS CONCERN IS: ✓Immediate ___Recurring ___Unique

DOES THE CONDITION IMMEDIATELY THREATEN DEATH OR SERIOUS HARM? ✓Yes ___No

NATURE OF CONCERN: (Check all that apply)
___Violation ___Willful ___Price-Anderson Violation ___Industrial Safety Hazard ✓Health Hazard
✓Environmental Concern ___Nuclear or Radiation Concern ___Construction ✓Other (specify): Willful Endangerment

EXACT LOCATION OF CONCERN: Oak Ridge K-25 Site

SUPERVISOR IN CHARGE OF WORK: (Supervisor)   SUPERVISOR'S PHONE NO. 576-0129

WHAT DO YOU BELIEVE MAY BE THE CONSEQUENCE(S) OF YOUR CONCERN IF IT REMAINS UNSOLVED?
___Loss of life or injury ✓Personnel Health Hazard ___Damage or loss of facilities or equipment
___Damage to the Environment ___Other(specify:)

WHERE ELSE AND WHEN HAVE YOU PREVIOUSLY REPORTED THIS CONCERN? (See Attached)
✓Immediate Supervisor ___Union/Mgt. Grievance ___DOE ___IG ___Nowhere ✓Other (specify) ✱ When? 12/11/95
Jerry (Last name removed) 574-9806 Employee Concern/Response Program (mo./day/yr.)
WHAT EFFORTS WERE MADE TO CORRECT IT? Incomplete and inadequate Survey by K-25 Site Industrial Hygiene

WHO IS YOUR EMPLOYER? (Name of company)
___DOE ___Contractor (specify:) Lockheed Martin   Other (specify:)
If this is your former employer, check here ___

IF YOU ARE A REPRESENTATIVE OF EMPLOYEES, GIVE YOUR POSITION AND THE NAME AND ADDRESS OF YOUR ORGANIZATION: N/A

(Continue on Reverse Side)
OR F 5480.29B (2-94)

✱ K-25 Site Health Services, Medical Incident Report, 12/11/95

A Breath of Cyanide

CONFIDENTIALITY REQUEST/RELEASE: (Check one)
___ I DO NOT WANT MY NAME DISCLOSED   ✓ I DO WANT MY NAME DISCLOSED

SIGNATURE: *Sherrie G. Farver*   DATE: January 23, 1996
(include your name only if anonymity is NOT desired)

YOUR 3 LETTER CODE _____ (include if you wish to remain anonymous; enter any 3 letters to identify yourself and keep a separate note of them for yourself; see instructions on reverse)

YOUR NAME (Please print): Sherrie G. Farver   YOUR JOB TITLE: Sr. Health Physics Tech.
(Include your name only if anonymity is NOT desired)

YOUR DIVISION, DEPT. OR WORK GROUP: K-25 Site Health & Safety Division (#76), Radiological Control Organization (#1207)

YOUR WORK MAILING ADDRESS: K-25 Site, P.O. Box 2003 (Building K-1020, MS 7404)
CITY, STATE, ZIP: Oak Ridge, TN 37831-7404

YOUR TELEPHONE NUMBER (work): (423) 576-4563

BEST DAYS AND TIMES TO CALL: Any day - Shift is 7:00 AM - 3:30 PM

DESCRIBE YOUR CONCERN HERE

Describe your concern as fully and explicitly as possible. Answer any of the following questions you think are important. What is the unsafe or unhealthful condition or practice and how often does it occur? What kind of work is being performed there? Have injuries, illnesses, property damage accidents, exposures, incidents, near-misses, or nonpermitted environmental (air, water, waste) releases occurred (what, when, and how often)? How many people are exposed to the condition and how often? How close do people work to the hazard? Include what you believe really caused the problem, and what actions can be taken to both correct it and prevent a recurrence. Is personal protective safety equipment available and used when needed? Is the condition a violation of a DOE, OSHA, EPA, State, contractor, or other requirement (Be specific)? What is your role with regard to the area of concern? What other people may be contacted regarding your concern? Are other serious hazards present? (Attach additional sheets to form if

Many K-25 Site personnel have elevated levels of urinary thiocyanate. These personnel range from clerical workers to maintenance workers and are located in several different buildings. Some of the spouses of those involved have been tested with no detectable levels of thiocyanate present in the urine.

A partial list of symptoms experienced by those affected:
  fatigue, depression, shortness of breath, eye irritation, confusion, heart palpitations, dizziness, muscle/joint paint headaches, short-term memory loss, extremity numbness/tingling

I am one of the personnel affected, and my husband was one of those who showed no urinary thiocyanate. I have above normal levels of urinary thiocyanate. Additionally, I have shown a toxic level of cyanide in my blood. The prospect of chronic exposure to cyanide and/or cyanide compounds in my workplace is extremely frightening. I have asked to be moved off-site until the source of exposure can be determined and evaluated. No one seems to care about the physical and mental toll that this situation is taking upon me. My health and the quality of my life is at stake. I suspect that I am hypersensitive to cyanide and/or cyanide compounds. I fear that I may be at risk for permanent, non-reversible health effects.

Please relocate me from the K-25 Site.

I have included the following items for your information and review:
  * Employee Concern/Response Program (UCN-19937)
  * Ethics complaint, "Oak Ridge/Medical/Ethics?"
  * Letter, "Sampling Results for Building K-1020" / Sample #444301
  * Original sampling data for building K-1020 / Sample #444302

Please feel free to contact me at which time I will work with you to explain this delimna more fully and provide additional sources of contact. For the sake of myself and my coworkers, this

pg 2 of 2

Timothy Swiss

(Attachment II)

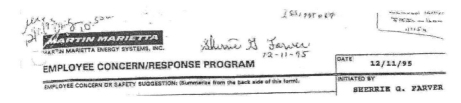

Sherrie Farver   **Employee #28222**
12/11/95

As per Lockheed Martin Employee Concern/Response Program please consider this a formal submission of UCN-19937.

Due to levels of thiocyanate in my urine (and urine of coworkers) and levels of cyanide in my blood which are elevated and above normal:

1.) Imminent concern for my own health, safety, and well-being.
2.) Imminent concern that cyanide intoxication is life-threatening for my coworker, Ann Orick.
3.) Concern that source(s) of toxin(s) be determined.
4.) Concern that source(s) of toxins(s) be eliminated.
5.) Concern that the K-25 Site does not have in-house technical ability or resources to alleviate items #2 and #3 above.
6.) Concern that the scope of the K-1020 survey for cyanide was extremely limited and inadequate.
7.) Concern for availability of a clinical toxicologist to evaluate past, present, and future health implications.
8.) Concern that toxins or heavy metals from past occupational exposure may still be stored in my body.
9.) Concern that past and present occupational exposure to toxins may have resulted in permanent damage to my person.
10.) Belief and fear that my health is being continually jeopardized and damaged at the K-25 Site.
11.) Belief that management of health, safety, and medical disciplines of the K-25 Site and of Lockheed Martin Corporate are

A Breath of Cyanide

involved in a cover-up due to the magnitude of the problem and legal implications.

12.) Concern and outrage of the ethics and "concern for people" exhibited by the K-25 Site Health Services Department.

13.) Concern as to why Lockheed Martin will not allow me an open and documented consultation with Dr. Timothy Oesch.

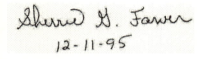

Sherrie Farver   **Employee #28222**
12/11/95

Proposed Corrective Action:

1.) I should be immediately removed from the K-25 Site.
2.) An Orick should be immediately removed from the K-25 Site.
3.) Lockheed Martin should locate the source of cyanide intoxication and determine whether it is at the workplace, at the home, or a combination of both.
4.) If the source of cyanide intoxication is occupational, Lockheed Martin should remove employees at risk and eliminate the source.
5.) Industrial, environmental, medical, and toxicological professionals should be subcontracted by Lockheed Martin to assess cyanide intoxication.
6.) Not limited to but to include – Pesticides? Wood? Concrete? Sewer? Drains? Ambient air? Occupational work history? Urine tests for other K-1020 occupants? Trending of affected personnel at the site? Sampling other buildings? History of disposal methods for cyanide and cyanide compounds? Inventory of all cyanide and cyanide compounds now at the site?
7.) Lockheed Martin physicians should be assisted in this matter by other physicians who are expertized in clinical toxicology.
8.) I and all employees suspected of cyanide intoxication should be sent for a medical/toxicological evaluation to determine body burdens of metals, toxins, chemicals, and etc.

9.) A complete evaluation by physicians (occupational and toxicological) who are competent to make this determination should be done as soon as possible.

10.) Remove me to an alternative work location, off-site, such as Jackson Plaza; 105 Mitchell Road; or 701 Scarboro while further evaluation of the K-25 Site continues.

11.) Medical and Health/Safety disciplines should address the subject of cyanide intoxication openly and honestly.

12.) Resolve the unethical and unprofessional behavior which was exhibited to me by the K-25 Site Health Services Department on 11/2/95. My laboratory reports and associated medical data should be placed in my medical file at the site.

13.) Dr. Oesch has a published paper on cyanide intoxication. He is a resource that I should be allowed to consult with on the record.

Sherrie D. Farver
12-11-95

(Note: the next two paragraphs, following this paragraph which I have added within parenthesis, are the response that Sherrie Farver was given per K-25 Site management. I received the contents of this *Attachment #2* from Sherrie Farver per an email on 6/5/2020; and with this email, she sent the following message: *Lockheed Martin knew what was going on with silencing you. Look these documents over. I had reported it to them. Also, look at the minimal response that I was given to my concerns. It's not even signed or dated!*)

As noted in a letter to the employee dated November 20, 1995, there is no evidence that cyanide compounds exist in the employee's work area. The survey performed for cyanide compounds in the K-1020 building was appropriate and included sampling of air, water, and soil. In addition to the initial survey, the Operational Safety and Health Department is continuing to evaluate whether cyanide compounds could exist at the K-25 Site.

The K-25 Site has a very knowledgeable and technically competent staff working on this issue. The site also has additional certified staff and other resources available to assist with this evaluation or any other health and safety matter, when needed. The K-25 Site Health and Safety Division (H&SD) has always operated in an open and honest manner and will continue to do so. Similarly, the H&SD conducts operations in an ethical manner and is committed to maintaining the highest standards of excellence.

(Attachment III)

```
00004520
OCCUPATIONAL HEALTH SERV                    SB SmithKline Beecham
3 W. TENN. AVE.                                 Clinical Laboratories
MEDICAL ARTS BLDG #408
OAK RIDGE  TN  37830-                        LABORATORY REPORT

Patient Name           Patient ID/Hospital ID    Room No.   Age  Sex  Physician
FARVER, SHERRIE                                             42   F                    , MD

Page  Requisition No.  Accession No.  Lab Ref No.  Collection Date & Time  Log-in Date   Report Date & Time
1     3020409          NS6313011      3020409      11/04/96 09:32          11/04/96      11/09/96 09:00

Remarks   TEST PERFORMED AT:
          NATIONAL MEDICAL SERVICES
          3450 STRATFORD AVENUE
          WILLOW GROVE, PA. 19090
          F. RIEDERS, Ph. D. DIRECTOR
Urine Volume: 1400/24

Report                        Result                                Reference       Site
Status  FINAL   Test    In Range    Out of Range    Units           Range           Code

THIOCYANATE (U)                                                                     EY
   THIOCYANATE                 NONE DETECTED       MCG/ML
                     REP. LIMIT: 1.0

   NORMAL: NON-SMOKERS: 1-4 MCG/ML
           SMOKERS:     7-17 MCG/ML

   THIOCYANATE                 NONE DETECTED       MG/G CREAT.
                     REP. LIMIT: 0.5
```

Following is an interoffice memorandum that Sherrie Farver sent on November 16, 1995, reaching out to Lockheed Martin Corporate to document ethics concerns:

INTEROFFICE MEMORANDUM
Date: 16-Nov-1995 03:38pm EST
From: Sherrie G Farver
        FARVERSG
Dept: 1207
Tel No: 6-4560

TO: John R. Bigelow   (PAPER MAIL)

CC: Sherrie G Farver   (FARVERSG)
CC: Gail Allen   (PAPER MAIL)

Timothy Swiss

Subject: Oak Ridge/Medical/Ethics?
File: OUTBOX

Mr. Bigelow,

I placed a call at approximately 10:45 A.M. this morning to the Bethesda, Maryland, Office of Ethics and Business Conduct for Lockheed Corporation. I spoke briefly with Gail Allen. She told me that you would be my contact for Energy Systems concerns and offered to take my concerns by telephone or by fax due to your unavailability today. I asked if I could communicate via e-mail to you and copy her on the transmittal so that my complaint would be fully documented, complete with date and time of receipt. She was agreeable. I did state my name to her.

As I prepare this correspondence, I am looking at the last paragraph on page 1 of the Lockheed Martin booklet, "Setting the Standard – Code of Ethics and Business Conduct." It is stated, "Lockheed Martin aims to 'set the standard' for ethical business conduct. We will achieve this through six virtues: Honesty, Integrity, Respect, Trust, Responsibility, and Citizenship." The following page elaborates on these six virtues. I will not restate them in this correspondence: I am sure that you have a copy of the same booklet.

May this correspondence serve as my method to document a formal ethics concern and complaint with Lockheed Martin. Please take it seriously, investigate it completely, and resolve it.

1.) The Oak Ridge K-25 Site Health Services Department has refused to receive and place in my medical records a copy of laboratory results which show elevated levels of thiocyanate in my urine. This laboratory report was provided to me by my private physician. It is my understanding that thiocyanate in the urine can be an indication of cyanide in the body.

2.) The Oak Ridge K-25 Site Health Services Department has refused to let me discuss symptoms or treatment of cyanide intoxication with a K-25 Site physician who has a published paper on this subject.

It is my understanding that Dr. (name omitted) Compliance Management, Corporation Occupational Health Services is responsible for the constraints placed upon my site health services department. It is my belief that Dr. Timothy R. Oesch, K-25 Health Services Department, has been placed in a precarious situation. As a physician, his first concern is human health. He is not able to help people, some of whom are very sick, because of directives from corporate. What a terrible dilemma for him. I fear for Dr. Oesch's job and feel that he will be forced to leave Lockheed Martin soon. I also fear for the loss of my job and feel that I too will be forced to leave Lockheed Martin, not by choice but because I expect to be treated with fairness and will pursue that fairness even at the risk of retaliation from management.

"Sensitive issue" and "controversial issue" are terms that have been recently used by the K-25 Site Health Services Department to myself and a coworker regarding environmental cyanide intoxication. If we are indeed working for a company who prides itself with honesty, integrity, and trust, why did I receive the treatment and rejection described above? If there is nothing to hide and no cover-up involved, why this type of treatment?

I am sick. A fellow coworker is much more serious. We need help. Our private physicians are having to dig and search for the answers to our questions and concerns. I do not understand at all, why a company whose slogan is "concern for people" has allowed the incident described above to take place with both myself and my coworker.

I do not know at this point in time where I am being exposed to cyanide. It could be from my home, it could be from my neighborhood, or it could be from the workplace. This determination remains to be seen. I intend to find the source. I have no choice for the sake of my personal health and well-being.

Address items #1 and #2 stated above:

Two weeks from today, 11/30/95, I will return to the K-25 Site Health Services Department with the same laboratory report and possibly additional ones pertaining to thiocyanate tests of my urine and blood. If this matter has been resolved to incorporate concern and ethics, then I fully expect for the laboratory report (s) to go in my medical files. Additionally, I fully expect to request to see Dr. Oesch and sit face to face with him, on the record, to have my questions and concerns addressed and recorded in the same fashion as he would any other ailment or illness. If Lockheed Martin Corporation practices the ethics that it teaches and distributes on paper to employees, then I and my coworker should be received in a totally different manner on 11/30/95.

Sincerely,

Sherrie Farver

Sherrie Farver

11/16/95

Of note, the above memorandum was written prior to the report date of Sherrie's positive blood cyanide test, which was 11/20/95. This is pertinent in regard to her statement in the memorandum that, at that point in time, she did not know where she was being exposed to cyanide. Also of note, Sherrie Farver was prohibited from meeting with me at the K-25 medical clinic on at least two occasions. The second time that she was prohibited from meeting with me, she was accompanied by a coworker named Ann Orick. Although I think that I eventually met with Sherrie Farver prior to her court trial, and although I think that I was one of Sherrie Farver's physicians at K-25 prior to any testing for cyanide exposure taking place, I do not remember Sherrie Farver ever being permitted to speak with me about cyanide intoxication at K-25 while I was still employed there.

And finally, pertaining to my recent communication with Sherrie Farver, are slides that she prepared and presented at the Joint House and Senate Conservation and Environment Committee Hearings in

A Breath of Cyanide

Nashville, TN on March 4, 1997. Several sick workers were in attendance and given brief time allotments to speak. The words that appear in parenthesis beneath three of the slides are my added comments, as is the statement that I make prior to Sherrie's last slide.

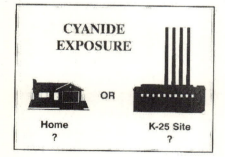

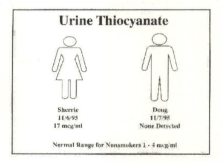

(Doug is Sherrie's husband.)

****

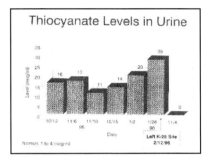

****

(The next slide was Sherrie's blood cyanide of 0.4mcg/ml. A scan of this lab report is previously shown in this chapter.)

(Sherrie was unaware that I had obtained a few urine thiocyanate tests on K-25 workers. To her knowledge, no biological testing was done after my testing was halted.)

****

I believe that the final three words in Sherrie's last slide speak on behalf of millions of persons who suffer from sensitivity to airborne cyanide across the surface of the earth.

> **The health and the lives of our coworkers, our families, and our community is at stake.**
>
> **.**
>
> **PLEASE HELP US**

Pictured below is the K-25 Toxic Substances Control Act Incinerator (TSCA Incinerator) in operation. Final demolition of the TSCA Incinerator was completed in September of 2018:

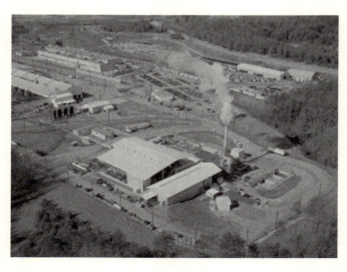

To this very day, Sherrie Graham Farver firmly believes that exposure to airborne acetonitrile from the TSCA Incinerator caused her illness as well as causing illness in many others at the K-25 Site. Acetonitrile converts to cyanide after being inhaled into the lungs and entering the body.

In regard to environmental investigations at K-25 during the time that I was treating patients for cyanide intoxication, testing for cyanide in the environment proved quite fruitless. After years of experience in dealing with cyanide pollution and the illness it causes, I am quite convinced that environmental testing for cyanide, in general, varies from fair or poor to worthless. If air testing for cyanide is attempted, I recommend testing for HCN (hydrogen cyanide), CNCl (cyanogen chloride), and acetonitrile (C_2H_3N), all of which can cause cyanide poisoning when inhaled.

Biological testing is notably better than environmental testing in regard to detecting and diagnosing environmental cyanide intoxication, especially pertaining to urine thiocyanate; but a trial of safe treatment in ill individuals has proven better and more sensitive than any sort of laboratory or environmental testing. If someone feels much, much better taking small doses of a salt every two or three hours, namely sodium thiosulfate pentahydrate, then such a positive response to treatment is a very powerful indication that the person's ailment likely results from airborne cyanide sensitivity. I take a small pinch of sodium thiosulfate pentahydrate every two hours throughout the day.

Following is a letter I've sent to a large number of ME (myalgic encephalomyelitis) and CFS (chronic fatigue syndrome) organizations. These organizations may receive a significant number of advertisements and advice, and I have not succeeded in acquiring much response from these organizations, although someone apparently gave the book that I recommended to these organizations, namely *Environmental Revelation*, a *one star* rating on Amazon. I've received very few Amazon ratings on books that I have written; but so far, all of the ratings on my fictional novels, such as *Princess Vayle*, are *five stars*; so I was disappointed to see the *one star* rating on the book that I hoped would bring relief to persons suffering from cyanide intoxication. And in addition, the email address that I was using to send information to different ME &/or CFS organizations was blocked so that I could not send emails to additional organizations (this pertained to organizations in Great Britain), and I had to circumvent this action by sending information from a different email address. Nonetheless, I've had at least a couple of interested persons from ME &/or CFS organizations respond to my letter, and I intend to send those persons this book, *A Breath of Cyanide*, as soon as it is published.

The letter that I've sent to these organizations follows:

Greetings,
I have been feeling well now (in regard to my chronic fatigue symptoms) for years, and I encourage anyone with CFS &/or ME to try a very inexpensive and safe dietary supplement. Just go to the free preview of an eBook on Amazon, namely *Environmental Revelation*, and then go to the table of contents, and then click on Sodium Thiosulfate Pentahydrate. This is a type of salt, and they sell it locally here in Oak Ridge, Tennessee as a *salt for quitting smoking*. The entire treatment with sodium thiosulfate pentahydrate, including how to obtain it and how to use it, is described in the free preview of *Environmental Revelation* (you do not need to purchase the book); and in addition, the eBook edition of *Environmental Revelation* is totally free of all copyright laws, so the entire book or any part thereof may be freely shared and disseminated without any concerns regarding copyright restrictions. I encourage you, of course, to ask your doctor if he or she thinks it would be okay to try some small doses of sodium thiosulfate and see if symptoms of CFS &/or ME improve, and to communicate any response with him or her. If sodium thiosulfate pentahydrate makes you feel a lot better (and it certainly made me feel a lot better, and it has made numerous other people feel a lot better), then your chronic fatigue syndrome &/or ME is likely from an air pollutant, namely cyanide, and you may hope to feel much, much better in the future. I consider a positive response to sodium thiosulfate pentahydrate to be the best test available for evaluating whether or not an individual's illness, such as ME or CFS, is from cyanide sensitivity. Generally, the response to treatment in cyanide-sensitive individuals is immediate, literally within minutes. Cyanide is a ubiquitous air pollutant with a half-life in the atmosphere measured in years, and I believe it may be the world's leading cause of ME/CFS, with some persons being much more sensitive or vulnerable to airborne cyanide exposure than other persons. In addition to

experiencing chronic fatigue myself, I became the world's pioneer researcher in airborne cyanide and its effects after first discovering the problem in 1981. I've been asked about how safe sodium thiosulfate pentahydrate is, and it's notably safe at the recommended doses, as is table salt: I generally go on to point out, then, that what sodium thiosulfate pentahydrate is treating, namely cyanide, is not safe—just google symptoms of cyanide poisoning and symptoms of ME/CFS and do a comparison, and see the comparable list of symptoms that I've pasted below. Some persons may cope with exposure to low levels of cyanide in the atmosphere without experiencing any notable symptoms of illness, while other persons suffer terribly from the same exposure (I speak from extensive experience). PS: I haven't missed a single day of taking the sodium thiosulfate pentahydrate since 1994, and I feel much, much better now in my sixties than I did in my late twenties when suffering from chronic fatigue. When my illness first started, I got sickly and tired. Before long I was having real bad memory problems, could no longer tolerate exercise (a big change for me), and was getting short of breath simply trying to sustain a note while singing in church. As time went by, I seemed to be wasting away, and lost about twenty pounds (down to 135 lbs.). The day I started taking sodium thiosulfate I got better—a lot better! I now exercise 4 days a week, roller-blade at the rink with folks much younger than me, and my personal doctor told me that I'm the healthiest person he knows. I truly thank God for all this, and I think a whole lot of other people should know about it. Feel free to email me if you have any questions, or to have your doctor email me with any questions.

PS: I have also seen some great results in treating fibromyalgia with the same products, though Vital B12 injections (the only product that cannot be acquired without a prescription) seem to be more important in regard to fibromyalgia.

Sincerely,
Timothy R. Oesch, M.D. (aka Tim)
Oak Ridge, Tennessee (USA)

Symptoms of Cyanide Poisoning (Cyanide is a Ubiquitous Air Pollutant) vs Symptoms of CFS/ME

A Breath of Cyanide

<u>Cyanide</u>	<u>CFS/ME (Myalgic Encephalomyelitis)</u>
1. general weakness	1.) muscle weakness
2. confusion	2.) cognitive impairment
3. bizarre behavior	3.) personality change
4. excessive sleepiness	4.) unrefreshing sleep
5. coma	5.) coma-like experiences
6. shortness of breath	6.) shortness of breath
7. headache	7.) headaches, either new or worsening
8. dizziness	8.) dizziness is common
9. vomiting	9.) digestive issues
10. abdominal pain	10.) irritable bowel syndrome
11. seizures	11.) seizures
12. lethargy	12.) fatigue
13. elevated lactic acid	13.) exercise increases lactate accumulation
14. anxiety	14.) anxiety
15. chest pain	15.) chest pain
16. joint and muscle aches and pains	16.) joint pain, muscle pain and aches
17. cyanide blocks the body's ability to use oxygen	17.) sore throat and tender lymph nodes (oxygen is important for the immune system to work properly)
18. tachycardia and abnormal ECG	18.) tachycardia and abnormal ECG
19. perspiration	19.) chills and night sweats

How Airborne Cyanide Causes the Inflammation of Brain and Nerve Tissue Seen in Myalgic Encephalomyelitis

The brain and nerve tissues are sensitive to hypoxia, with the brain being the most sensitive organ in the body to lack of oxygen. One form of hypoxia is histotoxic hypoxia, with cyanide being a prime example of an agent that causes histotoxic hypoxia. Hypoxia in neuronal tissue, in turn, causes inflammation. Thus, the encephalomyelitis noted in ME is consistent with cyanide being the most common underlying cause of ME.
(Note: anyone who would like a list of articles that support histotoxic hypoxia as a cause of encephalomyelitis may reply to this email with a request for that list.)

Sometime prior to May 6, 1992, I received a call at work from a researcher in Ann Arbor, Michigan who spoke with me almost an hour before I excused myself to return to duties as an occupational physician. This researcher had the hypothesis that Chronic Fatigue Syndrome results from viral interference with the physiologic metabolism of cyanide. He pointed out that mitochondrial and neurologic abnormalities shown in Chronic Fatigue Syndrome are consistent with effects of cyanide. I assured him that he might be pursuing one of the most important medical discoveries of the century; and I pointed out that lactic acidosis, fatigue, mental impedance, exercise intolerance, and basically the entire gamut of symptoms attributed to Chronic Fatigue Syndrome are consistent with cyanide intoxication. I want to clarify, to the reader, that I do not believe that any virus has to be involved for persons to become sensitive to cyanide, but I would certainly be open-minded to the possibility that a viral infection may sometimes be a trigger for an individual to develop cyanide sensitivity.

After my release from K-25 in 1998, I still remained in Oak Ridge. Years later, a lady came to the medical clinic where I was employed for a physical sponsored through the Worker Health Protection Program, which was established under Section 3162 of the 1993 Defense Authorization Act and is funded by a contract from the U.S. Department of Energy (DOE). This lady had severe chronic fatigue syndrome (CFS); in fact, I remember seeing her seated in my office, head down, and appearing pitifully debilitated. After speaking with this lady and performing her physical, I was convinced that her CFS was caused by airborne cyanide sensitivity, and I shared some information with her. I explained that she could try some treatments that are notably safe. She was more than willing to give the treatments a try.

The individual suffering from severe CFS responded dramatically to each of the three major antidotes that I recommend for airborne cyanide sensitivity. Remember that all of these antidotes, how to acquire them, and how to use them are described in detail in *Environmental Revelation* by *Timothy Swiss*, which is available through Amazon. What is exceptional about this lady is that she succeeded in having her claim accepted for exposure to hazardous chemicals while employed at a DOE site and her antidotes for cyanide are paid for through the Energy Employee Occupational Illness Compensation Program Act (EEOICPA). She now lives in Tennessee, but her illness first began while working at a DOE facility in another state where nuclear operations using cyanide were performed. Although airborne cyanide is ubiquitous, the poison is found at higher concentrations in some atmospheres than other atmospheres, and once an individual becomes sensitive to cyanide from exposures at higher levels, that person can then also suffer symptoms of cyanide intoxication when exposed to lower levels. This lady's response to treatment was conclusive—her diagnosis and compensation were totally appropriate, even without a single test for cyanide or thiocyanate.

In regard to the lady described in the two preceding paragraphs, I obtained her permission to include information about her in this book, and she even helped me edit the preceding two paragraphs. I also asked her if I could include her email response to my inquiry, and she was kind enough to grant her permission. The first two paragraphs of her email, an email sent March 1, 2020, read as follows:

> It's great to hear that you're able to fit in time to write around the demands of your new work position. Yes, you have my permission to talk about me in your book. You've made such huge difference in the quality of my life that I'm happy to do anything I can to assist you.

Timothy Swiss

> I'm an expert at internet searching due to the work I've done for DOE over the years, and from what I can determine, you are the only specialist on cyanide-induced CFS in the United States (possibly in the world). There is no doubt in my mind that a higher power arranged for me to be sent to your office in 2011 for my physical. No other physician would have recognized the cause of the fatigue, much less had the knowledge to treat it. You might not realize it, but your name is blessed daily by me and all the others you've treated for this condition. Thanks to you, we have our lives back!

At some point, years ago, I wrote a two-page article entitled, *AIRBORNE ENVIRONMENTAL CYANIDE POLLUTION*. In that article, I provided a succinct description of various symptoms that persons may experience with varying degrees of sensitivity to airborne cyanide. The description follows:

A.) <u>Mild Symptoms</u>: lethargy, lack of motivation, decreased exercise tolerance, and mental depression.

B.) <u>Moderate Symptoms</u>: headaches, anxiety, notable depression, gastrointestinal problems, rapid pulse, personality changes, easy bruising, dizziness, mild shortness of breath, excessive sleeping, and nagging fatigue.

C.) <u>More Severe Symptoms</u>: frightening shortness of breath, mild to severe chest pain, oppressive headaches and body aches, decreased appetite, salivation, weight loss, hair loss, and mental dysfunction.

D.) <u>Symptoms More Suggestive of CNCl than HCN</u>: burning eyes, burning or irritated mucous membranes, skin rashes, bronchitis, and pneumonia.

E.) <u>Fatal Intoxication</u>: may mimic a heart attack, stroke, SIDS, Reye's syndrome, or unexplainable suicide.

Well then, this book is now rather lengthy, and I've included data that sheds light on what occurred in Houston and Philadelphia in the 1980s, some more recent data from Tennessee, and data that will hopefully bring relief to persons suffering from sensitivity to airborne cyanide. Presently, I'm happily employed with an excellent occupational clinic. I've written previous books dealing with the morality; the politics; and the physical health effects that one may encounter when dealing with airborne cyanide, namely books such as *The Emissaries* and *Enchanting Emissary* by *Timothy Swiss*, but those books are written in a fictional format. Hopefully, this factual autobiography will accomplish more good in bringing light to a preponderant etiology of human suffering—an etiology that has escaped public recognition for far too long.

Before bringing this book to an end, I want to include a couple of updates that I've received from Marie Black in Houston. I emailed her and asked about the GE plant, and the first portion of her reply, received on February 21, 2020, was as follows:

> My husband and I just drove by the place where GE used to be. It has been empty for a long time. They have the buildings torn down and it looks like they are getting the ground ready to build on it.

I also asked Marie about Dr. Hitt, given that I've not been able to locate him. Her response, received on February 22, 2020, is quite revealing:

> Oh, I forgot that you asked about Dr. Hitt. I have not heard anything about him. I don't know if he is still living. I know he was very frightened about losing his life and his family. We had to go see him very secretly.
> It was very scary at that time. I didn't want anything to happen to such a wonderful man. I pray that he is ok.

In closing, I want to give sincere thanks to some persons who played major roles in the course of events presented in this novel. First, above all else, I thank God—for guidance, protection, and blessing. Next, my heartfelt thanks to the courageous young woman who served, fought, and suffered at my side, namely my wife Melody. Melody was only seventeen years old when we opened our first medical practice at Gulf Coast Bible College in Houston, Texas. Lieutenant Edward (Ted) O'Hanlan is deserving of deepest admiration and gratitude; I cannot help but think that the legal department of the U.S. Navy was overall improved, ethically and professionally, by his presence, provided that he chose to remain in the military. Special thanks, also, to the other members of the JAGC, USNR who worked along with Lt. O'Hanlan, and I would like to proffer an apology to Lt. Brooks and Lt. Norris (fictitious names) for the fact that I cannot remember their real names, and have not found their names on any of the reports that I have examined.

And then, my thanks to all of the persons, in Philadelphia and Houston, who bore testimony on my behalf. Thanks to all of the students and faculty of Gulf Coast Bible College who supported and encouraged my wife and me, including Eileen Bland, R.N., and the family of John Shearin (the first patient found with a positive blood cyanide). Thanks to the Deere family (fictitious name) in New Jersey, and to the courageous corpsman in Philadelphia who befriended me and who warned me of political corruption. Hearty thanks to Amy Klinkhamer (I hope that I spelled her name correctly), who I've given the name of Barbara Preston in this novel. This nutritionist was very involved with the cyanide pollution in Houston, and she called me during my legal struggles in the navy with advice on how to stay alive. Much gratitude to Bob and Verdi Daniels, who provided a temporary home for my wife and me in Houston; as well as to **James Marshall and Ben McHanly** who permitted us to rent a bedroom in their house in Katy, Texas. James Marshall's real name is **Max Argo**, and Ben McHanly's real name is **Ronald Newman**.

Then, thanks to a woman who provided information and support over the years, and who permitted me to stay with her family when I traveled back to Houston in 1988, and who has provided me with some of the latest reports from Houston—namely, Marie Black. Thanks also to Attorney Alan Lawrence Schechter and Plaintiff Bobbie J. Crawford who apparently provided worthy cause and adequate documentation to keep the legal case in Houston from being dismissed, albeit the court system failed to honor this request. And there are so many others worthy of mention, from Houston, from Philadelphia, and from New Jersey, including the chaplain and others at the Philadelphia Naval Hospital, as well as employees at the shipyard dispensary, plus David and Kay Thompson in Houston, and many others. My sincere thanks to everyone who assisted, defended, provided for, and prayed for my wife and me.

Finally, my sincere thanks to Mr. Walter Davis for his involvement and for the pertinent material sent to me in Tennessee—this was truly a momentous contribution. And it would be difficult to express the depth of my gratitude to Sherrie Farver for her willingness to assemble insightful and revealing data from East Tennessee.

Made in the USA
Columbia, SC
25 July 2020